Math Everywhere

G. Aletti   M. Burger   A. Micheletti   D. Morale
Editors

Math Everywhere

Deterministic and Stochastic Modelling
in Biomedicine, Economics and Industry.
Dedicated to
the 60th Birthday of Vincenzo Capasso

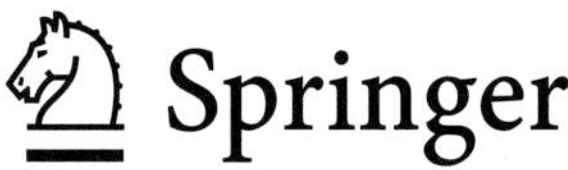
Springer

Giacomo Aletti
Alessandra Micheletti
Daniela Morale
ADAMSS & Department of Mathematics
University of Milano
Via C. Saldini 50
20133 Milano, Italy
E-mail: giacomo.aletti@unimi.it
         alessandra.micheletti@unimi.it
         daniela.morale@mat.unimi.it

Martin Burger
Institut für Numerische und
Angewandte Mathematik
Westfälische Wilhelms-Universität Münster
Einsteinstraße 62
48149 Münster, Germany
E-mail: martin.burger@jku.at

Mathematics Subject Classification (2000): 35Kxx, 60D05, 28A75, 62M30, 62G05, 60G17, 60H10, 65C30, 92B05

Library of Congress Control Number: 2006933717

ISBN-10 3-540-44445-9 Springer Berlin Heidelberg New York
ISBN-13 978-3-540-44445-9 Springer Berlin Heidelberg New York

Springer is a part of Springer Science+Business Media
springer.com
© Springer-Verlag Berlin Heidelberg 2007

Typesetting: by the authors and techbooks using a Springer LaTeX macro package
Cover design: *design & production* GmbH, Heidelberg

Printed on acid-free paper   SPIN: 11862000   46/techbooks   5 4 3 2 1 0

"Do you really want to
mathematize everything?"

Jacques-Louis Lions

Preface

The title of the book is a perfect way to synthesize the point of view of Vincenzo Capasso (VK) about the role played by mathematics in nature and all human activities, as mentioned by Willi Jäger in the Introduction. As VK mentioned in one of his speeches, "it is important that our scientific community appreciates the importance of theory and mathematics to face the enormous challenges which arise from the emerging fields of Biology and Medicine, Industry and Economics to improve the quality of Life." His enthusiasm and new ideas have brought him in this challenging mission. By transferring methods and tools from one field to another, by learning novel mathematical methods and ideas from the observation of real world phenomena and behavior, and by approaching real industrial problems, he has accepted to play a fundamental role in both the Italian and European community in the establishment and reinforcement of communication channels between Academia (methods) and Industry (applications), being himself a driving force of the scientific and technological progress that we are observing in our daily life.

This books collects the proceedings of the workshop *Math Everywhere: Deterministic and Stochastic Modelling in Biomedicine, Economics and Industry* which took place in Milano, Italy in the period September 4–6, 2005, and was organized in honor of the 60th birthday of Vincenzo Capasso (VK). It has been a successful meeting involving many prestigious scientists, in particular mathematicians from all over the world who have discussed, in a very friendly and relaxed atmosphere, relevant innovative mathematical methods which have been developed to solve mathematically complex systems arisen in connection with real industrial, economic and social problems. The main feature of the meeting has been the variety of the themes discussed both from the mathematical and the applied point of view, at an impressively high scientific level. It has reflected the wide spectrum of scientific interests of Vincenzo Capasso, which have been ranging from the first papers on the mathematical foundations of Quantum Mechanics in the early 70s, through his fundamental work on reaction-diffusion systems, including the qualitative behaviour, control problems and stochasticity of epidemic systems, published in many papers and a very cited book *"Mathematical structures of epidemic systems"* (an editorial success of the Lecture Notes in Biomathematics, published by Springer), up to the most recent work on time-and-space structured systems with evolving stochastic geometries. In this work, in which he has involved a number of students/collaborators from various universities in Europe, a series of open problems have been faced including the strong coupling of evolution equations for the (stochastic) geometries with the evolution equations of the underlying fields, at different scales. He has opened new mathematical problems at the interface of geometric measure theory, stochastic geometry, stochastic analysis, and statistics for evolution problems regarding densities, concentrations, i.e. relevant quantities describing the phenomena from an applied point of view, so to match one of the most important goals in VK's research, being useful to the applied sciences.

Along these lines, theoretically oriented papers have been presented in the field of reaction-diffusion systems, control theory, stochastic geometry, multi-parameter stochastic processes and stochastic interacting particles.

The workshop has been a mirror of VK's lively experience: from being the President of ESMTB, the European Society for Mathematical and Theoretical Biology and the President of ECMI, the European Consortium of Mathematics in Industry; by establishing at first MIRIAM, the Milan Research Centre for Industrial and Applied Mathematics, and more recently ADAMSS, the Interdisciplinary Centre for Mathematical Modelling, Statistical Analysis, and Computational Simulation for Scientific and Technological Innovation, aiming at a daily interaction between Mathematics and all other research areas, to further innovation in Industry, Finance, Medicine, public services, etc., in collaboration with a number of other centres, universities and public research bodies, companies, organically linked with similar activities at common levels of excellence in Europe, and elsewhere.

Here recent works in Biomathematics and Mathematical Medicine are presented: Structured Populations and interacting Individuals, Tumour Cords, Vascular Cancer, Vasculogenesis, Epidemics Models, Competition Models, Glucose-Insulin Homeostasis, Pattern Formation in Butterflies, Quiescent States, Reaction Diffusion System, and Neutron Lifetime Estimation are some of the main subjects investigated nowadays in the field. Furthermore in the industrial applications problems on the kinetics of nucleation and growth processes, crystallization phenomena and optimizing batch processes in the chemical industry have been investigated. Finally also the problem of optimal marketing in economics is presented here.

It is worth to mention here that the opening lecture and the closing lecture have been delivered by Grace Yang and Willi Jäger, respectively. Grace Yang has always been quoted by VK as his most influential scientific advisor, especially for introducing himself scientifically in one of the most prestigious Schools of Mathematical Statistics, the one lead by Jerzy Neyman and Lucien LeCam, whom, thanks to her, he had the chance to meet and discuss with.

Indeed his first relevant paper in probability was on the the asymptotics of the Neyman-Scott model of epidemics, a pioneering model of stochastic point processes; it was written by an enthusiastic and brilliant young scientist under the guidance of Grace, first during the Summer School on Biomathematics at the Scuola Normale Superiore in Pisa (1972), and later at the Department of Mathematics of the University of Maryland (1973). Willi Jäger has not only strongly influenced VK scientifically, by stimulating and encouraging him to face hard mathematical problems in the general area of nonlinear multiscale systems, but as Willi Jäger has reported, they have deeply shared such a view of Mathematics Everywhere, supported by a genuine interest in facing challenging problems in biomedicine of great relevance for the quality of life of human beings, by means of different mathematical methods and often creating problem-driven new ones.

With elation we are happy to state that everyone has very much enjoyed the very warm atmosphere, and the fantastic richness of scientific ideas that have pervaded the whole meeting.

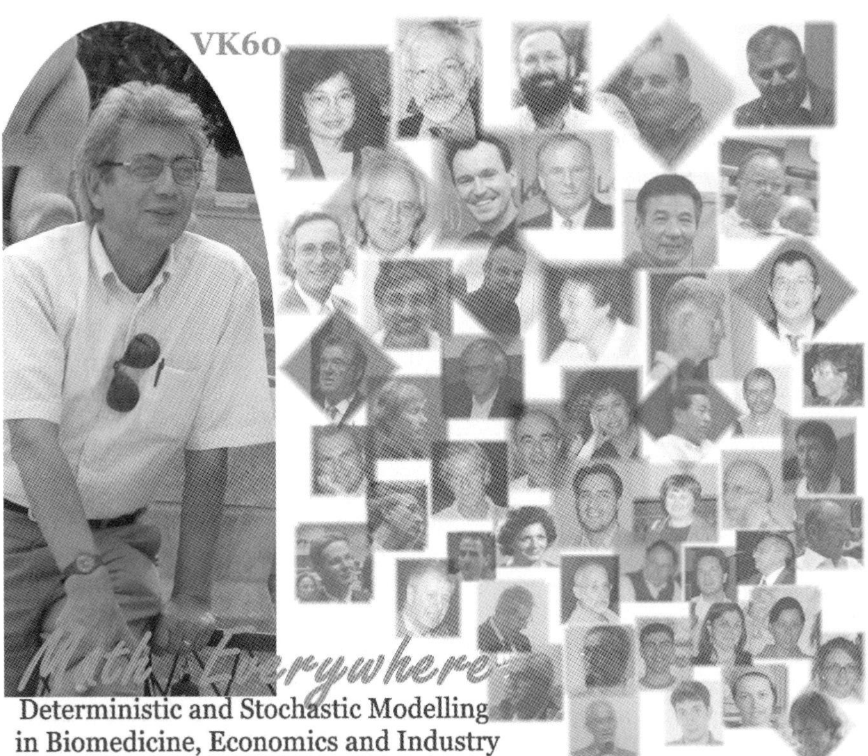

Here we would like to thank VK, for sharing with us his enthusiasm and this idea of a mathematics as a tool for a challenging mission. Your enthusiasm and happiness of being a mathematician, but first of all a human being have soaked in our being scientists. Thanks!

Milano, Linz,   *Giacomo Aletti*
July 2006   *Martin Burger*
                                                                  Alessandra Micheletti
                                                                       Daniela Morale

Contents

Part II Mathematical Problems in Biology, Medicine and Ecology

---

Part III Mathematical Problems in Industry and Economics

List of Contributors

Tomás Alarcón
Bioinformatics Unit, Department
of Computer Science, University
College London, Gower Street,
London WC1E 6BT, UK
t.alarcon@cs.ucl.ac.uk

Giacomo Aletti
ADAMSS & Dept. of Mathematics,
University of Milan, Via Saldini,
50, 20133 Milano, Italy
giacomo.aletti@unimi.it

Sebastian Aniţa
Institute of Mathematics, Romanian
Academy, Iaşi 700506,
Romania sanita@uaic.ro

Francesca Arrigoni
Dept. of Mathematics, University
of Trento, via Sommarive, 14,
38050 Povo (TN), Italy
arrigoni@science.unitn.it

Alessandro Bertuzzi
Istituto di Analisi dei Sistemi ed
Informatica "A. Ruberti",
CNR, Viale Manzoni 30, 00185
Roma, Italy
bertuzzi@iasi.cnr.it

Annamaria Bianchi
ADAMSS & Dept. of Mathematics,
University of Milan, Via Saldini,
50, 20133 Milano, Italy
abianchi@mat.unimi.it

Luis Bonilla
Universidad Carlos III de Madrid,
Avenida de la Universidad 30,
28911 Leganés, Spain
bonilla@ing.uc3m.es

Martin Burger
Institut für Industriemathematik,
Johannes Kepler Universität,
Altenbergerstr. 69, A 4040 Linz,
Austria martin.burger@jku.at

Rainer E. Burkard
Graz University of Technology
burkard@tugraz.at

Helen M. Byrne
Centre for Mathematical Medicine,
School of Mathematical Sciences,
University of Nottingham,
Nottingham NG7 2RD, UK
helen.byrne@nottingham.ac.uk

Sunčica Čanić
Department of Mathematics,
University of Houston, 4800 Calhoun
Rd., Houston TX 77204-3476, USA
canic@math.uh.edu

Vincenzo Capasso
ADAMSS & Dept. of Mathematics,
University of Milan, Via Saldini,
50, 20133 Milano, Italy
vincenzo.capasso@unimi.it

Alberto Carabarín-Aguirre
Department of Mathematics and
Statistics, University of Ottawa,
Ottawa K1N 6N5 Canada
acara553@science.uottawa.ca

Ana Carpio
Departamento de Matemática
Aplicada, Universidad Complutense
de Madrid, 28040 Madrid, Spain
ana_carpio@mat.ucm.es

Fausto Cavalli
Dipartimento di Matematica,
Università di Milano, via
Saldini 50, 20133 Milano, Italy
cavalli@mat.unimi.it

Marianna Cerasuolo
Dipartimento di Matematica e
Applicazioni "R. Caccioppoli",
Università degli Studi di Napoli
Federico II, Via Cintia, 80126
Napoli, Italy
marianna.cerasuolo@unina.it

Kevin J. Coakley
National Institute of Standards and
Technology, Boulder, Colorado,
USA 80305
kevin.coakley@nist.gov

Luigi De Cesare
Dipartimento di Scienze Economiche,
Matematiche e Statistiche,
Università di Foggia, Via IV
Novembre 1, 71100 Foggia, Italy
l.decesare@unifg.it

Andrea De Gaetano
Biomatlab of IASI-CNR, Università
Cattolica del Sacro Cuore,
Largo Gemelli 8, 00168 Roma, Italy
andrea.degaetano@biomatematica.it

Marcello De Giosa
Dipartimento di Matematica,
Università di Bari, via
Orabona 4, 70125, Bari, Italy
mdegiosa@dm.uniba.it

Andrea Di Liddo
Dipartimento di Scienze Economiche,
Matematiche e Statistiche,
Università di Foggia, Via IV
Novembre 1, 71100 Foggia , Italy
a.diliddo@unifg.it

Antonio Fasano
Dipartimento di Matematica
"U. Dini", Università di Firenze,
Viale Morgagni 67/A, 50134 Firenze,
Italy
fasano@math.unifi.it

Paolo Fergola
Dipartimento di Matematica e
Applicazioni "R. Caccioppoli",
Università degli Studi di Napoli
Federico II, Via Cintia, 80126
Napoli, Italy
paolo.fergola@dma.unina.it

Andrea Gamba
Dipartimento di Matematica,
Politecnico di Torino, Corso Duca
degli Abruzzi 24, 10129 Torino, Italy
andrea.gamba@polito.it

Alberto Gandolfi
Istituto di Analisi dei Sistemi ed
Informatica "A. Ruberti",
CNR, Viale Manzoni 30, 00185
Roma, Italy
gandolfi@iasi.cnr.it

Johannes Hatzl
Graz University of Technology
hatzl@opt.math.tu-graz.ac.at

Karl P. Hadeler
Universität Tübingen, Arizona State
University
hadeler@uni-tuebingen.de

Erick Herbin
Dassault Aviation, 78 quai Marcel
Dassault, 92552 Saint-Cloud
Cedex, France
erick.herbin@dassault-aviation.fr

Thomas Hillen
University of Alberta
thillen@ualberta.ca

Stefano Maria Iacus
Department of Economics, Business
and Statistics, University of
Milan, Via Conservatorio, 7, I-20122
Milan, Italy
stefano.iacus@unimi.it

B. Gail Ivanoff
Department of Mathematics and
Statistics, University of Ottawa,
Ottawa K1N 6N5 Canada
givanoff@uottawa.ca

Adriana Jordan
Department of Mathematics and
Statistics, University of Ottawa,
Ottawa, K1N 6N5 Canada
ajord687@science.uottawa.ca

Davide La Torre
Department of Economics, Business
and Statistics, University of
Milan, Via Conservatorio, 7, I-20122
Milan, Italy
davide.latorre@unimi.it

Philip K. Maini
Centre for Mathematical Biology,
Mathematical Institute,
University of Oxford, Oxford , UK
maini@maths.ox.ac.uk

Franklin Mendivil
Department of Mathematics and
Statistics, Acadia University,
Wolfville, Nova Scotia, Canada
franklin.mendivil@acadiau.ca

Ely Merzbach
Dept. of Mathematics, Bar Ilan
University, 52900 Ramat-Gan, Israel
merzbach@macs.biu.ac.il

Alessandra Micheletti
ADAMSS & Dept. of Mathematics,
University of Milan, Via Saldini,
50, 20133 Milano, Italy
Alessandra.Micheletti@unimi.it

Andro Mikelić
Institut Camille Jordan, UFR
Mathématiques, Université Claude
Bernard Lyon 1, Site de Gerland, Bt.
A, 50, avenue Tony Garnier,
69367 Lyon Cedex 07, France
Andro.Mikelic@univ-lyon1.fr

Daniela Morale
ADAMSS & Dept. of Mathematics,
University of Milano, Via
Saldini, 50, Milano, Italy
daniela.morale@mat.unimi.it

James Murphy
Centre for Mathematical Medicine,
School of Mathematical Sciences,
University of Nottingham,
Nottingham NG7 2RD, UK

Giovanni Naldi
Dipartimento di Matematica,
Università di Milano, via
Saldini 50, 20133 Milano, Italy
naldi@mat.unimi.it

John C. Neu
Department of Mathematics, Universidad de California at Berkeley, Berkeley, CA 94720; USA
neu@math.berkeley.edu

Filippo Notarnicola
Istituto per le Applicazioni del Calcolo, IAC-CNR Sezione di Bari, Via Amendola 122-D, 70126 Bari, Italy
f.notarnicola@ba.iac.cnr.it

Matteo Ortisi
ADAMSS & Dept. of Mathematics, University of Milano, Via Saldini, 50, Milano, Italy
ortisi@mat.unimi.it

Markus R. Owen
Centre for Mathematical Medicine, School of Mathematical Sciences, University of Nottingham, Nottingham NG7 2RD, UK
markus.owen@nottingham.ac.uk

Pasquale Palumbo
Istituto di Analisi dei Sistemi "A. Ruberti", IASI-CNR, Viale Manzoni 30, 00185 Roma, Italy
palumbo@iasi.cnr.it

Andrea Pugliese
Dept. of Mathematics, University of Trento, via Sommarive, 14, 38050 Povo (TN), Italy
pugliese@science.unitn.it

Diane Saada
Department of Statistics, Hebrew University, Jerusalem, Israel
dianes@mscc.huji.ac.il

Toshio Sekimura
Department of Biological Chemistry, College of Bioscience and Biotechnology, Chubu University, Kasugai, Aichi 487-8501, Japan
sekimura@isc.chubu.ac.jp

Matteo Semplice
Dipartimento di Matematica, Università di Milano, via Saldini 50, 20133 Milano, Italy
semplice@mat.unimi.it

Carmela Sinisgalli Istituto di Analisi dei Sistemi ed Informatica "A. Ruberti", CNR, Viale Manzoni 30, 00185 Roma, Italy sinisgalli@iasi.cnr.it

Elena Villa
ADAMSS & Dept. of Mathematics, University of Milan, Via Saldini, 50, 20133 Milano, Italy
villa@mat.unimi.it

Edward R. Vrscay
Department of Applied Mathematics, Faculty of Mathematics, University of Waterloo Waterloo, Ontario, Canada N2L 3G1
ervrscay@uwaterloo.ca

Grace L. Yang
Department of Mathematics, University of Maryland, College Park, Maryland, USA 20742
gly@math.umd.edu

Introduction

"Math Everywhere": this title of the conference dedicated to the sixtieth birthday of Vincenzo Capasso just summarizes an evaluation of the role of mathematics in science and society. Mathematics has always been an important part of culture and is respected as a basic discipline for natural sciences, medicine, engineering, economics and social sciences. The rapid progress of computer systems as well as new concepts and methods in mathematical modelling and simulation have strengthened the position of Mathematics. They offer a large potential and new perspectives for solving complex problems and for tackling important technological, medical, environmental, social, economical, and political challenges. The achievements of Mathematics in theory and methods are playing a central and still growing role in setting up models and analyzing their characteristic properties, designing fast and reliable algorithms for the numerical solution of model equations, designing and optimizing processes, validating and up-scaling the models with respect to real situations. Mathematics, imbedded in an interdisciplinary concept, has itself become a key technology. A main feature of mathematical methods is their portability, that means they are structure-oriented and thus independent of special applications. E.g. partial differential equations arising as model equations for option prices belong to the same class of mathematical systems, used to model spatial spread of chemical sub-stances or epidemics respectively to smoothen noisy images. This feature demands a special approach in developing mathematical tools and promoting research in mathematical technology.

During the last decade, mathematics opened up to other sciences and to real world problems. The German poet Hans Magnus Enzensberger, who can be considered to be a fan of mathematics, describes in an essay *"Zugbrücke außer Betrieb. Die Mathematik im Jenseits der Kultur. Drawbridge up - A cultural Anathema."* (Natick (MA): A K Peters Ltd. 1998) the relation of mathematicians, sitting in a castle cut off by a moat, and the society, and the consequences for mathematics. However, the drawbridge is being lowered more and more. This development is strongly influenced by mathematicians with visions and ideas like Vincenzo Capasso, contributing and promoting top quality mathematical research as well as building bridges to Sciences, Industry and Economics. Capasso is one of the pioneers in transfer of mathematics to real life applications.

These proceedings are reporting on the conference *"Math Everywhere"*, a successful event celebrating a leading scientist, promoting ideas he pursued and sharing the open atmosphere he is known for. The broad spectrum of contributions to this volume illustrates that its title is correct, despite the fact that mainly those areas were selected, to which Vincenzo Capasso gave his most important contributions:

1. Deterministic and Stochastic Systems.
2. Mathematical Problems in Biology, Medicine and Ecology.
3. Mathematical Problems in Industry and Economics.

Disciplinarity is basic for interdisciplinarity. This statement seems to be trivial, however, everyone, not influenced by fashionable trends and buzzwords entering more and more also science, will find out that it is nontrivial at all in practice. Competence in mathematics and the field of application are both needed. The relevance of mathematical theory is getting more obvious the more one faces the challenges of real life applications. It is a well-known fact that mathematical modelling of real problems very often leads to frontiers of mathematical theory and requires new mathematical methods. This conference combined competence in mathematical theory and methods with competence in the fields of applications.

One of the main challenges to mathematics arises due to the fact that real systems very often lead to stochastic processes in random geometry or to huge systems with multiple scales. The analytical, numerical and statistical investigations in these areas based on advanced mathematical theory are in great demand. Whereas research in stochastic geometry is developed to a large extent, processes like diffusion, transport or reactions are not treated well enough in case of stochastic geometry. Biochemical and biophysical processes in cells and tissues, growth, birth and spread in bio-systems have to be modelled taking into account the stochastic effects both in the dynamics and the geometry. The same statement holds true for many other areas of applications e.g. in material sciences or technology. Integrating stochastic and deterministic processes, stochastic geometry and statistics in an extent and a quality, which is needed for theory as well as for applications, is the strength distinguishing Capasso and his Milanese team.

Chapter I presents contributions focused on recent developments of theoretical results and mathematical methods, guided by test problems like growth, diffusion or birth-growth processes in population dynamics.

Chapter II covers the analysis and the simulation of model equation for the spread of epidemics, for tumour dynamics and growth, blood flow including mechanics of the walls of the vessels and vasculogenesis. These are all problems where mathematical modelling and simulations are decisive tools for further biomedical and clinical research. Due to the fact that experimental research is providing more precise and reliable information on all system scales, these topics are posing new challenges to mathematics and will attract more mathematical research.

Chapter III contains several examples of industrial applications in polymer chemistry and nucleation, of control of chemical reactors and bio-remediation in soil. The portability of mathematical concepts and methods to economic and social problems has been proven in many cases. Here, one example in optimal market decisions is given. In the future, more detailed mathematical modelling of processes will be used e.g. to replace unspecific "background" processes. Concepts and methods, developed by Capasso and his team for spatial growth and spatial pattern formation or for the dynamics of a communicating and interacting population of ants, can be used in modelling and simulation of economic and social networks. This fact has already been demonstrated with great success.

Vincenzo Capasso deserves great recognition for his important scientific contributions to mathematics and its applications especially in biosciences, medicine and industry, but also for initiatives and achievements in promoting these fields.

Mathematics has become a key technology important for the progress of science, technology and society. Computers can only replace that part of mathematics, which can be reduced to automatic operations. Leonardo da Vinci expressed his respect for mathematics in statements, which have not lost their truth despite the revolutions caused by modern information technology.
"O studianti, studiate le matematiche, e non edificate sanza fondamenti."

(Fogli di Windsor Royal Library (Windsor) 19066)

"Chi biasima la somma certezza delle matematiche si pasce di confusione!"
(Fogli di Windsor Royal Library (Windsor) 19084)

Heidelberg, *Willi Jäger*
July 2006

Part I

Deterministic and Stochastic Systems

Coupled Dynamics and Quiescent Phases

Karl P. Hadeler[1] and Thomas Hillen[2]

[1] Universität Tübingen, Germany & Arizona State University
  hadeler@uni-tuebingen.de
[2] University of Alberta thillen@ualberta.ca

Summary. We analyze diffusively coupled dynamical systems, which are constructed from two dynamical systems in continuous time by switching between the two dynamics. If one of the vector fields is zero we call it a *quiescent phase*. We present a detailed analysis of coupled systems and of systems with quiescent phase and we prove results on scaling limits, singular perturbations, attractors, gradient fields, stability of stationary points and amplitudes of periodic orbits. In particular we show that introducing a quiescent phase is always stabilizing.

1 Introduction

Two different dynamics acting on the same space can be coupled in several ways, e.g. by using the *Lie-Trotter approach* of periodically switching between the two dynamics or by *diffusive coupling*. Diffusive coupling has the advantage that the resulting system is autonomous. Whereas the limiting system of the Lie-Trotter approach leads to a convex combination of the two vector fields, diffusive coupling leads to another limiting system. In the general non-linear situation the two limiting systems are not equivalent. Here diffusive coupling is studied in terms of singular perturbation theory and in terms of second order systems.

If one of the two vector fields vanishes then a given dynamics is coupled to a quiescent phase. While one could conjecture that adding a quiescent phase should have similar effects as a delay, e.g. cause oscillations in negative feedback situations, the opposite is true. Introducing quiescent phases damps oscillations or even causes them to disappear. Quiescent phases occur in population models in various ways and under various names such as quiescent state [19], [12], dormancy [9], [17], resting phase [6], ecological refuge. It is generally understood that such phases may have drastic effects on the dynamics.

We show a general linear stability theorem for systems with quiescent phases near an equilibrium, another theorem on how a quiescent phase decreases the amplitude of a periodic orbit away from equilibrium, and we show

some preliminary results on the global behavior of such systems. To our best
knowledge these results are new.

In Section 2 we compare diffusive coupling to the Lie-Trotter approach,
establish the connection to second order equations, and give examples. We
cast the problem into the framework of singular perturbations in Section 2.3
and prove results on global behavior in Section 2.4. In Section 3 we introduce
the concept of quiescent phases, study local stability of stationary points in
Section 3.1, then periodic orbits in Section 3.2, and global behavior of systems with quiescent phases in Section 3.3. Finally, in Section 4 we prove the
generalized Lie-Trotter approximation (Theorem 1).

2 Coupled Systems

Let f and g be smooth vector fields on $\mathbb{R}^m$. The differential equations

$$\dot{v} = f(v), \quad \dot{w} = g(w)$$

have unique local solutions. One way to couple these two equations is the
classical Lie product formula, the other is diffusive coupling. Here we compare
both approaches.

2.1 The Lie-Trotter Approach

Let $\chi : \mathbb{R} \to [0, 1]$ be a piecewise continuous function of period 1. For $\delta > 0$
consider the periodic system with period δ

$$\dot{u}_\delta = \chi(t/\delta)f(u_\delta) + (1 - \chi(t/\delta))g(u_\delta) \tag{1}$$

with the initial datum $u_\delta(0) = u_0$. For a fixed time horizon T consider the
solution $u_\delta(t)$ for $0 \leq t \leq T$ for $\delta \to 0$. The limiting function $u(t)$ satisfies the
autonomous equation

$$\dot{u} = \rho_1 f(u) + \rho_2 g(u) \tag{2}$$

with $\rho_1 = \int_0^1 \chi(s)ds$, $\rho_2 = 1 - \rho_1$, and the initial datum $u(0) = u_0$. Although
this statement it intuitively obvious, the proof is not that obvious, in particular as the important special case, i.e., the Lie product formula for matrices
$\exp\{A+B\} = \lim_{k\to\infty}(\exp\{A/k\}\exp\{B/k\})^k$ (Lie 1875) is usually proved via
estimates for matrix products, see [1], p. 254, and [8], p. 496. In the following
$\| \ \|$ is the maximum norm on $\mathbb{R}^m$ and the corresponding operator norm.

Theorem 1. *Let $\|f(u)\|$, $\|g(u)\|$, $\|f'(u)\|$, $\|g'(u)\|$ be bounded by some const-
ant M uniformly in u. Let $T > 0$ be a fixed time. Then for $\delta \to 0$ the solutions
of (1) converge to the solution of (2) uniformly on $[0, T]$.*

The proof is given in Section 4. A special case arises for

$$\chi(t) = \begin{cases} 1, & 0 \le t < \rho_1 \\ 0, & \rho_1 \le t < 1 \end{cases}$$

with some $\rho_1 \in (0,1)$ and $\rho_2 = 1 - \rho_1$. The vector field (2) is a convex combination of the vector fields f and g. The standard case is $\rho_1 = 1/2$. Extensions to infinite dimensions and operator semigroups are called Lie-Trotter and Trotter-Kato formulae (Trotter 1959, Kato 1978). For extensions to infinite-dimensional non-linear systems see, e.g. [15]. The Lie-Trotter approach is well suited for numerical schemes (e.g. fractional steps, alternating directions (ADI), splitting methods) because it simplifies the design of consistent schemes. From the view point of dynamical systems it has the disadvantage that the coupled system becomes non-autonomous.

The theorem can be generalized to the case of $N \ge 2$ vector fields f_i in R^m, $i = 1, \ldots, N$. Given piece-wise continuous functions χ_i which are periodic with period 1, and $\chi_i \ge 0$, $\sum_{k=1} \chi_k = 1$, Lie-Trotter coupling

$$\dot{u}_\delta = \sum_{i=1}^{N} \chi_i(t/\delta) f_i(u_\delta)$$

leads to the limiting equation

$$\dot{u} = \sum_{i=1}^{N} \rho_i f_i(u) \quad \text{with} \quad \rho_i = \int_0^1 \chi_i(s)ds.$$

2.2 Diffusive Coupling

Let γ_1, γ_2 be positive coupling constants. Then consider the system in $\mathbb{R}^{2m}$

$$\begin{aligned} \dot{v} &= f(v) - \gamma_2 v + \gamma_1 w \\ \dot{w} &= g(w) - \gamma_1 w + \gamma_2 v. \end{aligned} \tag{3}$$

With particle density u and flux z as new variables

$$u = v + w, \quad z = \gamma_2 v - \gamma_1 w, \tag{4}$$

the system assumes the form

$$\begin{aligned} \dot{u} &= f(\rho_1 u + \tau z) + g(\rho_2 u - \tau z) \\ \tau \dot{z} &= \rho_2 f(\rho_1 u + \tau z) - \rho_1 g(\rho_2 u - \tau z) - z \end{aligned} \tag{5}$$

where the time constant τ and proportions ρ_1, ρ_2, with $\rho_1 + \rho_2 = 1$, are given by

$$\tau = 1/(\gamma_1 + \gamma_2), \quad \rho_i = \tau \gamma_i, \quad i = 1, 2.$$

If we let τ go to zero then we arrive at the limiting system

$$\dot{u} = f(\rho_1 u) + g(\rho_2 u) \tag{6}$$

which is rather different from the limiting equation (2). The equations (6) and (2) are equivalent if at least one of the functions f, g is homogeneous of degree 1. If $g = f$ then (2) yields $\dot{u} = f$ while (6) is not that simple except in the symmetric case $\gamma_1 = \gamma_2$.

The difference between the two limiting equations can be interpreted in terms of particles in a variable environment. In the Lie-Trotter approach (2) the particle ensemble is subject to a changing environment (switching between two environments in the classical case) while in the situation of diffusive coupling (6) each particle switches between two phases according to Poisson processes with rates γ_1, γ_2. Another interpretation of (6) versus (2): In (6) the functions f and g act on the corresponding fraction of the total population while in (2) the weighted mean of f and g acts on the total population.

We connect the first order system for two variables (3) to a second order system for one variable (for smooth f). Differentiate the equations,

$$\ddot{v} = f'(v)\dot{v} - \gamma_2\dot{v} + \gamma_1\dot{w}$$
$$\ddot{w} = g'(w)\dot{w} - \gamma_1\dot{w} + \gamma_2\dot{v}$$

and in the first equation replace $\dot{w}$ using the second equation of (3) and then replace w from the first equation of (3). We get a second order system in $\mathbb{R}^m$ for the variable v,

$$\tau\ddot{v} + (1 - \tau f'(v))\dot{v} = \rho_1 f(v) + \rho_1 g\left(\left(\frac{\rho_2}{\rho_1}\right)v + \frac{\tau}{\rho_1}(\dot{v} - f(v)) \right). \tag{7}$$

If v is a solution of (7) then the solution of (3) can be recovered by putting $w = (\dot{v} - f(v) + \gamma_2 v)/\gamma_1$. Hence (3) and (7) are equivalent.

In the limiting case of strong coupling, $\gamma_i = \gamma_i/\varepsilon$, $\varepsilon \to 0$, we get a first order system

$$\dot{v} = \rho_1 f(v) + \rho_1 g(\frac{\rho_2}{\rho_1}v). \tag{8}$$

The function $u = v/\rho_1$ satisfies (6).

Example 1. For Verhulst equations $f(v) = a_1 v(1 - v/K_1)$, $g(w) = a_2 w(1 - w/K_2)$ the limiting equation via diffusive coupling is

$$\dot{u} = au(1 - \frac{u}{K})$$

where $a = \rho_1 a_1 + \rho_2 a_2$ is the effective growth rate and

$$K = \frac{\rho_1 a_1 + \rho_2 a_2}{\frac{\rho_1^2 a_1}{K_1} + \frac{\rho_2^2 a_2}{K_2}}$$

is the effective carrying capacity. The growth rate is an arithmetic mean of growth rates while the carrying capacity can be written as a harmonic mean of the carrying capacities times some factor independent of the K_i. The Lie-Trotter approach (2) yields the same value for the growth rate a but the effective capacity is a simple harmonic mean

$$K = \frac{\rho_1 a_1 + \rho_2 a_2}{\frac{\rho_1 a_1}{K_1} + \frac{\rho_2 a_2}{K_2}}.$$

Example 2. The ideas can be carried over to infinite-dimensional systems, e.g., reaction-diffusion equations. The system

$$v_t = D\Delta v - \mu v - \gamma_2 v + \gamma_1 w$$
$$w_t = f(w) - \gamma_1 w + \gamma_2 v$$

describes a situation where the v particles diffuse and are subject to mortality while the w particles interact and do not move. In

$$v_t = D\Delta v + f(v) - \gamma_2 v + \gamma_1 w$$
$$w_t = -\gamma_1 w + \gamma_2 v$$

a reaction-diffusion equation is coupled to a quiescent phase. For more details on coupled reaction-diffusion equations and quiescent transport equations see the references [11], [5], [6]. In [2] this approach is applied to a problem in protein dynamics. In [14] a coupled system has been used to understand the so-called river drift paradox in spread and persistence of species in stream ecosystems.

Example 3. The example of a delay equation $\dot{u}(t) = f(u(t - \theta))$ shows that one has to be careful with diffusive coupling. The system

$$\dot{v}(t) = f(v(t - \theta)) - \gamma_2 v(t) + \gamma_1 w(t)$$
$$\dot{w}(t) = \gamma_2 v(t) - \gamma_1 w(t)$$

may be of some interest but it is *not* the system one gets from coupling the dynamical system to the zero vector field. The reason is that the state space of the delay equation is not $\mathbb{R}$ but $C[-\tau, 0]$.

Example 4. Coupled dynamics is particularly relevant in epidemic modeling, when individuals switch between phases of different behavior, e.g., in core-non core situations or in public health education campaigns. In [4] coupling of moving and resting infected has been used to present the two classical approaches for epidemic spread, via diffusion and via contact distributions, within the same framework.

Again consider the case of $N \geq 2$ vector fields f_i (notice that v_i are vectors and not components of one vector)

$$\dot{v}_i = f_i(v_i) + \frac{1}{\tau} \sum_{k=1}^{N} \gamma_{ik} v_k$$

The matrix $\Gamma = (\gamma_{ik})$ has non-negative off-diagonal entries and column sums equal to 0. Let Γ be irreducible. Let $\rho = (\rho_i)$ with $\rho_i > 0$, $\sum_{i=1}^{N} \rho_i = 1$, be the unique stationary distribution. The "total particle density"

$$u = \sum_{i=1}^{N} v_i$$

satisfies the equation

$$\dot{u} = \sum_{i=1}^{N} f_i(w_i u)$$

whereby $w_i = v_i/u$. For $\tau \to 0$ the limiting equation becomes

$$\dot{u} = \sum_{i=1}^{N} f_i(\rho_i u).$$

2.3 Singular Perturbation Approach

In the language of singular perturbation theory the system (5) is a slow system with τ as a small parameter [10]. Its solutions are called the outer solutions. Scaling the time variable as $\vartheta = t/\tau$ gives the fast system

$$\begin{aligned}
\dot{u} &= \tau(f(\rho_1 u + \tau z) + g(\rho_2 u - \tau z)) \\
\dot{z} &= \rho_2 f(\rho_1 u + \tau z) - \rho_1 g(\rho_2 u - \tau z) - z
\end{aligned} \tag{9}$$

which describes the dynamics in the initial layer, the so-called inner solution. It provides initial data for the outer solution. For the outer solution we solve the slow system (5) with initial conditions

$$u(0) = u_0, \quad z(0) = \rho_2 f(\rho_1 u_0) - \rho_1 g(\rho_2 u_0). \tag{10}$$

We expand u and z as $u(t) = U_0(t) + \tau U_1(t) + \tau^2 U_2(t) + \cdots$ and $z(t) = Z_0(t) + \tau Z_1(t) + \tau^2 Z_2(t) + \cdots$. To leading order we get from (5)

$$\dot{U}_0 = f(\rho_1 U_0) + g(\rho_2 U_0) \tag{11}$$
$$0 = \rho_2 f(\rho_1 U_0) - \rho_1 g(\rho_2 U_0) - Z_0. \tag{12}$$

Equation (12) describes the *slow manifold*

$$\mathcal{M}_0 = \{(u, z) : z = \rho_2 f(\rho_1 u) - \rho_1 g(\rho_2 u)\}$$

whereas the first equation (11) describes the dynamics on that manifold. Note that this dynamics is the same as in (6) whereby the formal limit (8) is justified. The inner solution approximates the slow manifold $\mathcal{M}_0$ as $\vartheta \to \infty$ and then the *matching* initial conditions in $\mathcal{M}_0$ as given in (10).

To apply Fenichel's geometric singular perturbation theory ([10]) we show that $\mathcal{M}_0$ is normally hyperbolic.

Lemma 1. *The manifold $\mathcal{M}_0$ is normally hyperbolic with respect to the flow of the fast system at $\tau = 0$.*

Proof. Linearize the fast system at $(\bar{u}, \bar{z}) \in \mathcal{M}_0$,

$$\frac{d}{d\vartheta} \begin{pmatrix} u \\ z \end{pmatrix} = A_\tau \begin{pmatrix} u \\ z \end{pmatrix} \quad \text{with} \quad A_0 = \begin{pmatrix} 0 & 0 \\ a & -I_m \end{pmatrix}$$

whereby $a = \rho_1 \rho_2 (f'(\rho_1 \bar{u}) - g'(\rho_2 \bar{u}))$, and f' and g' denote the Jacobians of f, g and I_m is the $m \times m$ identity. Hence the eigenvalues are 0 and -1 with eigenvectors $(0, 1)^T$ and $(1, a)^T$. $\quad \square$

Fenichel's first theorem (Theorem 1 and 2 in [10]) gives

Theorem 2. *For $\tau > 0$ small enough there exists a locally invariant manifold $\mathcal{M}_\tau$ (the critical manifold) with the following properties:*
i) $\mathcal{M}_\tau$ is τ-close to $\mathcal{M}_0$.
ii) $\mathcal{M}_\tau$ is locally invariant for the fast system.
iii) $\mathcal{M}_\tau = \{(u, z) : z = h^\tau(u)\}$ is a graph with $h^0(u) = \rho_2 f(\rho_1 u) - \rho_1 g(\rho_2 u)$.

From the linearization in Lemma 1 one sees that $\mathcal{M}_0$ has a stable manifold of dimension m. From Fenichel's second theorem (Theorem 3 in [10]) it follows that $\mathcal{M}_\tau$ has an m-dimensional stable manifold and solutions approach $\mathcal{M}_\tau$ exponentially fast. In the present case the exponent is -1.

2.4 Global Behavior

We cannot expect that the dynamics of the coupled system (3) is largely determined by the dynamics of the two constituents (15), not even in the linear case $f(v) = Av$, $g(w) = Bw$ there are useful results for general matrices A, B. The only immediate observation is concerned with gradient fields.

Proposition 1. *Assume the vector fields f and g are gradient fields. Then the system (3) is equivalent to a system with a gradient field.*

Proof. By substituting $v = \sqrt{\gamma_1}\tilde{v}$, $w = \sqrt{\gamma_2}\tilde{w}$ and then dropping the tildes the system (3) becomes

$$\dot{v} = \frac{1}{\sqrt{\gamma_1}} f(\sqrt{\gamma_1}v) - \gamma_2 v + \sqrt{\gamma_1 \gamma_2}w$$

$$\dot{w} = \frac{1}{\sqrt{\gamma_2}} g(\sqrt{\gamma_2}w) - \gamma_1 w + \sqrt{\gamma_1 \gamma_2}v. \tag{13}$$

Let $f = F'$, $g = G'$. Then (13) has the potential

$$\frac{1}{\gamma_1}F(\sqrt{\gamma_1}v) + \frac{1}{\gamma_2}G(\sqrt{\gamma_2}w) - \frac{1}{2}\|\sqrt{\gamma_2}v - \sqrt{\gamma_1}w\|^2. \tag{14}$$

$\square$

Even this result is not generally applicable: If F, G are bounded below then the potential (14) need not be bounded below. To compensate for the negative term for large w the functionals F, G must grow at least quadratically. However, the result is strong enough for space dimension one.

Corollary 1. *If the space dimension is $m = 1$ then every bounded trajectory of (3) converges to an equilibrium.*

This result could also have been concluded from the theory of cooperative systems [7] since for $m = 1$ the system (3) is cooperative. Our next observations are concerned with global attractors.

Suppose it is known that the limiting system (6) has a (local or global) attractor. We will show that, for τ small enough, the system (9) has a local attractor as well. Let $\mathcal{A}_0$ denote the attractor of (6) in question. Then define

$$\tilde{\mathcal{A}}_0 = \{(u, z) : u \in \mathcal{A}_0, z = h^0(u)\}$$

where $h^0(u)$ has been defined in Theorem 2. From the general theory of attractors (see, e.g. Temam [18] or Robinson [16]) we obtain the following result.

Theorem 3. *Assume the system (6) in $\mathbb{R}^m$ has a compact local or global attractor $\mathcal{A}_0$. For $\tau > 0$ small enough the system (9) in $\mathbb{R}^{2m}$ has a compact attractor $\mathcal{A}_\tau \subset \mathbb{R}^{2m}$ near $\tilde{\mathcal{A}}_0$ in the sense that $\mathcal{A}_\tau$ is upper semi-continuous at $\tilde{\mathcal{A}}_0$ for $\tau = 0$, i.e., $\lim_{\tau \to 0} \mathrm{dist}\,(\mathcal{A}_\tau, \tilde{\mathcal{A}}_0) = 0$ where*

$$\mathrm{dist}\,(X, Y) = \sup_{x \in X} \inf_{y \in Y} \|x - y\|.$$

Moreover, if in addition

$$\mathcal{A}_0 = \cup_{\xi \in \mathcal{E}}\overline{W^u(\xi)}$$

where $\mathcal{E}$ consists of a finite number of equilibria, then the attractors are lower semi-continuous as well, i.e. $\lim_{\tau \to 0} \mathrm{dist}\,(\tilde{\mathcal{A}}_0, \mathcal{A}_\tau) = 0$.

Note that in Theorem 3 the attractor $\mathcal{A}_\tau$ need not be a global attractor, see the following example.

Example 5. Let $m = 1$, $\rho_1 = \rho_2$, $f(x) = x(x - 1)$, $g(x) = -x(x + 1)$. Then the limiting system (6) reads $\dot{u} = -u$ which has the compact global attractor $\mathcal{A}_0 = \{0\}$. The coupled system (5) reads

$$\dot{u} = (-1 + \tau z), \quad \tau\dot{z} = \frac{u^2}{4} + (\tau z)^2 - 2z.$$

From the second equation it is evident that solutions with large $z(0) > 0$ blow up in finite time. But $\mathcal{A}_\tau\{(0, 0)\} = \tilde{\mathcal{A}}_0$ is an asymptotically stable node and hence it is still a local attractor.

3 Quiescent Phases

Probably the most interesting special case of equation (3) arises if the vector field g vanishes. Then we can interpret w as a resting or quiescent phase. Let the dynamics in $\mathbb{R}^m$ be given by

$$\dot{u} = f(u). \tag{15}$$

Then the corresponding system with quiescent phase is

$$\begin{aligned}
\dot{v} &= f(v) - \gamma_2 v + \gamma_1 w \\
\dot{w} &= -\gamma_1 w + \gamma_2 v
\end{aligned} \tag{16}$$

and the second order system (7) reads $\tau \ddot{v} + (1 - \tau f'(v))\dot{v} = \rho_1 f(v)$. For $\tau \to 0$ we recover the dynamics (15) with a different time scale. Also the limiting system (6) recovers the original system (15) on a different time scale $\dot{u} = f(\rho_1 u)$.

Example 6. If the Verhulst equation $\dot{u} = au(1 - u/K)$ is coupled to a quiescent phase, then the limiting equation reads

$$\dot{u} = a\rho_1 u \left(1 - \rho_1 \frac{u}{K}\right).$$

The exponent is decreased to $a\rho_1$ and the carrying capacity is increased to K/ρ_1 saying that the population grows slower and the habitat can support a larger population.

The equation with Allee effect $\dot{u} = u(1 - u)(u - \alpha)$, with $0 < \alpha < 1$, if coupled to a quiescent phase, yields the limiting equation

$$\dot{u} = \rho_1 u(1 - \rho_1 u)(\rho_1 u - \alpha).$$

The carrying capacity is increased and also the threshold.

3.1 Stabilization by Quiescent Phases

Introducing a quiescent phase does not essentially change the equilibria.

Lemma 2. *The stationary points of the system (16) with quiescent phase are essentially the same as those of the simple dynamics (15), i.e., they have the form $(\bar{v}, (\gamma_2/\gamma_1)\bar{v})$ where $f(\bar{v}) = 0$.*

In the view of interacting particles a quiescent phase should act as a delay. Introducing a delay into a dynamical system with negative feedback in general causes oscillatory instability if the delay is large. But introducing a quiescent phase does not lead to oscillatory instability, quite on the contrary, it is stabilizing. This fact can be seen from the following theorem which has been proved in [3]. In (16), with $m \geq 1$, assume $f(\bar{v}) = 0$. Then $(\bar{v}, \bar{w})$ with $\bar{w} = \gamma_2 \bar{v}/\gamma_1$ is a stationary state. The eigenvalues μ of $f'(\bar{v})$ and the corresponding eigenvalues λ of the Jacobian at $(\bar{v}, \bar{w})$ are connected by the equation

$$\varphi(\lambda) \equiv \lambda^2 + \lambda(\gamma_1 + \gamma_2 - \mu) - \mu\gamma_1 = 0.$$

We describe the relationships between these eigenvalues in detail.

Theorem 4. *Let μ be an eigenvalue of the linearization of (15) at a steady state $\bar{u}$. Then the linearization of (16) at $(\bar{u}, \gamma_2\bar{u}/\gamma_1)$ has two corresponding eigenvalues λ_1, λ_2 with $\Re\lambda_2 \leq \Re\lambda_1$. The eigenvalues μ and λ_1, λ_2 are related as follows:*
(a) Let $\mu = \alpha \in \mathbb{R}$. Then λ_1, λ_2 are real.
(a.i) If $\alpha < 0$ then $\lambda_2 < \alpha < \lambda_1 < 0$.
(a.ii) If $\alpha = 0$ then $\lambda_2 = -(\gamma_1 + \gamma_2) < 0 = \lambda_1$.
(a.iii) If $\alpha > 0$ then $\lambda_2 < 0 < \lambda_1 < \alpha$.
(b) Let $\mu = \alpha \pm i\beta$, $\beta > 0$. Then $\Re\lambda_2 < 0$.
(b.i) If $\alpha \leq 0$ then $\Re\lambda_1 < 0$.
(b.ii) If $\alpha > 0$ then $\Re\lambda_1 < \alpha$.
(b.iii) If $\alpha \leq 0$ and
$$\beta^2 + (\gamma_1 + \gamma_2 + \alpha)^2 + 4\alpha\gamma_2 > 0 \text{ and } \beta^2(\gamma_1 + \alpha) + \alpha(\gamma_1 + \gamma_2 + \alpha)^2 > 0,$$
then $\Re\lambda_1 < \alpha$.
(b.iv) If $\alpha > 0$ and
$$\beta^2 > 4\alpha\gamma_1 - (\gamma_1 + \gamma_2 - \alpha)^2 \text{ and } \beta(\gamma_2 - \alpha) > \alpha(\gamma_1 + \gamma_2 - \alpha)^2,$$
then $\Re\lambda_1 < 0$.

With respect to the leading eigenvalue λ_1 the theorem says that a zero eigenvalue is maintained while non-zero real eigenvalues maintain their sign and move closer towards zero. For conjugate complex eigenvalues in general the real part decreases, in particular if the imaginary part is large (in absolute value). Purely imaginary eigenvalues are always carried into eigenvalues with negative real parts. The property (b.i) was also proven in Neubert et al. [13]. Properties (b.iii) and (b.iv) say that if $\gamma_i >> |\alpha|$ and β^2 is large then oscillations are damped.
A proof of Theorem 4 is given in [3].

Example 7 (Paradox of enrichment). The MacArthur-Rosenzweig model for a prey-predator population exhibits a Hopf bifurcation when the capacity of the prey exceeds a certain threshold. We extend the model by a quiescent phase for the prey only. The extended system for active prey x, predators y and quiescent prey z reads

$$\dot{x} = ax\left(1 - \frac{x}{K}\right) - \frac{bxy}{A + x} - \gamma_2 x + \gamma_1 z$$
$$\dot{y} = cy\left(\frac{x}{A + x} - \frac{B}{B + A}\right)$$
$$\dot{z} = \gamma_2 x - \gamma_1 z.$$

There are stationary states $(0,0,0)$, $(K,0,0)$ and the coexistence state $(\bar{x},\bar{y},\bar{z})$ with $\bar{x} = B$, $\bar{y} = (a/b)(1 - B/K)(A+B)$, $\bar{z} = \gamma_2 B/\gamma_1$. Notice that $\bar{x},\bar{y}$ do not depend on γ_1,γ_2. The coexistence state is feasible (positive) if $B < K$. In the absence of a quiescent phase the coexistence state is stable if $B > (K - A)/2$ and unstable if $B < (K - A)/2$.

The characteristic polynomial of the Jacobian at the coexistence state is

$$\lambda^3 + (\gamma_1 + \gamma_2 - T)\lambda^2 + (S - T\gamma_1)\lambda + S\gamma_1 = 0$$

where

$$T = \frac{aB}{K(A+B)}(K - A - 2B), \qquad S = \frac{acAB}{K(A+B)^2}(K - B).$$

Because of $S > 0$ the Routh-Hurwitz criterion for stability reduces to the single inequality

$$(\gamma_1 + \gamma_2 - T)(S - \gamma_1 T) > S\gamma_1. \tag{17}$$

For the system with a quiescent phase we have stability for $T < 0$. In that case also (17) is satisfied for any choice of $\gamma_1, \gamma_2 > 0$. On the other hand, if $T > 0$ then the system can be stabilized by first choosing $\gamma_1 < S/T$ and then γ_2 so large that (17) is satisfied. Hence the system can be stabilized by making the exit rate from the quiescent compartment small and the entrance rate to that compartment large. We find that the system becomes stabilized against oscillations when the prey has a refuge in the form of a quiescent phase.

3.2 Periodic Orbits and Quiescent Phases

We know that near a stationary point a quiescent phase tends to suppress oscillations. Now we ask what effect a quiescent phase has on existing "large" periodic orbits expecting that in some sense the "amplitude" is decreased or that the periodic orbit disappears. We choose the model problem in the plane

$$\dot{r} = rg(r), \quad \dot{\varphi} = 1$$

where $g \in C^1(\mathbb{R})$ is strictly decreasing from $g(0) > 0$ to negative values, and $g(\bar{r}) = 0$, $g'(\bar{r}) < 0$. In cartesian coordinates the system reads, with $r^2 = u_1^2 + u_2^2$,

$$\dot{u}_1 = g(r)u_1 - u_2$$
$$\dot{u}_2 = g(r)u_2 + u_1.$$

We define a system with an active phase v and a quiescent phase w as before (a system in $\mathbb{R}^4$). We return to polar coordinates $v = (r,\varphi)$, $w = (\rho,\psi)$ and get a four-dimensional system

$$\dot{r} = rg(r) - \gamma_2 r + \gamma_1 \rho \cos(\varphi - \psi)$$
$$\dot{\varphi} = 1 - \gamma_1 (\rho/r) \sin(\varphi - \psi)$$
$$\dot{\rho} = -\gamma_1 \rho + \gamma_2 r \cos(\varphi - \psi)$$
$$\dot{\psi} = \gamma_2 (r/\rho) \sin(\varphi - \psi). \tag{18}$$

Finally we introduce the displacement angle $\theta = \varphi - \psi$ and get a three-dimensional system

$$\dot{r} = rg(r) - \gamma_2 r + \gamma_1 \rho \cos \theta$$
$$\dot{\theta} = 1 - (\gamma_1 (\rho/r) + \gamma_2 (r/\rho)) \sin \theta$$
$$\dot{\rho} = -\gamma_1 \rho + \gamma_2 r \cos \theta. \tag{19}$$

For this system we prove the following result.

Theorem 5. *Consider the model problem (19). Define $\bar{\beta} = \bar{\beta}(\gamma_1, \gamma_2)$ as the unique positive solution of the cubic equation*

$$\beta(\beta - \gamma_2 - \gamma_1)^2 + \beta - \gamma_2 = 0, \tag{20}$$

and let $\bar{\kappa}$ be the unique positive solution of the equation

$$\frac{\gamma_1^2}{\gamma_2^2} \kappa + \frac{\kappa}{(\gamma_1 \kappa + \gamma_2)^2} = 1. \tag{21}$$

If $g(0) > \bar{\beta}$ then let R be defined by $g(R) = \bar{\beta}$. In this case the system has a periodic orbit with constant radius $r = R < \bar{r}$, whereby $\rho = R\bar{\kappa}$. If $g(0) \le \bar{\beta}$ then there is no such orbit.

Proof. We look for a solution of (19) along which r, ρ and θ are constant. Then the time derivatives are zero and we have three equations for r, ρ, θ. From the last two equations we find

$$\cos \theta = \frac{\gamma_1 \rho}{\gamma_2 r}, \quad \sin \theta = \left(\gamma_1 \frac{\rho}{r} + \gamma_2 \frac{r}{\rho} \right)^{-1}$$

and hence we get two equations for r and $\kappa = (\rho/r)^2$,

$$g(r) - \gamma_2 + \frac{\gamma_1^2}{\gamma_2} \kappa = 0, \tag{22}$$

and (21). If κ runs from 0 to ∞ then the left hand side of (21) is strictly increasing from 0 to ∞. Hence there is a unique solution $\bar{\kappa} > 0$ which depends only on γ_1 and γ_2. Furthermore the left hand side of (21) is greater than 1 at $\kappa = \gamma_2^2/\gamma_1^2$, hence we have

$$\bar{\kappa}(\gamma_1, \gamma_2) < \frac{\gamma_2^2}{\gamma_1^2}. \tag{23}$$

Now $\bar{\kappa}$ has been determined and equation (22) becomes $g(r) = \bar{\beta}$ whereby

$$\bar{\beta} = \gamma_2 - \frac{\gamma_1^2}{\gamma_2}\bar{\kappa}(\gamma_1, \gamma_2).$$

We have $\bar{\beta} > 0$ in view of (23).

Now we express $\bar{\kappa}$ in terms of $\bar{\beta}$ which gives $\bar{\kappa} = (\gamma_2 - \bar{\beta})\gamma_1/\gamma_1^2$, we insert this expression into (21), and get an equation for $\bar{\beta}$ in terms of γ_1, γ_2 which is (20). This equation has a unique positive solution.

Now there are two cases.

Case 1: $g(0) > \bar{\beta}$. Then there is a unique value R with $g(R) = \bar{\beta}$. Determine $\bar{\theta}$ from

$$\cos\bar{\theta} = (\gamma_1/\gamma_2)\sqrt{\bar{\kappa}}, \quad (\gamma_1\sqrt{\bar{\kappa}} + \gamma_2(1/\sqrt{\bar{\kappa}}))\sin\bar{\theta} = 1.$$

Finally go back to (18) and find a solution $r = R$, $\rho = \sqrt{\bar{\kappa}}R$, $\dot{\varphi} = \dot{\psi} = 1 - \gamma_1\sqrt{\bar{\kappa}}\sin\bar{\theta}$. The equation (21) for $\kappa = \bar{\kappa}$ ensures that indeed $\dot{\varphi} = \dot{\psi}$. The period of the orbit is $T = 2\pi(\gamma_1\bar{\kappa}/\gamma_2 + 1)$.

Case 2: $g(0) \le \bar{\beta}$. Then the equation $g(r) = \bar{\beta}$ has no solution. $\square$

3.3 Global Behavior of Systems with Quiescent Phases

We further explore the connection between (15) and (16). If (15) has a compact global attractor then one can ask whether (16) has a compact global attractor. Such a general result is perhaps not true. We show a weaker result using the Lyapunov function $v^T v$. Even for space dimension 1 the problem of global existence is not trivial.

Lemma 3. *Let $m = 1$. Assume that all solutions of (15) exist for all times $t \ge 0$. Then all solutions of (16) exist for all positive times.*

Proof. Assume that $(v, w) \to \infty$ in finite time. Then $v \to \infty$ in finite time. For if v would stay bounded then w would be bounded in finite time (variation of constants applied to the second equation of (16)). Since the system is cooperative, the tangent vector $(\dot{v}, \dot{w})$ can switch the orthant at most once and eventually stays in one of the four orthants [7]. We distinguish several cases according to the orthant.

Case 1: $\dot{v} \ge 0$, $\dot{w} \ge 0$. Let $v \to \infty$ in finite time. Then $\gamma_1 v - \gamma_2 w \ge 0$ and $\dot{v} \le f(v)$. Hence $v(t) \le u(t)$ where u is the solution of (15) with the same initial value. Hence $u \to \infty$ in finite time which is a contradiction.

Case 2: $\dot{v} \ge 0$, $\dot{w} < 0$. Let v go to infinity in finite time. From

$$\dot{w}(t) = \left(\gamma_2 v(0) - \gamma_1 w(0) + \gamma_2\int_0^t e^{\gamma_1 s}\dot{v}(s)ds\right)e^{-\gamma_1 t}$$

it follows that $\dot{w}$ becomes eventually positive. Hence this case is impossible. The preceding formula follows easily from $\ddot{w} = \gamma_2\dot{v} - \gamma_1\dot{w}$, but it holds also if w is only C^1.

The other two orthants are treated similarly, $\dot{v} \le 0$, $\dot{w} \le 0$ as in case 1, $\dot{v} \le 0$, $\dot{w} \ge 0$ as in case 2. $\square$

We do not know whether a similar statement holds in several dimensions. However, we show the following:

Theorem 6. *Let $v^T f(v) < 0$ hold for large $\|v\|$. Then for any choice of $\gamma_1, \gamma_2 > 0$ the system (16) has a compact global attractor.*

Proof. We show that for some large R the ball $\gamma_2 v^2 + \gamma_1 w^2 \leq R^2$ is positively invariant. We write $v^2 = v^T v$. Along trajectories of (16) we have

$$\frac{1}{2}\frac{d}{dt}(\gamma_2 v^2 + \gamma_1 w^2) = \gamma_2 v^T f(v) - (\gamma_2 v - \gamma_1 w)^T(\gamma_2 v - \gamma_1 w).$$

Choose $r > 0$ such that $v^T f(v) < 0$ for $\|v\| \geq r$. Choose $m > 0$ such that $v^T f(v) \leq m$ for $\|v\| \leq r$. Finally choose $R > \sqrt{(\sqrt{\gamma_2 m} + \gamma_2 r)^2/\gamma_1 + \gamma_2 r^2}$. We want to show $\frac{1}{2}d/dt(\gamma_2 v^2 + \gamma_1 w^2) < 0$ for $\gamma_2 v^2 + \gamma_1 w^2 \geq R^2$. Let (v, w) such that $\gamma_2 v^2 + \gamma_1 w^2 \geq R^2$.
Case 1: $\|v\| \geq r$. Then $v^T f(v) < 0$ by assumption and hence the desired inequality is evident.
Case 2: $\|v\| < r$. From $\gamma_2 v^2 + \gamma_1 w^2 \geq R^2$ it follows that

$$w^2 \geq \frac{1}{\gamma_1}(R^2 - \gamma_2 v^2) \geq \frac{1}{\gamma_1}(R^2 - \gamma_2 r^2)$$

and the right hand side is positive by assumption on R. Hence

$$\|w\| \geq \frac{1}{\sqrt{\gamma_1}}\sqrt{R^2 - \gamma_2 r^2},$$

$$\|\gamma_1 w - \gamma_2 v\| \geq \gamma_1 \|w\| - \gamma_2 \|v\| \geq \sqrt{\gamma_1}\sqrt{R^2 - \gamma_2 r^2} - \gamma_2 r.$$

Finally

$$\frac{1}{2}\frac{d}{dt}(\gamma_2 v^2 + \gamma_1 w^2) \leq \gamma_2 m - [\sqrt{\gamma_1}\sqrt{R^2 - \gamma_2 r^2} - \gamma_2 r]^2$$

which is negative by the assumption on R. $\square$

Corollary 2. *Let the space dimension be $m = 1$. If the original system (15) has a bounded global attractor then for any choice of γ_1, γ_2 the system with a quiescent phase (16) has a bounded global attractor. This global attractor consists of the stationary states and their unstable manifolds.*

Proof. In space dimension 1 the condition $vf(v) < 0$ for large $|v|$ is necessary and sufficient for the existence of a global attractor. The remainder of the proof follows from Theorem 6. $\square$

4 Proof of Theorem 1

The difference $u_\delta - u$ satisfies

$$
\begin{aligned}
\dot{u}_\delta - \dot{u} &= \chi(t/\delta)f(u_\delta) + (1 - \chi(t/\delta))g(u_\delta) - \rho_1 f(u) - (1 - \rho_1)g(u) \\
&= \chi(t/\delta)f(u_\delta) + (1 - \chi(t/\delta))g(u_\delta) - \chi(t/\delta)f(u) - (1 - \chi(t/\delta))g(u) \\
&\quad + \chi(t/\delta)f(u) + (1 - \chi(t/\delta))g(u) - \rho_1 f(u) - (1 - \rho_1)g(u) \\
&= \chi(t/\delta)(f(u_\delta) - f(u)) + (1 - \chi(t/\delta))(g(u_\delta) - g(u)) \\
&\quad + (\chi(t/\delta) - \rho_1)(f(u) - g(u)).
\end{aligned}
$$

We integrate

$$
\begin{aligned}
u_\delta(t) - u(t) &= \int_0^t [\chi(s/\delta)(f(u_\delta) - f(u)) + (1 - \chi(t/\delta))(g(u_\delta) - g(u))]ds \\
&\quad + \int_0^t (\chi(s/\delta) - \rho_1)(f(u) - g(u))ds + u_\delta(0) - u(0)
\end{aligned}
$$

and get a first estimate

$$
\begin{aligned}
\|u_\delta(t) - u(t)\| &\leq \|u_\delta(0) - u(0)\| + 2M \int_0^t \|u_\delta - u\|ds \\
&\quad + \left\| \int_0^t (\chi(t/\delta) - \rho_1)\phi(s)ds \right\|
\end{aligned}
\tag{24}
$$

where ϕ is the fixed continuous vector function $\phi(s) = f(u(s)) - g(u(s))$. The other factor in the integral is a scalar function which is rapidly oscillating around zero. Hence the integral should be small. It is sufficient to show this for the case where ϕ is a scalar function.

Let $\epsilon > 0$ be given. Choose a step function $\psi(s)$ with finitely many steps such that
$$
|\phi(s) - \psi(s)| < \epsilon e^{-2MT}/2
$$
for $0 \leq s \leq T$. Let $N = N(\epsilon)$ be the number of steps, let the N step intervals be denoted by I_k, $k = 1, \ldots, N$, and the values of the step function by ψ_k.

Then choose $t \in [0, T]$ fixed. Let $N' \leq N$ be the largest number such that $I_k \cap [0, T) \neq \emptyset$ for $k = 1, \ldots, N'$, and let $I'_k = I_k \cap [0, t]$. Of course $I'_k = I_k$ for $k < N'$. Then we have

$$
\int_0^t (\chi(s/\delta) - \rho_1)\psi(s)ds = \sum_{k=1}^{N'} \int_{I'_k} (\chi(s/\delta) - \rho_1)ds\psi_k.
$$

Consider the k-th step. The length of the k-th interval can be expressed in multiples of δ as $|I'_k| = n_k\delta + r_k$ with $0 \leq r_k < \delta$. Since the integral of $\chi(s/\delta) - \rho_1$ over an interval of length δ vanishes, from the k-th term remains only an integral over an interval of length r_k which can be estimated by $r_k|\psi_k| \leq \delta 2M$. Hence

$$\left| \int_0^t (\chi(s/\delta) - \rho_1)\psi(s)ds \right| \le 2MN'\delta \le 2MN\delta.$$

Now choose δ_0 such that

$$4MNe^{2MT}\delta_0 < \epsilon.$$

Then

$$\left| \int_0^t (\chi(\frac{s}{s}) - \rho_1)\psi(s)ds \right| \le \epsilon e^{-2MT}/2$$

for all $\delta < \delta_0$ and hence (returning to the vector case)

$$\left\| \int_0^t (\chi(s/\delta) - \rho_1)\phi(s)ds \right\| \le \epsilon e^{-2MT}$$

for all $\delta < \delta_0$. From (24) we find

$$\|u_\epsilon(t) - u(t)\| \le \|u_\epsilon(0) - u(0)\| + 2M \int_0^t \|u_\epsilon - u\|ds + \epsilon e^{-2MT}. \tag{25}$$

A Gronwall argument gives

$$\int_0^t \|u_\epsilon(s) - u(s)\|ds \le \frac{\|u_\epsilon(0) - u(0)\| + \epsilon e^{-2MT}}{2M}(e^{2MT} - 1).$$

Introduce this expression into (25) and get

$$\|u_\epsilon(t) - u(t)\| \le \|u_\epsilon(0) - u(0)\|e^{2MT} + \epsilon.$$

Hence, for $u_\epsilon(0) = u(0)$ we get for $0 \le t \le T$

$$\|u_\epsilon(t) - u(t)\| \le \epsilon$$

which shows uniform convergence for $\epsilon \to 0$.

References

1. R. Bathia, Matrix Analysis, Springer 1996.
2. G. Carrero, D. McDonald, E. Crawford, G. de Vries, and M. Hendzel, Using FRAP and mathematical modeling to determine the in vivo kinetics of nuclear proteins. *Methods*, 29:14–28, 2003.
3. K.P. Hadeler, Quiescent phases and stability. submitted.
4. K.P. Hadeler, The role of migration and contact distribution in epidemic spread. In C. Castillo-Chavez and H.T. Banks, editors, *Frontiers Appl. Math.*, *28, Bioterrorism*, pages 188–210. SIAM, 2003.
5. K.P. Hadeler and M.A. Lewis, Spatial dynamics of the diffusive logistic equation with a sedentary compartment. *Canadian Appl. Math. Quart.*, 10:473–499, 2002.
6. T. Hillen, Transport equations with resting phases. *Europ. J. Appl. Math.*, 14:613–636, 2003.

7. M.W. Hirsch, H.L. Smith, Monotone dynamical systems. pp. 239–357 In: Handbook of Differential Equations. Ordinary Differential Equations, Vol. 2 (eds. A Cañada, P. Drábek A. Fonda) Elsevier 2005.

8. R.A. Horn, C. Johnson, Topics in Matrix Analysis. Cambridge U. Press 1994.

9. W. Jäger, S. Krömker, and B. Tang, Quiescence and transient growth dynamics in chemostat models. *Math. Biosci.* 119:225–239, 1994.

10. C.K.R.T. Jones, Geometric singular perturbation theory. In J. Russell, editor, *Dynamical Systems*, CIME Lectures Montecatini Terme, Italy, 1994. Lect. Notes Math. 1609, 44–118 1995.

11. M.A. Lewis and G. Schmitz, Biological invasion of an organism with separate mobile and stationary states: Modeling and analysis. *Forma*, 11:1–25, 1996.

12. T. Malik, H.L. Smith, A resource-based model of microbial quiescence. *J. Math. Biol.*, 53, 231–252, 2006

13. M.G. Neubert, P. Klepac, and P. van den Driessche, Stabilizing dispersal delays in predator-prey metapopulation models. *Theor. Popul. Biol.*, 61:339–347, 2002.

14. E. Pachepsky, F. Lutscher, R.M. Nisbet, M. Lewis, Persistence, spread and the drift paradox. *Theor. Pop. Biol.* 67:61–73, 2005.

15. A. Pazy, *Semigroups of Linear Operators and Applications to Partial Differential Equations.* Springer, New York, 1983.

16. J.C. Robinson, *Infinite-Dimensional Dynamical Systems.* Cambridge Texts in Applied Mathematics. Cambridge University Press, Cambridge, 2001.

17. B. Tang, Mathematical models of microbial competition in laboratory cultures incorporating environmental heterogeneities: coexistence. *Surveys Math. Indust.* 3, 49–70, 1993.

18. R. Temam, *Infinite–Dimensional Dynamical systems in Mechanics and Physics.* Springer, 1988.

19. G. Webb, Structured population dynamics. Mathematical modelling of population dynamics, 123–163, Banach Center Publ., 63, Polish Acad. Sci., Warsaw, 2004.

Long Time Behavior of a System of Stochastic Differential Equations Modelling Aggregation

Vincenzo Capasso, Daniela Morale, and Matteo Ortisi

ADAMSS (Advanced Applied Mathematical and Statistical Sciences) &
Department of Mathematics, University of Milano, Via C. Saldini, 50, Milano, Italy
{capasso,morale,ortisi}@mat.unimi.it

Summary. In many biological settings it is possible to observe phenomena of pattern formation and clustering by cooperative individuals of a population. In biology and medicine there is a wide spectrum of examples which exhibit collective behavior, leading to self organization, with pattern formation. Aggregation patterns are usually explained in terms of forces, external and/or internal, acting upon individuals. Over the past couple of decades, a large amount of literature has been devoted to the mathematical modelling of self-organizing populations, based on the concepts of short-range/long-range "social interaction" at the individual level. The main interest has been in catching the main features of the interaction at the lower scale of single individuals that are responsible, at a larger scale, for a more complex behavior that leads to the formation of aggregating patterns.

Here we analyze the long time behavior of a system of N stochastic differential equations. We show that a condition for stable aggregation is the presence of a suitable "confining" potential.

1 Introduction

In many biological settings it is possible to observe phenomena of pattern formation and clustering by cooperative individuals of a population. In biology and medicine there is a wide spectrum of examples which exhibit collective behavior, leading to self organization, with pattern formation. This may happen at any scale: from the cellular scale of embryonic tissue formation, wound healing or tumor growth, and vasculogenesis, the microscopic scale of life cycles of bacteria or social amoebae, to the larger scale of animal grouping; indeed animals may form *swarms*, characterized by a cohesive but unorganized aggregation (e.g. midges), or *schools* with a cohesive and synchronized organization (e.g. in fish schooling, individuals are oriented so that distances are uniform), or *shoals* (e.g. for fish) and *flocks* (e.g. for birds) in which animals are gathered together for social aims, in a synchronized or asynchronized way, or *herds, congregation*, and so on.

Aggregation patterns are usually explained in terms of forces, external and/or internal, acting upon individuals. Over the past couple of decades, a large amount of literature has been devoted to the mathematical modelling of self-organizing populations, based on the concepts of short-range/long-range "social interaction" at the individual level. The main interest has been in catching the main features of the interaction at the lower scale of single individuals that are responsible, at a larger scale, for a more complex behavior that leads to the formation of aggregating patterns. A classical widespread approach has been based on PDE's [3, 12, 15, 16, 19]; this is due, above all, to the wider spread knowledge on nonlinear PDE's. The disadvantages of this approach include especially the fact that the identity of individuals is compromised. As pointed out by Durrett and Levin [7] and by Grünbaum and Okubo [8], an individual-based approach is useful in deriving the correct limiting equation, also in the case when the use of a continuum model can be justified, because of the large number of individuals in the population [2, 13, 14, 15].

In [2, 15] the authors analyzed the asymptotics of a system of N stochastic differential equations (SDEs) subject to McKean-Vlasov and moderate interaction as the size N of the system tends to infinity, on a fixed time interval $[0, T]$. In this way a nonlinear partial integral differential equation for the asymptotic mean field was obtained.

Here we wish to analyze the long time behavior of a (stochastic) generalized system for a fixed N. Our interest is to analyze mechanisms that are responsible for stable aggregation.

We consider a population of constant size $N \in \mathbb{N} - \{0\}$. From the Lagrangian point of view, we assume that the "state" of the k-th particle is described by a random vector $X_N^k(t) \in \mathbb{R}^d, t \geq 0$. Hence, for each $k \in \{1, .., N\}$, $\{X_N^k(t), t \in \mathbb{R}_+\}$ is a stochastic process in the state space $(\mathbb{R}^d, \mathcal{B}_{\mathbb{R}^d})$, on a common probability space $(\Omega, \mathcal{F}, P)$. Notice that X_N^k may describe the spatial position, but may also describe any state of the k-th particle. We consider the case of continuous time evolution, and the dynamics is described by a system of stochastic differential equations subject to additive noise

$$dX_N^k(t) = \left[f(X_N^k(t)) + F_N \left[X_N(t) \right] \left(X_N^k(t) \right) \right] dt$$
$$+ \sigma dW^k(t), \quad k = 1, \ldots, N. \tag{1}$$

In equation (1) $\{W^k, k = 1, \ldots\}$ is a family of independent standard Wiener processes, $f : \mathbb{R}^d \to \mathbb{R}$, and the functional F_N is defined on $\mathcal{M}_{\mathcal{P}}(\mathbb{R}^d)$, the space of all probability measures on $\mathbb{R}^d$, and depends on the empirical measure

$$X_N(t) = \frac{1}{N} \sum_{k=1}^{N} \epsilon_{X_N^k(t)} \in \mathcal{M}_P(\mathbb{R}^d). \tag{2}$$

The measure (2) describes the system by an Eulerian approach: the collective behavior of the discrete (in the number of particles) system is given in terms of the spatial distribution of particles at time t.

Equation (1) describes a system of N individuals whose evolution is due to a stochastic individual component coupled with an advection term. Advection is due to both an interaction dynamics among the particles (aggregation, repulsion) and an individual one.

The individual dynamics

The advection term $f : \mathbb{R}^d \to \mathbb{R}$, which describes the individual dynamics of a particle, may depend on external information. Indeed we will consider the case in which f is of the form

$$f(x) = -\gamma_1 \nabla U(x), \tag{3}$$

due to a non negative smooth even potential $U : \mathbb{R}^d \to \mathbb{R}_+ \in C^2(\mathbb{R}^d)$; $\gamma_1 \in \mathbb{R}_+$ is a suitable weight. From the modelling point of view the transport term (3) represents some external information from the environment which drives any individual particle along the flow due to U.

The interaction dynamics

The interaction term F_N depends on the relative location of the specific individual $X_N^k(t)$ with respect to the other individuals, via the empirical measure of the whole system. The interaction we consider is due to different phenomena: aggregation and repulsion. These two different "forces" compete but act at different scales.

Aggregation acts at the macroscale and is modelled by a suitably chosen McKean-Vlasov interaction kernel

$$G : \mathbb{R}^d \longrightarrow \mathbb{R}_+;$$

the interaction of a particle located in $X_N^k(t)$ at time t with the others is then described by a "generalized" gradient operator (as discussed in [3, 15]) acting on the empirical measure

$$(\nabla G * X_N(t)) \left(X_N^k(t) \right). \tag{4}$$

Repulsion acts at the mesoscale; the mesoscale is introduced as in [13, 15, 17] rescaling kernel V_1, chosen as a symmetric (with respect to zero) probability density

$$V_N(z) = N^\beta V_1(N^{\beta/d} z), \quad \beta \in (0, 1).$$

The repelling force exterted on the k-th (out of N) particle located at $X_N^k(t)$ is then given by

$$-\sum_{i=1}^{N} N^{\beta-1}\nabla V_1\left(N^{\beta/d}\left(X_N^k(t)-X_N^i(t)\right)\right) = -(\nabla V_N * X_N(t))(X_N^k(t)) \quad (5)$$

In (5) it is clear how the choice of β may determine the range and the strength of the influence of neighboring particles; indeed, any particle interacts (repelling) with $O\left(N^{1-\beta}\right)$ other particles in a small volume $O\left(N^{-\beta}\right)$.

From (4) and (5), the advection interaction term $F[X_N]$ is given by

$$F[X_N](x) = \gamma_2\left(\nabla(G-V_N)*X_N(t)\right)(x), \quad (6)$$

with $\gamma_2 \in \mathbb{R}_+$.

The stochasticity

The stochastic component in equation (1) may describe both a lack of information about the environment or the particle itself, and the need of each particle to interact with the others, so that particles move randomly with a mean free path σ until they meet other particles and interact. In [3, 15] the authors have chosen $\sigma = \sigma_N$ decreasing with N in order to express the decreasing need of each particle to move randomly in order to meet other particles as N increases; since N is now fixed, we may not explicit the possible dependence of σ upon N.

By (1), (3), and (6) the system we study is the following

$$dX_N^k(t) = -\left[\gamma_1\nabla U(X_N^k(t)) + \gamma_2\left(\nabla\left(V_N-G\right)*X_N\right)\left(X_N^k(t)\right)\right]dt$$
$$+\sigma dW^k(t), \qquad k=1,\ldots,N. \quad (7)$$

In previous papers [3, 13, 15] the authors have taken $\gamma_1 = 0$, so that the system was

$$dX_N^k(t) = \gamma_2\left[(\nabla G*X_N(t))(X_N^k(t)) - (\nabla V_N*X_N(t))(X_N^k(t))\right]dt$$
$$+\sigma dW^k(t), \qquad k=1,\ldots,N. \quad (8)$$

They have focused their attention on the convergence of the system as the number of particles N increases to infinity. Via a "law of large numbers" it was shown the convergence of the empirical measure to a probability measure, whose density evolves according to a suitable integro-differential equation. In [3] the existence and uniqueness of the solution of such a PIDE has been investigated.

In this work we focus our attention on system (7); we analyze the long time behavior of the system with a fixed size N. In particular we study the existence of an invariant measure of the system. Our interest about these topics has been addressed by a wide-through-years literature by several authors interested in modelling aggregation behavior, and studying existence and convergence to an invariant distribution [1, 6, 10, 21, 22].

In Section 3 we show that system (8) cannot admit a nontrivial invariant distribution. On the other hand in Section 4 we prove that system (7), under suitable conditions on the "confining" potential U does admit a nontrivial invariant distribution to which the system converges. We notice that, by applying recent results by Veretennikov [21, 22], the requirement on U are less restrictive about its convexity as required in previous literature [5, 10, 11, 21].

To conclude we show the need of a localizing potential for the existence of an asymptotic in time nontrivial distribution of the interacting particle system.

2 Existence and Uniqueness of the Solution

Let us consider the following assumptions on the kernel involved in system (7)

$$G, V_1 \in C_b^2(\mathbb{R}^d, \mathbb{R}_+) \cap L^1(\mathbb{R}^d, \mathbb{R}_+) \tag{9}$$

$$U \in C^2(\mathbb{R}^d, \mathbb{R}_+) \tag{10}$$

$$|\nabla U(\mathbf{x}) - \nabla U(\mathbf{y})|^2 \leq k|\mathbf{x} - \mathbf{y}|^2, \quad \forall(\mathbf{x}, \mathbf{y}) \in \mathbb{R}^d \times \mathbb{R}^d \tag{11}$$

$$|\nabla U(\mathbf{x})|^2 \leq k^*(|\mathbf{x}|^2 + 1), \quad \forall \mathbf{x} \in \mathbb{R}^d \tag{12}$$

where k and k^* are positive constants.

By standard arguments [4] we can prove the following.

Proposition 2.1 ([9]) *If G, V_1, U satisfy assumptions (9)-(12) then system (7) admits a unique solution $X = (X_1, \cdots, X_N) \in C[\mathbb{R}_+, \mathbb{R}^d]$.*

Note that the hypothesis (11) may be substituted by a condition of local lipschitzianity of the gradient of U with polynomial growth

$$|\nabla U(\mathbf{x}) - \nabla U(\mathbf{y})| \leq |\mathbf{x} - \mathbf{y}|| P(\mathbf{x}) - P(\mathbf{y})|, \quad \forall(\mathbf{x}, \mathbf{y}) \in \mathbb{R}^d \times \mathbb{R}^d,$$

where P is a polynomial [9].

For the required interpretation of G as aggregating kernel, we impose the following assumptions

$$G(x) = \tilde{G}(|x|), \quad x \in \mathbb{R}^d,$$

with $\tilde{G}$ is an increasing real valued function defined on $\mathbb{R}_+$.

3 Systems without Individual Dynamics: Non-existence of Invariant Distributions

Consider system (7) without the potential U, i.e. with $\gamma_1 = 0$. This means that we consider system (8), where the drift is due only to interaction among particles.

Figure 1 shows the result of numerical simulations of system (8) with $V_1 = \alpha_1 \mathcal{N}(0,1)$ and $G = \alpha_2 \mathcal{N}(0,1)$, for different values of α_1 and α_2.

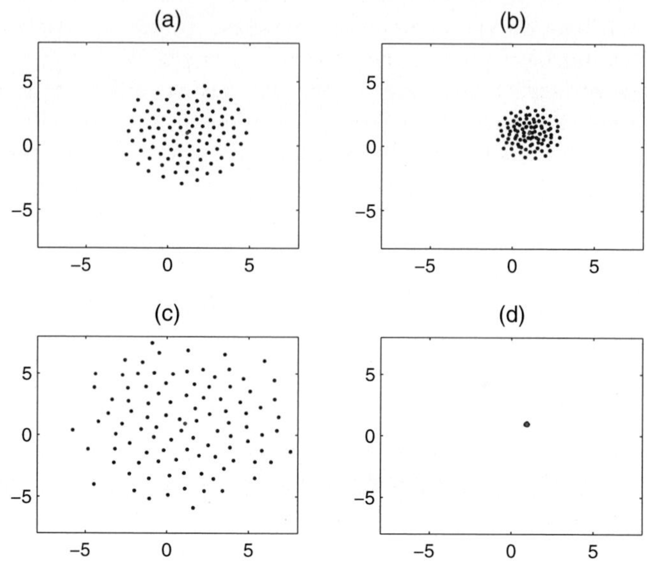

Fig. 1: Configuration of 100 particles at T=2000 for different values of parameters: (a) $\alpha_1 = \alpha_2 = 1$; (b) $\alpha_1 = 1; \alpha_2 = 2$; (c) $\alpha_1 = 1; \alpha_2 = 0$; (d) $\alpha_1 = 0; \alpha_2 = 1$. $\sigma = 0.02$, $\beta = 0.5$ and $\gamma_2 = 1$.

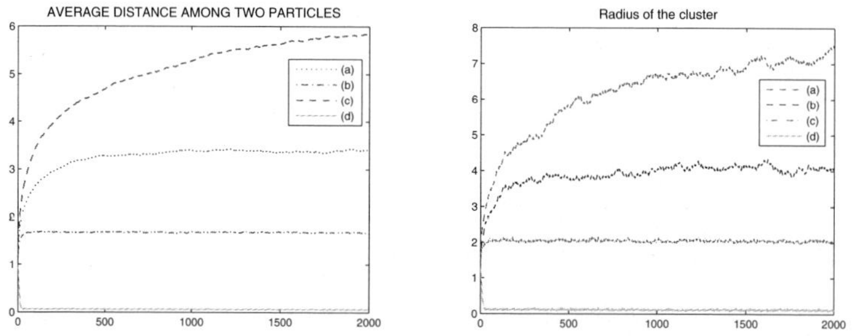

Fig. 2: Comparison among the evolution of the radius of the cluster and the average distance among particles for different values of parameters: (a) $\alpha_1 = \alpha_2 = 1$; (b) $\alpha_1 = 1; \alpha_2 = 2$; (c) $\alpha_1 = 1; \alpha_2 = 0$; (d) $\alpha_1 = 0; \alpha_2 = 1$. See also Plate 1 on page 337

We may observe a space-time behavior which is coherent with the meaning of V_1 and G; clustering is more evident as the force of aggregation is larger with respect to the force of repulsion.

Furthermore from Figure 2 we notice that, as t increases, the mean distance between two particles and consequently the radius of clusters fluctuates around an asymptotic value which is finite, but in the case of pure repulsion.

On the other hand, following [10], for the position of the center of mass of the N particles,

$$\bar{X}_N(t) = \frac{1}{N} \sum_{k=1}^{N} X_N^k(t),$$

we have

$$d\bar{X}_N(t) = -\frac{1}{N^2} \sum_{k,j=1}^{N} \nabla (V_N - G)(X_N^k(t) - X_N^j(t))dt + \sigma d\bar{W}(t),$$

where $\bar{W}(t) = \frac{1}{N} \sum_{k=1}^{N} W^k(t)$; by the symmetry properties of V_1 and G, the first term on the right hand side vanishes and we get

$$d\bar{X}_N(t) = \sigma d\bar{W}(t),$$

i.e. $\bar{X}_N(t)$ is a Brownian motion. Hence, its distribution is

$$\mathcal{L}\left(\bar{X}_N(t)|\bar{X}_N(0)\right) = \mathcal{L}\left(\bar{X}_N(0), \sigma^2 \bar{W}(t)\right) = \mathcal{N}\left(\bar{X}_N(0), \frac{\sigma^2}{N}t\right);$$

with variance $\frac{\sigma^2}{N} t$, which, for any fixed N, increases as t tends to infinity.

Consequently we may claim that the probability law of the system does not converge to any probability law, since otherwise the same would happen for the law of the center of mass.

We may obtain an explicit result in the following way. Let $\mathbf{Y} = (y_1, \ldots, y_N) \in (\mathbb{R}^d)^N$ and define

$$H_N(\mathbf{Y}) = \frac{1}{N} \sum_{i,l=1}^{N} (V_N - G)(y_i - y_l).$$

As a consequence system (8) can be rewritten in the form

$$d\mathbf{X}_N(t) = -\frac{1}{2} \nabla \cdot H_N(\mathbf{X}_N(t))dt + \sigma d\mathbf{W}(t). \tag{13}$$

For each N let ρ_N be the density of the joint probability distribution of the X_N^k, $k = 1, \ldots, N$. We know that (13) admits an invariant distribution if and only if the density $\rho_{N,\infty}$ of the invariant distribution is a steady state of the Fokker-Plank equation, i.e. if it satisfies the following equation,

$$\frac{1}{2}\sum_{k=1}^{N}\left\{\nabla_{X_N^k}\cdot\left[(\nabla_{X_N^k}H_N)\rho_{N,\infty}\right]+\sigma^2\Delta_{X_N^k}\rho_{N,\infty}\right\}=0. \tag{14}$$

Furthermore it is a well known result that, in the case of regularity of the kernel, a solution $\rho_{N,\infty}$ of (14) must have the following form [18]

$$\rho_{N,\infty}:=\frac{1}{Z_N}\exp\left\{-\sigma^{-2}H_N(\mathbf{X}_N)\right\},$$

where Z_N is a normalizing constant.

For the case $\gamma_1=0$, $Z_N=\int_{(\mathbb{R}^d)^N}\exp\left\{-\sigma^{-2}H_N(\mathbf{X}_N)\right\}d\mathbf{X}_N=\infty$, so that $\mu_N(\infty)$ is trivial.

In other models where the interaction potential $K=V_N-G$ is strictly convex, i.e.

$$\exists\lambda>0,\forall x,v\in\mathbb{R}^d,\quad\langle\mathrm{Hess}K(x)v,v\rangle\geq\lambda\langle v,v\rangle, \tag{15}$$

the same situation occurs, whenever the potential is symmetric. Indeed it can be shown that in all these cases the system

$$d\mathbf{X}_N(t)=-\nabla\cdot K(\mathbf{X}_N(t))dt+\sigma d\mathbf{W}(t),\quad\mathbf{X}_N(t)\in\mathbb{R}^d,\forall t,$$

does not admit an invariant distribution. In order to claim this result, in [10], a reduced system is considered for the relative coordinates

$$Y_N^j(t)=X_N^j(t)-\bar{X}_N$$

where $\bar{X}_N(t)=\frac{1}{N}\sum_{i=1}^N X_N^i(t)$ is again the location of the center of mass of the system. It was shown that under the assumption (15), the reduced system

$$Y_N^k(t)=Y_N^k(0)-\frac{1}{N}\sum_{l=1}^N\int_0^t\nabla K(Y_N^k(s)-Y_N^l(s))ds$$

$$+\sigma W^k(t)-\frac{\sigma}{N}\sum_{l=1}^N W^l(t)\qquad k=1,\ldots,N,$$

which is still a diffusion on the manifold

$$\mathcal{M}=\left\{(x_1,\ldots,x_n):\sum_i x_i=0\right\}, \tag{16}$$

does admit an invariant measure, while the center of mass follows a pure Brownian motion, which does not admit a non trivial invariant distribution (because of the symmetry of K).

Roughly speaking, due to the strict convexity, each particle is attracted by any other one in the whole space, and so does the center of mass.

The mathematical reason is that the reduced system evolves on the manifold (16), not in $\mathbb{R}^d$, and on $\mathcal{M}$ the dominant eigenvalue of the Hessian of the potential is strictly negative. This also implies a Sobolev inequality with parameter λ, and as a consequence we have a convergence from any initial distribution $\mu_N(t)$ to the invariant one $\mu_N(\infty)$, in terms of the relative entropy

$$S(\mu_N(t)|\mu_{N,\infty}) = \int \frac{d\mu_N(t)}{d\mu_{N,\infty}} \log \frac{d\mu_N(t)}{d\mu_{N,\infty}} d\mu_{N,\infty}.$$

For further results we refer to [10] and references therein.

4 Systems with a Confining Potential: Existence of the Invariant Distribution

Here we consider the more realistic model (7), with $\gamma_1 > 0$ including, in addition to a long range attraction and short range repulsion, a confining potential U, centered at some point $x_0 \in \mathbb{R}^d$. Here for technical convenience we choose the origin, i.e. $x_0 = 0 \in \mathbb{R}^d$.

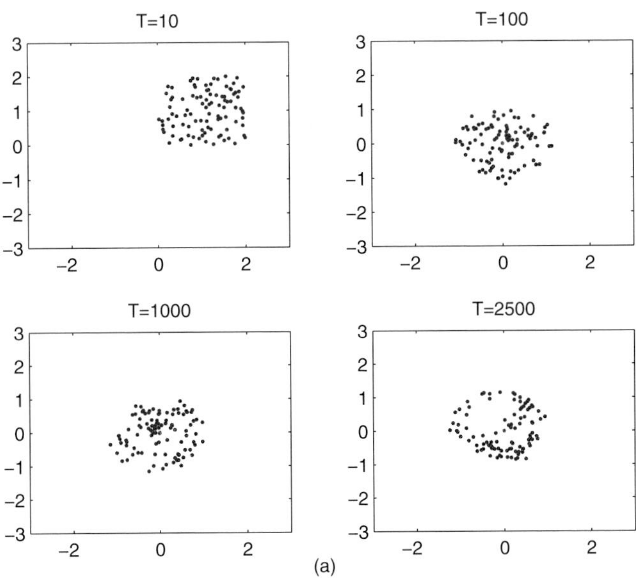

Fig. 3: Configuration of 100 particles for the following values of parameters: (a) $\alpha_1 = \alpha_2 = 1$. $\sigma = 0.02$, $\beta = 0.5$ and $\gamma_2 = 1$.

Consider now the potential P associated with a measure on $\mathbb{R}^d$, $\mu \in \mathcal{M}(\mathbb{R}^d)$

$$P(\mu)(x) = \gamma_1 U(x) - \gamma_2 \left((V_N - G) * \mu\right)(x), \quad x \in \mathbb{R}^d,$$

so that system (7) can be rewritten as

$$dX_N^k(t) = -\nabla P(X_N(t))(X_N^k(t)) + \sigma dW^k(t), \qquad k = 1, \ldots, N. \quad (17)$$

In Figures 3-4 the simulated behavior of system (17) with respect to time and space is shown.

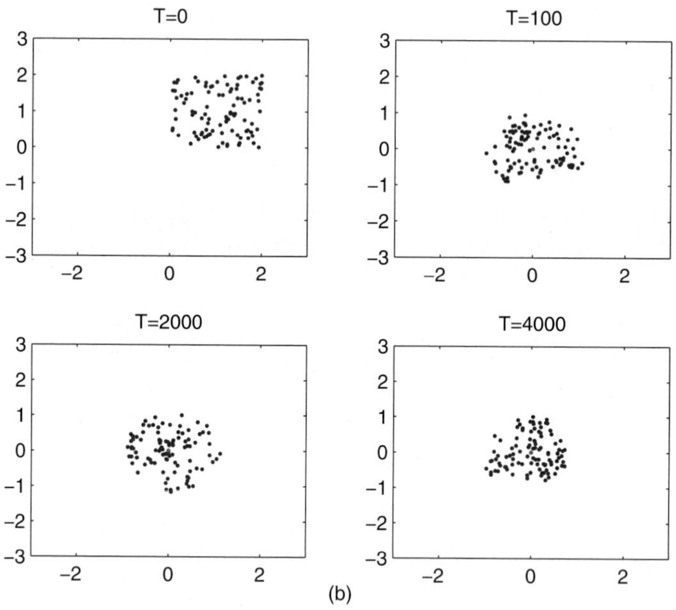

Fig. 4: Configuration of 100 particles for the following values of parameters: (b) $\alpha_1 = 1$; $\alpha_2 = 2$. $\sigma = 0.02$, $\beta = 0.5$ and $\gamma_2 = 1$.

System (17) has been thoroughly analyzed in literature under the sufficient condition (15) of strictly convexity on U ; it has been shown [5, 10, 11] that if this condition applies, system (17) does admit a nontrivial invariant distribution. From a biological point of view a strictly convex confining potential is difficult to explain; it would mean an infinite range of attraction, with an at least constant, drift even far from origin.

A weaker sufficient condition for the existence of a unique invariant measure has been more recently suggested by Veretennikov [21, 22], following Has'minski [9], there exist constants $M_0 \geq 0$ and $r > 0$ such that for $|x| \geq M_0$

$$\left(-\nabla P(\mu)(x), \frac{x}{|x|} \right) \leq -\frac{r}{|x|}. \tag{18}$$

Without any further condition on the interaction kernels V_N and G, for (18) to hold it is sufficient to assume that
there exist constants $M_0 \geq 0$ and $r > \frac{1}{N\gamma_1}(\frac{Nd}{2} + 1)$ such that for $|x| \geq M_0$

$$\left(-\nabla U(x), \frac{x}{|x|} \right) \leq -\frac{r}{|x|}. \tag{19}$$

We wish to remark that condition (19) means that ∇U may decay to zero as $|x|$ tends to infinity, provided that its tails are sufficiently "fat".

Proposition 4.1 *If the confining potential U satisfies condition (19), then (17) admits a unique invariant measure.*

Proof. Let $\pi_i(\mathbf{x}) = x_i, i = 1, ..., N$ be the i-th projection of $\mathbf{x} \in (R^d)^N$, $\tilde{U}(\mathbf{x})$ and $\tilde{K}(\mathbf{x})$ the vector function defined by

$$\tilde{U}(\mathbf{x}) = (U \circ \pi_i(\mathbf{x}))_{1 \leq i \leq N}, \quad \tilde{K}(\mathbf{x}) = \left((G - V_N) * \frac{1}{N} \sum_i \epsilon_{\pi_i(\mathbf{x})} \circ \pi_i(\mathbf{x}) \right)_{1 \leq i \leq N}$$

In order to apply Theorem 2 in [20], we have to prove that there exist constants $M \geq 0$ and $\tilde{r} > (\frac{Nd}{2} + 1)$ such that for all $\mathbf{x} \in (R^d)^N : |x| \geq M$

$$\left(-\gamma_1 \nabla \tilde{U}(\mathbf{x}) + \gamma_2 \nabla \tilde{K}(\mathbf{x}), \frac{\mathbf{x}}{|\mathbf{x}|} \right) \leq -\frac{\tilde{r}}{|\mathbf{x}|}. \tag{20}$$

We have

$$\left(-\gamma_1 \nabla \tilde{U}(\mathbf{x}) + \gamma_2 \nabla \tilde{K}(\mathbf{x}), \frac{\mathbf{x}}{|\mathbf{x}|} \right) = -\gamma_1 \sum_{k=1}^{N} \nabla U(x_k) \frac{x_k}{|\mathbf{x}|}$$

$$+ \gamma_2 \frac{1}{N} \sum_{k=1}^{N} \sum_{i=1}^{N} \nabla(G - V_N)(x_i - x_k) \frac{x_k}{|\mathbf{x}|}$$

$$\leq -\gamma_1 \sum_{k=1}^{N} \nabla U(x_k) \frac{x_k}{|\mathbf{x}|}$$

$$+ \gamma_2 \frac{1}{N} \sum_{k=1}^{N} \sum_{i=1}^{N} \nabla(G - V_N)(x_i - x_k)$$

$$= -\gamma_1 \sum_{k=1}^{N} \nabla U(x_k) \frac{x_k}{|\mathbf{x}|} \leq -\frac{\gamma_1 r N}{|\mathbf{x}|}$$

The last two inequalities derive from the symmetry of the G and V_N and (19). So if for $\tilde{r} = \gamma_1 r N$ and condition on r in (19), we have condition (20). $\square$

Remark 1. An interpretation of the fact that system (8) without U (i.e. with $\gamma_1 = 0$) cannot admit an invariant distribution, even though we knew that there exist constants $M_0, r > 0$, s.t.

$$\left(-\nabla(G - V_N)(x), \frac{x}{|x|} \right) \leq -\frac{r}{|x|}$$

for $|x| > M_0$, is the following; in such case the drift in (8) would be $\gamma_2 \nabla \tilde{K}(\mathbf{x})$ and so we would have

$$\left(\gamma_2 \nabla \tilde{K}(\mathbf{x}), \frac{\mathbf{x}}{|\mathbf{x}|} \right) = \gamma_2 \frac{1}{N} \sum_{k=1}^{N} \sum_{i=1}^{N} \nabla(G - V_N)(x_i - x_k) \frac{x_k}{|\mathbf{x}|},$$

from which we can claim that $(-\nabla((G - V_N) * X_N(t))(x), x/|x|)$ is negative but we cannot get any control on the tails.

Let now $P_N^{x_0}(t)$ denote the joint distribution of the N particles at time t, conditional upon a non random initial condition x_0, and let P_S denote the invariant distribution.

As far as convergence of $P_N^{x_0}(t)$, for t tending to infinity, is concerned, we may state that [21]

Theorem 1. *Under assumption* (19), *for any* k, $0 < k < \tilde{r} - \frac{Nd}{2} - 1$ *with* $m \in (2k + 2, 2\tilde{r} - Nd)$ *and* $\tilde{r} = \gamma_1 N r$, *there exists a positive constant* c *such that*

$$\left| P_N^{x_0}(t) - P_N^S \right| \leq c(1 + |x_0|^m)(1 + t)^{-(k+1)},$$

where $\left| P_N^{x_0}(t) - P_N^S \right|$ *denotes the total variation distance of the two measures, i.e.*

$$\left| P_N^{x_0}(t) - P_N^S \right| = \sup_{A \in \mathcal{B}_{\mathbb{R}^d}} \left[P_N^{x_0}(t)(A) - P_N^S(A) \right].$$

and x_0 *the initial data.*

Acknowledgments

It is a pleasure to acknowledge Annamaria Bianchi of the University of Milano, for fruitful discussions.

VC acknowledges the warm hospitality of the Austrian Academy of Sciences at RICAM (Radon Institute for Computational and Applied Mathematics) in Linz, chaired by Prof. H. Engl.

References

1. Bodnar M., Velazquez J.J.L. (2005) Derivation of macroscopic equations for individual cell-based models: A formal approach. Math. Meth. Appl. Sci., **28**, 1757–1779, 2005.
2. Boi S., Capasso V., Morale D. Modeling the aggregative behavior of ants of the species Polyergus rufescens. Spatial heterogeneity in ecological models. Nonlinear Anal. Real World Appl., **1**, 163–176, 2000.
3. Burger M., Capasso V., Morale D., On an aggregation model with long and short range interactions, Nonlinear Anal. Real World Appl.,(2006), in press.
4. Capasso V., Bakstein D. An Introduction to Continuous-Time Stochastic Processes - Theory, Models and Applications to Finance, Biology and Medicine. Birkhäuser, Boston, 2004.
5. Carrillo J.A., McCann R.J., Villani C. Kinetic equilibration rates for granular media and related equations: entropy dissipation and mass transportation estimates. Rev. Mat. Iberoamericana, **19**, 971–1018, 2003.
6. Dawson D.A., Gärtner J. Large deviations, free energy functional and quasi-potential for a mean field model of interacting diffusions. Memoirs of the American Mathematical Society, **78**, N. 398, 1989.
7. Durrett, R., Levin, S.A. "The importance of being discrete (and spatial)." Theor. Pop. Biol., **46**, 1994, 363–394.
8. Grünbaum, D., Okubo, A. "Modelling social animal aggregations" In "Frontiers of Theoretical Biology" (S. Levin Ed.), Lectures Notes in Biomathematics, 100, Springer Verlag, New York, 1994, 296–325.
9. Has'minski, R.Z. Stochastic stability of differential equations. Sijthoff & Noordhoff, Alphen aan den Rijn, The Netherlands and Rockville, Maryland, USA, 1980.
10. Malrieu, F. Convergence to equilibrium for granular media equations and their Euler schemes. The Annals of Applied Probability, **13**, 540–560, 2003.
11. Markowich P.A., Villani C. On the trend to equilibrium for the Fokker-Planck equation: an interplay between physics and functional analysis. Mathematica Contemporanea **19**, 1–31, 2000.
12. Mogilner A., L. Edelstein-Keshet, A non-local model for a swarm, J. Math. Bio. **38**, 534–549, 1999.
13. Morale, D. Cellular automata and many-particles systems modeling aggregation behaviour among populations, Int. J. Appl. Math. & Comp. Sci.**10**, 157–173, 2000.
14. Morale, D. A stochastic particle model for vasculogenesis: a multiple scale approach In Mathematical Modelling & Computing in Biology and Medicine. 5th Conference of the ESMTB 2002, (V. Capasso, Ed.), ESCULAPIO, Bologna, 616–622, 2003.
15. Morale, D., Capasso V., Oelschläger K. An interacting particle system modelling aggregation behavior: from individuals to populations. J. Mathematical Biology, **50**, 49–66, 2005.
16. Nagai, T., Mimura, N. Asymptotic behavior for a nonlinear degenerate diffusion equation in population dynamics, SIAM J. Appl. Math. **43**, 449–464, 1983.
17. Oelschläger K. On the derivation of reaction-diffusion equations as limit dynamics of systems of moderately interacting stochastic processes. Prob. Th. Rel. Fields, **82**, 565–586, 1989.

18. Soize, C. The Fokker-Planck equation for stochastic dynamical systems and its explicit steady state solutions. Series on Advances in Mathematics for Applied Sciences, Vol. 17. World Scientific, Singapore, 1993.
19. Topaz, C., Bertozzi, A.L. Swarming patterns in a two-dimensional kinematic model for biological groups, SIAM J. Appl. Math. **65**,152 - 174, 2004.
20. Veretennikov, A.Y. On polynomial mixing bounds for stochastic differential equations. Stochastic Processes and their Applications, **70**, 115–127, 1997.
21. Veretennikov, A.Y. On polynomial mixing and convergence rate for for stochastic differential equations. Theory Probab. Appl., **44**, 361–374, 1999.
22. Veretennikov, A.Y. On subexponential mixing rate for Markov processes. Theory Probab. Appl., **49**, 110–122,, 2005.

Invariant Density Estimation
for Multidimensional Diffusions

Annamaria Bianchi

ADAMSS & Department of Mathematics, University of Milan, Via C. Saldini 50,
20133 Milano, Italy
abianchi@mat.unimi.it

Summary. We consider an $\mathbb{R}^d$ dimensional homogeneous diffusion process with a
unique invariant density f. We construct a kernel type estimator for the invariant
density and study its mean–square convergence. We find that this estimator reaches
in a specific minimax sense a rate that is slower than parametric but faster than
in classical d-dimensional estimation problems. Finally we examine the almost sure
(pointwise and uniform) behavior of the estimator and we give examples.

1 Introduction

Let us consider an $\mathbb{R}^d$-dimensional homogeneous diffusion

$$\mathrm{d}X_t = S(X_t)\mathrm{d}t + \mathrm{d}W_t , \quad X_0 , \quad 0 \leq t \leq T , \tag{1}$$

where $\{W_t, t \geq 0\}$ is a standard d-dimensional Wiener process and $S : \mathbb{R}^d \to
\mathbb{R}^d$ is an (unknown) bounded drift coefficient. We assume the diffusion coeffi-
cient to be the identity matrix. The function $S(\cdot)$ is such that there exists a
unique strong solution to equation (1) (see [5]). X_0 is the initial value of X_t
and it is supposed to be independent of the Wiener process.

We assume that the process $\{X_t, t \geq 0\}$ has a unique invariant probability
density $f(\cdot)$. We assume also the existence of the transition density $p_u(x,y)$,
$u \neq 0$; notice that if the initial value X_0 has density function $f(\cdot)$ then the
process $\{X_t, t \geq 0\}$ is stationary in the strict sense (see, for example, [12]).
It follows that the process $\{X_t, t \geq 0\}$ possesses a two-dimensional density
$f_{(X_0,X_u)}(x,y) = f(x)p_u(x,y)$. Hence we can define for $u > 0$ the local measure
of dependence as follows

$$g_u(x,y) = f_{(X_0,X_u)}(x,y) - f(x)f(y) = f(x)p_u(x,y) - f(x)f(y) .$$

The statistical theory for scalar diffusions is very well developed. Kutoyants has studied it thoroughly in the minimax context in [10]. Also Veretennikov in [14] has studied the problem of invariant density estimation and

has proved the classical Castellana and Leadbetter condition ([7]) for such a process

$$\int_0^{+\infty} \sup_{x,y} |g_u(x,y)|du < +\infty .$$

This condition in particular implies that the kernel type density estimators reach in mean square the so-called parametric rate of convergence T^{-1} as $T \to +\infty$. Unfortunately it is not possible to prove the Castellana and Leadbetter condition for multidimensional diffusion processes. The problematic part is in zero; indeed, the following bound ([11])

$$C_1 u^{-d/2} \le p_u(x,y) \le C_2 u^{-d/2} , \quad 0 < u \le 1 ,$$

with C_1 and C_2 positive constants, combined with $\sup f(x) < \infty$ implies that

$$\int_0^1 \sup_{x,y} |g_u(x,y)|du = +\infty .$$

The fact that the Castellana and Leadbetter condition is not valid may be one of the reasons why inference problems in the multidimensional case have been much less studied.

We only know about a preprint by Dalalyan and Reiß [8] in which they estimate the invariant density and study the mean–square rate of convergence. With respect to our work they impose different assumptions; in particular, they ask the drift to be only locally bounded and to be the gradient of a potential. Under these and other assumptions they find slightly different rates with respect to the ones that we find and not in the minimax sense.

Concerning the almost sure behavior we know that Van Zanten [13] gives the uniform strong consistency (without rates) of density estimators for scalar ergodic processes. For the multidimensional case we only know of the recent work by Bandi and Moloche [1], where they study the strong consistency of the discretized kernel density estimator.

The rest of the paper is organized as follows; in Sect. 2 we estimate $f(\cdot)$ from the observation of a trajectory of the process $\{X_t, 0 \le t \le T\}$. A weaker condition is adopted here with respect to the one by Castellana and Leadbetter. Blanke and Bosq [2] introduce a weaker condition for general multidimensional processes, which brings us intermediate rates of convergence of the density estimator in the mean–square sense. They also prove that these rates are minimax in a specific sense. We will show that, under suitable assumptions, process (1) satisfies their hypotheses.

In Sect. 3 we provide almost sure (pointwise and uniform) rates of convergence of the kernel density estimator to $f(\cdot)$. The result has been given for the general case by Blanke [3]. We show that also our process satisfies all her conditions.

In Sect. 4 we give examples of diffusions which satisfy all our assumptions.

2 Mean–Square Convergence

In this section we show that for process (1) the classical kernel density estimator reaches the intermediate rates in the mean–square context presented by Blanke and Bosq [2]. We will see that these rates strongly depend upon the dimension of the process.

Let $\mathcal{S}_{d/2}$ be the class of functions $S(\cdot)$ such that

(A1) S is bounded and Lipschitz continuous, i.e. there exists a constant $A > 0$ such that
$$\|S(x) - S(y)\| \le A\|x - y\| , \quad \forall x , y \in R^d ;$$

(A2) there exist constants $M_0 \ge 0$ and $r > 0$ such that
$$(S(x), x) \le -r\|x\| , \quad \|x\| \ge M_0 .$$

Notice that assumption (A1) guarantees the existence of a unique strong solution to equation (1) and assumption (A2) implies the existence of an invariant measure for the process. Moreover from (A1) we deduce that the invariant measure admits a density $f(\cdot)$ with respect to the Lebesgue measure. From now on we assume that the initial value X_0 follows the invariant law ensuring thus the strict stationarity of the process.

The kernel density estimator for $f(\cdot)$ is defined by

$$f_T(x) = \frac{1}{Th_T^d} \int_0^T K\left(\frac{x - X_t}{h_T}\right) dt , \quad x \in R^d ,$$

where $h_T \to 0^+$ as $T \to +\infty$ and $K : \mathbb{R}^d \to \mathbb{R}$ is a bounded probability density function such that

(K1) $\int_{R^d} K(u_1, \ldots, u_d) u_1^{\alpha_1} \ldots u_d^{\alpha_d} du_1 \ldots du_d = 0;$
(K2) $\int_{R^d} \|u\| |u_1|^{\alpha_1} \ldots |u_d|^{\alpha_d} K(u_1, \ldots, u_d) du_1 \ldots du_d < +\infty,$

where $\alpha_1, \ldots, \alpha_d \in N$ and $\alpha_1 + \ldots + \alpha_d = 1$.

For the reader's convenience we briefly formulate Blanke and Bosq's general result [2]. Let $\{X_t, t \ge 0\}$ be an $\mathbb{R}^d$-valued and measurable process and denote by $C_{2,d}(b)$ the class of real densities $f(\cdot)$ defined on $\mathbb{R}^d$, twice continuously differentiable and such that $\|f\|_\infty \le b$ and $\|\partial^2 f/\partial x_i \partial x_j\|_\infty \le b$ for $i, j = 1, \ldots, d$. They introduce the family of processes $\mathcal{X}_{\gamma_0}$ satisfying

(i) $g_{s,t} = g_{|t-s|}$ does exist for $t \neq s$,

(ii) $f \in C_{2,d}(b)$, $f_{(X_0,X_u)}$ is continuous at (x,x) for $u > 0$,

(iii) $\displaystyle \sup_{x,y} \int_{u_0}^{+\infty} |g_u(x,y)| du \leq M_1$ for some $u_0 > 0$

$$\sup_{x,y} f_{(X_0,X_u)}(x,y) \leq M_2 u^{-\gamma_0} \ , \gamma_0 > 0 \text{ and } u \in (0,u_0) \ , \tag{2}$$

(iv) there exists a positive function $\Psi_u(\cdot,\cdot)$ such that

$$f_{(X_0,X_u)}(x,y) \geq \frac{\Psi_u(x,y)}{u^{\gamma_0}} \quad \text{for } u \in (0,u_0) \ ,$$

and

$$\liminf_{T \to +\infty} \ \inf_{u \in [\varepsilon_T^{d/\gamma_0}, u_0)} \Psi_u(x - \varepsilon_T v, x - \varepsilon_T w) \geq \Psi_0(x,v,w) \ ,$$

where Ψ_0 is a positive function non $-$ identically null and $\varepsilon_T \overset{T \to +\infty}{\longrightarrow} 0$.

Notice that the Castellana and Leadbetter condition has been replaced by the weaker condition (iii). In particular, (2) and (iv) are related to local regularity of sample paths and they mean that $f_{(X_0,X_u)}$ explodes when $u \to 0$ but not too fast. The parameter γ_0 is related to the behavior of $f_{(X_0,X_u)}$ in a neighborhood of $u = 0$ and we will see that in our case it depends strongly on the dimension of the process.

For processes belonging to the family $\mathcal{X}_{\gamma_0}$ Blanke and Bosq find the exact rate of convergence of the kernel density estimator.

Theorem 1. *For all* $X \in \mathcal{X}_{\gamma_0}$

1) if $\gamma_0 = 1$ *and* $h_T = c\,(\ln T/T)^{1/4}$ *(c > 0)*

$$\limsup_{T \to +\infty} \frac{T}{\ln T} \mathrm{E}(f_T(x) - f(x))^2 < +\infty \ ;$$

2) if $\gamma_0 > 1$ *and* $h_T = cT^{-\gamma_0/(d(\gamma_0-1)+4\gamma_0)}$ *(c > 0)*

$$\limsup_{T \to +\infty} T^{4\gamma_0/(d(\gamma_0-1)+4\gamma_0)} \mathrm{E}(f_T(x) - f(x))^2 < +\infty \ .$$

Theorem 2. *For all* $X \in \mathcal{X}_{\gamma_0}$

1) if $\gamma_0 = 1$ *and* $h_T = c\,(\ln T/T)^{1/4}$ *we have*

$$\liminf_{T \to +\infty} \frac{T}{\ln T} \mathrm{E}(f_T(x) - f(x))^2 > 0 \ ;$$

2) if $\gamma_0 > 1$ *and* $h_T = T^{-\gamma_0/(d(\gamma_0-1)+4\gamma_0)}$ *we have*

$$\liminf_{T \to +\infty} T^{4\gamma_0/(d(\gamma_0-1)+4\gamma_0)} \mathrm{E}(f_T(x) - f(x))^2 > 0 \ .$$

By the previous theorems it follows that the kernel density estimator reaches exactly the rate $(\ln T/T)^{1/2}$ in the case $\gamma_0 = 1$, and the rate $T^{-2\gamma_0/(d(\gamma_0-1)+4\gamma_0)}$ in the case $\gamma_0 > 1$.

In the current section our purpose is to show that under assumptions (A1) and (A2), the multidimensional diffusion process (1) satisfies hypotheses (i)–(iv) and so it reaches the intermediate rates presented before.

Theorem 3. *For all* $S \in \mathcal{S}_{d/2}$, *process (1) satisfies conditions (i)–(iv).*

Proof. Let $\mu_t^x(\cdot)$ be the distribution of X_t, x being the initial data. Assumption (A1) implies the existence of a transition density $p_t(\cdot, \cdot)$ (see [9], page 251). Hence we can write

$$\mu_t^x(\mathrm{d}y) = p_t(x, y)\mathrm{d}y , \quad \forall x , y \in R^d .$$

In order to prove condition (iii) we need the convergence of the transition measure to an invariant measure. We formulate the result from [15] which gives us all the technical means that we need now. Denote μ^{inv} the invariant measure of the process, var the total variation metric and $\mathcal{F}_A^X = \sigma(X_t : t \in A)$. Recall the definition of the β-mixing coefficient for stationary processes

$$\beta_t := \sup_{s \geq 0} \mathrm{E} \sup_{B \in \mathcal{F}_{\geq t+s}^X} \left| P(B | \mathcal{F}_{\leq s}^X) - P(B) \right| ,$$

where E is the expectation with respect to the invariant measure.

Theorem 4. *Let (A2) hold. Then for any* $c_1 > 0$ *small enough there exist* $c_0, c_2 > 0$, *and vice versa, for any* $c_2 > 0$ *small enough there exist* $c_0, c_1 > 0$ *such that*

$$\mathrm{var}(\mu_t^x - \mu^{\mathrm{inv}}) \leq c_0 \exp\left(c_1 \|x\| - c_2 t \right) ,$$
$$\beta_t \leq c_0 \exp\left(-c_2 t \right) .$$

In particular μ^{inv} *does exist, it is unique and* $\int \exp\left(c_1 \|x\| \right) \mu^{\mathrm{inv}}(\mathrm{d}x) < +\infty.$

We see that assumption (A2) implies the existence of an invariant measure for process (1). Taking into account (A1), it follows immediately that

$$\mu^{\mathrm{inv}}(\mathrm{d}y) = f(y)\mathrm{d}y ,$$

where $f(\cdot)$ is the invariant probability density of the process. Since we have assumed that X_0 admits density function $f(\cdot)$, the process is stationary (see, for example, [12]); therefore condition (i) holds, i.e. there exists $g_{s,t} = g_{|t-s|}$ for $t \neq s$.

Now for any multi-index $m = (m_1, \ldots, m_d) \in N^d$ we set $|m| = m_1 + \ldots + m_d$. Under assumption (A1) we have that the transition density $p_u(\cdot, \cdot)$ satisfies the following inequality (see [9] on pages 251, 255)

$$\left| \frac{\partial^{|m|} p_u}{\partial x_1^{m_1} \cdots \partial x_d^{m_d}}(y, x) \right| \leq b_1 u^{-(|m|+d)/2} \exp\left(-c\frac{\|x-y\|^2}{u} \right) ,$$

with $0 \leq |m| \leq 2$ and b_1, c positive constants. So we can conclude that $p_1(x, \cdot) \in C_{2,d}(b_1)$. By using the Chapman-Kolmogorov identity

$$f(y) = \int f(x) p_1(x, y) \mathrm{d}x$$

we can see that also $f(\cdot) \in C_{2,d}(b_1)$; indeed,

$$\sup_{y \in \mathbb{R}^d} f(y) \leq \sup_{x,y \in \mathbb{R}^d} p_1(x, y) \leq b_1$$

$$\sup_{y \in \mathbb{R}^d} \left| \frac{\partial f}{\partial y_i}(y) \right| \leq \sup_y \int f(x) \left| \frac{\partial p_1}{\partial y_i}(x, y) \right| \mathrm{d}x \leq b_1$$

and

$$\sup_y \left| \frac{\partial^2 f}{\partial y_i \partial y_j}(y) \right| \leq \sup_y \int f(x) \left| \frac{\partial^2 p_1}{\partial y_i \partial y_j}(x, y) \right| \mathrm{d}x \leq b_1 ,$$

for $i, j = 1, \ldots, d$. Moreover $f_{(X_0, X_u)}$ is continuous at (x, x) for $u > 0$ and so we have also condition (ii).

Concerning condition (iii), we can take $u_0 = 1$ and see that

$$\sup_{x,y} \int_1^{+\infty} |g_u(x, y)| \mathrm{d}u \leq \int_1^{+\infty} \sup_{x,y} f(x) |p_u(x, y) - f(y)| \mathrm{d}u .$$

We will prove that the last term is finite. First we estimate for $u > 1$

$$|p_u(x, y) - f(y)| = \left| \int [p_{u-1}(x, z) - f(z)] p_1(z, y) \mathrm{d}z \right|$$

$$\leq b_1 \int |p_{u-1}(x, z) - f(z)| \mathrm{d}z$$

$$= b_1 \mathrm{var}(\mu_{u-1}^x - \mu^{\mathrm{inv}})$$

$$\leq b_1 c_0 \exp\left(c_1 \|x\| - c_2 u \right) ,$$

where in the first inequality we have used the boundedness of $p_1(\cdot, \cdot)$ and in the second inequality we have applied Theorem 4.

Since $\int \exp\left(c_1 \|x\| \right) f(x) \mathrm{d}x < \infty$ (see Theorem 4) and $f \in C_{2,d}(b_1)$, it follows that $\exp\left(c_1 \|x\| \right) f(x) \to 0$ as $\|x\| \to \infty$. So finally we obtain

$$\int_1^{+\infty} \sup_{x,y} f(x) |p_u(x, y) - f(y)| \mathrm{d}u \leq C \int_1^{+\infty} \sup_x \exp\left(c_1 \|x\| \right) f(x) \exp\left(-c_2 u \right) \mathrm{d}u$$

$$= C \int_1^{+\infty} \exp\left(-c_2 u \right) \mathrm{d}u =: M_1 < \infty .$$

In order to prove the other conditions we use the following result by Qian et al. (see [11]):

Theorem 5. *Let* $S = \sum_{i=1}^{d} S^i \partial/\partial x_i$ *be a bounded vector field on* $\mathbb{R}^d$. *Suppose*

$$|S^i(x)| \le \beta_i \quad for \ all \ x \in \mathbb{R}^d$$

for some non-negative constants β_i, $i = 1, \ldots, d$, *then*

$$\frac{1}{(2\pi t)^{d/2}} \prod_{i=1}^{d} \left(\int_{|x^i - y^i|/\sqrt{t}}^{\infty} z e^{-(z+\beta_i t)^2/2} \mathrm{d}z \right) \le p_t(x, y)$$

and

$$p_t(x, y) \le \frac{1}{(2\pi t)^{d/2}} \prod_{i=1}^{d} \left(\int_{|x^i - y^i|/\sqrt{t}}^{\infty} z e^{-(z-\beta_i t)^2/2} \mathrm{d}z \right) .$$

Since we have assumed S to be bounded, we can apply the second inequality to obtain for $u \in (0, 1)$:

$$p_u(x, y) \le \frac{1}{(2\pi u)^{d/2}} \prod_{i=1}^{d} \left(\int_{|x^i - y^i|/\sqrt{u}}^{\infty} z e^{-(z-\beta_i u)^2/2} \mathrm{d}z \right)$$

$$\le \frac{1}{(2\pi u)^{d/2}} \prod_{i=1}^{d} 2 \left(\int_{0}^{+\infty} (z + \beta_i u) e^{-z^2/2} \mathrm{d}z \right) = M u^{-d/2} .$$

Since $f \in C_{2,d}(b_1)$ we can prove condition (2):

$$\sup_{x,y} f_{(X_0, X_u)}(x, y) = \sup_{x,y} f(x) p_u(x, y) \le M_2 u^{-d/2} .$$

Let us now prove the last condition:

$$f_{(X_0, X_u)}(x, y) = f(x) p_u(x, y)$$

$$\ge f(x) \frac{1}{(2\pi u)^{d/2}} \prod_{i=1}^{d} \left(\int_{|x^i - y^i|/\sqrt{u}}^{\infty} z e^{-(z+\beta_i u)^2/2} \mathrm{d}z \right)$$

$$=: u^{-d/2} \Psi_u(x, y) .$$

So we have that

$$\inf_{u \in [\varepsilon_T^2, 1)} \Psi_u(x - \varepsilon_T v, x - \varepsilon_T w) =$$

$$= \inf_{u \in [\varepsilon_T^2, 1)} f(x - \varepsilon_T v) \frac{1}{(2\pi)^{d/2}} \prod_{i=1}^{d} \left(\int_{\varepsilon_T |v^i - w^i|/\sqrt{u}}^{\infty} z e^{-(z+\beta_i u)^2/2} \mathrm{d}z \right)$$

$$= f(x - \varepsilon_T v) \frac{1}{(2\pi)^{d/2}} \prod_{i=1}^{d} \left(\int_{|v^i - w^i|}^{\infty} z e^{-(z+\beta_i)^2/2} \mathrm{d}z \right)$$

$$\overset{T \to +\infty}{\longrightarrow} f(x) \frac{1}{(2\pi)^{d/2}} \prod_{i=1}^{d} \left(\int_{|v^i - w^i|}^{\infty} z e^{-(z+\beta_i)^2/2} \mathrm{d}z \right) =: \Psi_0(x, v, w) ,$$

where we have used the continuity of $f(\cdot)$ at the point x. $\qquad \square$

So we have proved that the multidimensional diffusion process (1) with $S \in \mathcal{S}_{d/2}$ belongs to the family $\mathcal{X}_{d/2}$. Hence the kernel density estimator has rate $(\ln T / T)^{1/2}$ for $d = 2$ and rate $T^{-2\gamma_0/(d(\gamma_0 - 1) + 4\gamma_0)} = T^{-2/(d+2)}$ for $d > 2$. Notice that the rate of convergence of the estimator decreases as the dimension increases.

Since we have proved Theorems 1 and 2, it follows immediately from [2] that the rates we have found are also minimax in the sense that if the kernel estimator reaches an intermediate rate over a class of processes, than this rate turns out to be minimax. This means that no better estimator exists over that class.

Theorem 6. *Let $\mathcal{F}_T$ be the set of all measurable density estimators built from data $(X_t, t \in [0, T])$. Then for $x \in \mathbb{R}^d$*

1) if $d = 2$

$$\liminf_{T \to +\infty} \inf_{\tilde{f}_T \in \mathcal{F}_T} \sup_{S \in \mathcal{S}_1} \frac{T}{\ln T} \mathrm{E}(\tilde{f}_T(x) - f(x))^2 > 0 \,,$$

2) if $d > 2$

$$\liminf_{T \to +\infty} \inf_{\tilde{f}_T \in \mathcal{F}_T} \sup_{S \in \mathcal{S}_{d/2}} T^{4/(d+2)} \mathrm{E}(\tilde{f}_T(x) - f(x))^2 > 0 \,.$$

3 Almost Sure Convergence

In this section we establish the almost sure convergence of the estimator f_T to f. This ensures that, asymptotically, one has a precise information about the general shape of the density. We will apply the results by Blanke ([3], Corollary 2.3), where she proves the almost sure pointwise convergence for all processes in $\mathcal{X}_{\gamma_0}$ satisfying the additional assumption

(v) $\{X_t\}$ is a geometric strongly mixing process, with coefficient α_X such that $\alpha_X(u) \le \alpha_0 \rho^u$, $0 < \rho < 1$, $u > 0$, $\alpha_0 > 0$,

and for kernels $K(\cdot)$ satisfying (K1) and

(K2') $\int_{R^d} \|u\| |u_1|^{\beta_1} \ldots |u_d|^{\beta_d} K(u_1, \ldots, u_d) du_1 \ldots du_d < +\infty$, for integers β_i such that $\beta_1 + \ldots + \beta_d = 2$;

(K3) $K^{(i)} = \frac{\partial K}{\partial x_i}$ exists and is continuous everywhere for $i = 1, \ldots, d$;

(K4) $\|K^{(i)}\|_\infty < \infty$, $i = 1, \ldots, d$.

Theorem 7. *For all $S \in \mathcal{S}_{d/2}$ and for all kernels $K(\cdot)$ satisfying conditions (K1), (K2'), (K3) and (K4) and $h_T = c \left((\log T)^2 / T\right)^{1/(2+d)}$, $c > 0$*

$$\limsup_{T \uparrow +\infty} \left(\frac{T}{(\log T)^2}\right)^{2/(2+d)} |f_T(x) - f(x)| < +\infty \quad \text{a.s.}$$

Proof. The only condition that we have to prove is the strongly mixing property. It follows directly from Theorem 4

$$\alpha_u \le \beta_u \le c_0 \exp\left(-c_2 u\right). \qquad \square$$

In order to establish the corresponding uniform result over the whole $\mathbb{R}^d$ we have to prove the following further assumptions ([3], Corollary 2.4):

(vi) $\{X_t\}$ is a strictly stationary process such that $\sup_{0\le t\le T}\|X_t\|$ is measurable for all T and $E(\sup_{0\le t\le 1}\|X_t\|) < \infty$, moreover f is ultimately decreasing.

Theorem 8. *For all $S \in \mathcal{S}_{d/2}$ and for all kernels $K(\cdot)$ satisfying conditions (K1), (K2'), (K3) and (K4) and $h_T = c\left((\log T)^2/T\right)^{1/(2+d)}$, $c > 0$*

$$\limsup_{T\uparrow+\infty} \left(\frac{T}{(\log T)^2}\right)^{2/(2+d)} \sup_{x\in R^d} |f_T(x) - f(x)| < +\infty \quad \text{a.s.}$$

Proof. It suffices to prove assumption (vi). The process $\{X_t\}$ is stationary in the strict sense since we have supposed that X_0 follows the invariant measure. Secondly, since $\{X_t\}$ has continuous trajectories

$$\sup_{t\in[0,T]} \|X_t\| = \sup_{t\in[0,T]\cap Q} \|X_t\|$$

and therefore the previous quantity is measurable for all T.

In order to show that $E\left(\sup_{0\le t\le 1}\|X_t\|\right) < \infty$, it suffices to show that $E\left(\sup_{0\le t\le 1}|X_t^i|^2\right) < \infty$ for all $i = 1,\ldots,d$, where we have denoted by X_t^i the i-th component of the process. Since

$$X_t^i = X_0^i + \int_0^t S^i(X_s)ds + \int_0^t dW_s^i$$

we have that

$$|X_t^i|^2 \le 3|X_0^i|^2 + 3\left(\int_0^t |S^i(X_s)|ds\right)^2 + 3\left|\int_0^t dW_s^i\right|^2$$

and so

$$E\left(\sup_{0\le t\le 1} |X_t^i|^2\right)$$

$$\le 3E\left[|X_0^i|^2\right] + 3E\left[\int_0^1 |S^i(X_s)|ds\right]^2 + 3E\left[\sup_{0\le t\le 1}\left|\int_0^t dW_s^i\right|^2\right].$$

By applying the Doob's martingale inequality (see, for example, [5]) we obtain that

$$\mathrm{E}\left(\sup_{0\leq t\leq 1}|X_t^i|^2\right) \leq 3\mathrm{E}\left[|X_0^i|^2\right] + 3\|S^i\|_\infty^2 + 12 < \infty.$$

Finally, instead of proving that f is ultimately decreasing we will prove directly that

$$\left(\frac{T}{(\log T)^2}\right)^{2/(2+d)} \sup_{\|x\|>c_{(d)}T^a} f(x) \to 0 \quad \text{as} \quad T \uparrow +\infty,$$

where $c_{(d)}$ and a are positive constants. Please refer to [3] (Corollary 2.4) for all the details. We may write

$$\left(\frac{T}{(\log T)^2}\right)^{2/(2+d)} \sup_{\|x\|>c_{(d)}T_n^a} f(x) \leq \left(\frac{T}{(\log T)^2}\right)^{2/(2+d)} \frac{1}{c_{(d)}T^a} \sup_{\|x\|>c_{(d)}T^a} \|x\|f(x).$$

For T sufficiently large

$$\sup_{\|x\|>c_{(d)}T^a} \|x\|f(x) \leq \sup_{\|x\|>c_{(d)}T^a} \exp\left(c_1\|x\|\right) f(x)$$

and the last quantity is bounded since $\int \exp\left(c_1\|x\|\right)\mu^{\mathrm{inv}}(dx) < +\infty$ (see Theorem 4) and f is continuous. Clearly

$$\left(\frac{T}{(\log T)^2}\right)^{2/(2+d)} \frac{1}{c_{(d)}T^a} \to 0 \quad \text{as } T \to +\infty$$

for all $a > 2$. $\square$

4 Examples

Let us consider the process

$$\begin{pmatrix} dX_1 \\ dX_2 \end{pmatrix} = \begin{pmatrix} \beta_{11} & \beta_{12} \\ \beta_{21} & \beta_{22} \end{pmatrix} \begin{pmatrix} \frac{X_1}{1+\alpha(|X_1|+|X_2|)} \\ \frac{X_2}{1+\alpha(|X_1|+|X_2|)} \end{pmatrix} dt + \begin{pmatrix} dW_1 \\ dW_2 \end{pmatrix} \tag{3}$$

with $\beta_{11}, \beta_{22} < 0$ and $\alpha > 0$. For simplicity we consider the bi-dimensional case, but it is easy to see that this process can be extended to the case $d > 2$. Notice that (3) is a sort of approximation of the Ornstein-Uhlenbeck process: varying the parameter α, the drift can become as big as we want. Since in practice all processes are bounded, this is not a big restriction. Models of this kind are used in biology (see [6]) and also in economy.

Let us now verify that this process satisfies conditions (A1) and (A2). In order to prove (A1) it is sufficient to prove that all the first partial derivatives of S are bounded. Due to the symmetry of S we prove it for $\frac{\partial S_1}{\partial x_1}$:

$$\left|\frac{\partial S_1}{\partial x_1}(x_1, x_2)\right| = \left|\frac{\beta_{11}(1+\alpha(|x_1|+|x_2|)) - \alpha(\beta_{11}x_1 + \beta_{12}x_2)\mathrm{sgn}(x_1)}{(1+\alpha(|x_1|+|x_2|))^2}\right|$$

$$\leq |\beta_{11}| + \frac{\max(|\beta_{11}|, |\beta_{12}|)}{\alpha} < \infty.$$

Concerning condition (A2), without loss of generality we take $\beta_{12} = \beta_{21}$.

$$\left(S(x_1, x_2), \begin{pmatrix} x_1 \\ x_2 \end{pmatrix} \right) = \frac{\beta_{11}x_1^2 + 2\beta_{12}x_1 x_2 + \beta_{22}x_2^2}{1 + \alpha(|x_1| + |x_2|)} \leq \frac{\tilde{\beta}\|x\|^2}{1 + \alpha\|x\|} \leq \frac{\tilde{\beta}}{\alpha}\|x\| \,,$$

with $\tilde{\beta} < 0$ and $\|x\| > M_0$, $M_0 = M_0(\beta_{11}, \beta_{12}, \beta_{22})$. So we have proved condition (A2) with $r = \frac{\tilde{\beta}}{\alpha}$ and $p = 0$.

Another similar example is the following mean reverting process

$$\begin{pmatrix} \mathrm{d}X_1 \\ \mathrm{d}X_2 \end{pmatrix} = \begin{pmatrix} \beta_{11} & \beta_{12} \\ \beta_{21} & \beta_{22} \end{pmatrix} \left[\begin{pmatrix} \alpha_1 \\ \alpha_2 \end{pmatrix} - \begin{pmatrix} \frac{X_1}{1+\gamma(|X_1|+|X_2|)} \\ \frac{X_2}{1+\gamma(|X_1|+|X_2|)} \end{pmatrix} \right] \mathrm{d}t + \begin{pmatrix} \mathrm{d}W_1 \\ \mathrm{d}W_2 \end{pmatrix} \,,$$

with $\beta_{11}, \beta_{22} < 0$, $\alpha_1, \alpha_2 > 0$ and $\gamma > 0$.

Acknowledgments

We are thankful to Prof. Denis Bosq and Prof. Vincenzo Capasso for their continuous advice and relevant discussions.

References

1. Bandi, F.M., Moloche, G.: On the functional estimation of multivariate diffusion processes. Preprint (2002), available under `http://gsbwww.uchicago.edu/fac/federico.bandi/research/`
2. Blanke, D., Bosq, D.: A family of minimax rates for density estimators in continuous time. Stoch. Anal. Appl., **18**, 6, 871–900 (2000)
3. Blanke, D.: Sample paths adaptive density estimator. Math. Methods Statist., **13**, 2, 123–152 (2004)
4. Bosq, D.: Nonparametric statistics for stochastic processes. Springer-Verlag, New York (1998)
5. Capasso, V., Bakstein, D.: An Introduction to Continuous–time Stochastic Processes. Birkhäuser, Boston (2005)
6. Capasso, V.: Mathematical structures of epidemic systems. Springer-Verlag, Berlin (1993)
7. Castellana, J.V., Leadbetter, M.R.: On smoothed probability density estimation for stationary processes. Stoch. Processes Appl., **21**, 179–193 (1986)
8. Dalalyan, A., Reiß, M.: Asymptotic statistical equivalence for ergodic diffusions: the multidimensional case. Preprint (2005), available under `http://www.proba.jussieu.fr/pageperso/dalalyan/Links/AD.html`
9. Friedman, A.: Partial Differential Equations of Parabolic Type. Prentice-Hall, Englewood Cliffs, N.J. (1964)
10. Kutoyants, Yu.A.: Statistical Inference for Ergodic Diffusion Processes. Springer Series in Statistics, New York (2004)
11. Qian, Z., Russo, F., Zheng, W.: Comparison theorem and estimates for transition probability densities of diffusion processes. Probab. Theory Related Fields **127**, 388–406 (2003)

12. Soize, C.: The Fokker-Planck equation for stochastic dynamical systems and its explicit steady state solutions. World Scientific, Singapore (1994)
13. Van Zantan, J.H.: On the uniform convergence of the empirical density of an ergodic diffusion. Statist. Inf. Stoch. Proc., **3**, 251–262 (2000)
14. Veretennikov, A.Yu.: On Castellana-Leadbetter's Condition for Diffusion Density Estimation. Statist. Inf. Stoch. Proc., **2**, 1–9 (1999)
15. Veretennikov, A.Yu.: On subexponential mixing rate for Markov processes. Theory Probab. Appl., **49(1)**, 110–122 (2005)

First Contact Distribution Function Estimation for a Partially Observed Dynamic Germ-Grain Model with Renewal Dropping Process

Marcello De Giosa

Dipartimento di Matematica, Università di Bari, via Orabona 4, 70125, Bari, Italy.
`mdegiosa@dm.uniba.it`

Summary. We consider a partially observed dynamic germ-grain model $\Theta = \{\Theta(t) : t \geq 0\}$ whose grains drop on the plane $\mathbb{R}^2$ at times of a renewal process. The first contact distribution at time t is the distribution function of the distance from a fixed point 0 to the nearest point of $\Theta(t)$, where the distance is measured using scalar dilations of a fixed test set B. Due to partial observation of the model, an estimation problem arises for the first contact distribution function. We propose a product integral type estimator. Its asymptotic properties are studied.

1 Introduction

Suppose that, at random times, discs of random bounded sizes drop on the plane $\mathbb{R}^2$ with centers randomly distributed in a convex region C. The union of discs dropped up to time t forms a germ-grain model $\Theta(t)$ (see [8]). As a function of t, and because of its evolution in time, we call $\Theta = \{\Theta(t) : t \geq 0\}$ *dynamic germ-grain model* (*dggm*).

The *first contact distribution function* (*fcdf*) of Θ is defined by (see [6]):

$$F_B(r, t) := \mathbb{P}\left\{\rho_B\left(0, \Theta(t)\right) \leq r\right\}, \quad r \geq 0, \quad t \geq 0,$$

where

$$\rho_B\left(0, \Theta(t)\right) := \inf\left\{d \geq 0 \; : \; \Theta(t) \cap dB \neq \emptyset\right\}$$

is the shortest distance from 0 to $\Theta(t)$, and

$$dB := \{db \; : \; b \in B\}$$

is the scalar dilation of B by d.

If the realization of Θ is completely observable, F_B is (more or less easily) computable. Furthermore, if Θ is spatially partially observable within a bounded windows, F_B may be estimated using methods of spatial statistics

52   Marcello De Giosa

(see [6]). However, having in mind the following examples, we consider a different situation. That is we suppose that the dropping times and the areas of the dropping discs are observable but the positions of the dropped discs are not.

Example 1 (Bombing model with obscuring object). Suppose that, during a bombing, bombs have been dropped on a region C. Because of the presence of obscuring objects (clouds, hills, ...) it is not possible to observe the hitting points of the bombs. It is assumed that each bomb destroys a circular region around it proportional to its destructive power, and that the destructive power and the dropping times of each bomb is known. It is useful an estimation of the *fcdf* of the destroyed region.

Example 2 (Sources of pollution). Suppose it is known that, at random observable times, sources of pollution entered a region C but the positions of them are unknown. Suppose further that the polluting power of each source is known and that each source damages a circular region around it proportional to its polluting power. It is interesting to estimate the *fcdf* of the damaged part of the region.

So that, for any $r \geq 0$, a new estimation problem arises for the function $F_B(r, \cdot)$.

For notational convenience, for any $r \geq 0$, we will face the equivalent estimation problem for the *first contact survival function (fcsf)*

$$\omega(t) := 1 - F_B(r, t), \quad t \geq 0,$$

where r is fixed. Note that:

$$\omega(t) := \mathbb{P}\left\{0 \notin \Theta(t) \oplus r\check{B}\right\} = \mathbb{P}[\tau > t], \quad t \geq 0,$$

where

$$r\check{B} := \{-rb \,:\, b \in B\},$$

$$\Theta(t) \oplus r\check{B} := \{x + y \,:\, x \in \Theta(t), \, y \in r\check{B}\},$$

and τ is the hitting time (see [8]) of the point 0 by the *dggm* $\Theta \oplus r\check{B} := \{\Theta(t) \oplus r\check{B} \,:\, t \geq 0\}$. So ω is a kind of survival function of the position 0.

Following standard methods of Survival Analysis, one could think of estimating ω by a Kaplan-Meier type estimator. The point is that the needed data, that is the hitting times $\tau_1, ..., \tau_n$ of conveniently chosen test points $0_1, ..., 0_n$, are not observable in our model. So we have to find another estimation method.

In this paper we consider the case of a renewal type dropping process.

The problem is studied in $\mathbb{R}^2$, but all results may be extended to $\mathbb{R}^d$, $d \geq 2$.

We are looking for an estimator of ω that enjoys good asymptotic properties as the region C grows. Note that, when C is big enough, assuming that the disc areas are bounded, the edge effects may be considered negligible.

The paper is organized as follows. In Section 2 we describe the model in detail. First we prove a result and then derive from it the *fcsf* estimator. Section 3 is devoted to asymptotic properties. Uniform Consistency and Asymptotic Gaussianity of the estimator are proved. Furthermore, an estimator of the variance function is defined and its Uniform Consistency proved. In Section 4, the results of Section 3 are used to find Confidence Bands.

We assume all random variables considered in the paper are defined on the same probability space $(\Omega, \mathcal{F}, P)$.

In what follows, the symbol $\Longrightarrow$ will denote the weak convergence of sequences of random processes or random variables, see [2].

2 Model, Notations and Preliminary Results

As already mentioned, we are looking for an estimator of ω with good asymptotic properties as the region of interest increases. So we fix the time interval for observations to be, say, $[0, T]$ and, as usual in Spatial Statistics, consider a convex averaging sequence $\{C_n : n \geq 1\}$, as defined in [3, p. 332], that is:

1. $C_n \subset \mathbb{R}^2$ is a convex Borel set;
2. $C_n \subset C_{n+1}$, for $n = 1, 2, ...$;
3. $r(C_n) \to \infty$, as $n \to \infty$,
    where $r(C_n) := \sup\{r > 0 : C_n \text{ contains a ball of radius } r\}$.

Note that $c_n := \ell(C_n) \longrightarrow \infty$, as $n \to \infty$, where ℓ denotes Lebesgue measure on $\mathbb{R}^2$.

We have in mind a model in which the mean interdropping time is inversely proportional to the area of the region C_n. That is, on a bigger region there is a bigger dropping rate.

The dropping process on C_n is a renewal process $N_n = \{N_n(t) : t \geq 0\}$ defined by

$$N_n(t) := N(c_n t), \quad t \geq 0,$$

where N is an underlying renewal process whose interarrival times have mean μ_U and variance σ_U^2.

It is not difficult to prove that (see [4], [2] and [7]):

$$\sup_{0 \leq t \leq T} \left| \frac{N_n(t)}{c_n} - \frac{t}{\mu_U} \right| \Longrightarrow 0, \qquad \text{as } n \to \infty, \tag{1}$$

and that, for any $t \in [0, T]$:

$$\frac{\mathbb{E}[N_n(t)]}{c_n} = t \cdot \frac{\mathbb{E}[N(c_n t)]}{c_n t} \longrightarrow \frac{t}{\mu_U}, \qquad \text{as } n \to \infty. \tag{2}$$

At any renewal time T_{ni} of N_n a disc $D_{ni} = B\left(X_{ni}, \sqrt{A_{ni}/\pi}\right)$ of random area A_{ni} drops on $\mathbb{R}^2$ with random center $X_{ni} \in C_n$.

About disc centers and areas, we assume that, for any $n \geq 1$:

(A1) $X_{n1}, ..., X_{nm}, ...$ is a sequence of i.i.d. random variables uniformly distributed on C_n.

(A2) $A_{n1}, ..., A_{nm}, ...$ is a sequence of i.i.d. bounded random variables with finite first four moments.

(A3) The families of random variables $\{X_{nm} : m \geq 1\}$, $\{A_{nm} : m \geq 1\}$ and $\{N_n(t) : t \geq 0\}$ are independent of each other.

For any $t \geq 0$, we denote by $\Theta_n(t) = \{\Theta_n(t, \omega), \omega \in \Omega\}$ the random closed set (germ-grain model) composed by the union of the random discs dropped up to time t,

$$\Theta_n(t) := \bigcup_{1 \leq i \leq N_n(t)} D_{ni} = \bigcup_{T_{ni} \leq t} D_{ni}.$$

In the following, we consider $r \geq 0$ fixed and $w_n(t)$ will denote the *fcsf* of $\Theta_n(t)$ evaluated at r. That is

$$w_n(t) := \mathbb{P}\left\{0 \notin \Theta_n(t) \oplus r\check{B}\right\},$$

where

$$\Theta_n(t) \oplus r\check{B} = \bigcup_{T_{ni} \leq t} \left(D_{ni} \oplus r\check{B}\right).$$

Theorem 1 below gives an insight into a possible approach in estimating $w_n(t)$. Let's first assume the following notations. Define, for any $n \geq 1$ and $t \geq 0$:

$$A_r^{ni} := \ell\left(D_{ni} \oplus r\check{B}\right), \qquad \mu_A := \mathbb{E}\left[A_r^{ni}\right],$$

$$\mathcal{S}_n(t) := \left(1 - \frac{\mu_A}{c_n}\right)^{N_n(t)}, \qquad \mathcal{S}(t) := \exp\left(-\frac{\mu_A}{\mu_U}t\right).$$

Theorem 1. *With the previous notations, the following hold:*
a) $w_n(t) = \mathbb{E}[\mathcal{S}_n(t)]$, *for any* $t \geq 0$;
b) $\sup_{0 \leq t \leq T} |w_n(t) - \mathcal{S}(t)| \longrightarrow 0$, *as* $n \to \infty$.

Proof. *a)* Because of the independence assumption,

$$w_n(t) = \mathbb{E}\left[\mathbb{P}\left[0 \notin \Theta_n(t) \oplus rB | N_n(t)\right]\right] =$$

$$= \mathbb{E}\left[\left(1 - \frac{\mu_A}{c_n}\right)^{N_n(t)}\right] = \mathbb{E}[\mathcal{S}_n(t)],$$

and hence *a)* is proved.

b) Since, for any $t \geq 0$,

$$\mathcal{S}_n(t) := \exp\left(\frac{N_n(t)}{c_n} \cdot \frac{ln(1 - \mu_A/c_n)}{\mu_A/c_n} \cdot \mu_A\right),$$

in view of (1) and equicontinuity of the exponential in $[-T, 0]$, we have

$$\sup_{0 \le t \le T} |\mathcal{S}_n(t) - \mathcal{S}(t)| \implies 0, \quad \text{as} \quad n \longrightarrow \infty. \tag{3}$$

Since

$$\sup_{0 \le t \le T} |\mathcal{S}_n(t) - \mathcal{S}(t)| \le 1$$

and

$$\sup_{0 \le t \le T} |\omega_n(t) - \mathcal{S}(t)| \le \mathbb{E}\left[\sup_{0 \le t \le T} |\mathcal{S}_n(t) - \mathcal{S}(t)| \right],$$

b) follows by dominated convergence arguments. $\square$

We now deduce from Theorem 1 a possible approach for estimating the fcsf ω_n. Note that we may write

$$\mathcal{S}(t) = e^{-\Lambda(t)} = \prod_{s \le t} (1 - d\Lambda(s)), \quad 0 \le t \le T,$$

where $\prod$ denotes the product integral (see [1, II.6] or [5]), and

$$\Lambda(s) = \frac{\mu_A}{\mu_U} s.$$

Statement b) in Theorem 1 suggest an estimator for $\omega_n(t)$ of the following type:

$$\widehat{\mathcal{S}}_n(t) := \prod_{s \le t} (1 - d\widehat{\Lambda}_n(s)), \quad 0 \le t \le T, \tag{4}$$

where $\widehat{\Lambda}_n$ is an estimator for Λ. A natural estimator for Λ is the normalized cumulative sum process $\widehat{\Lambda}_n = \left\{ \widehat{\Lambda}_n(t) : 0 \le t \le T \right\}$ defined by:

$$\widehat{\Lambda}_n(t) := \frac{1}{c_n} \sum_{i=1}^{N_n(t)} A_r^{ni}, \quad 0 \le t \le T.$$

Note that, with $\widehat{\Lambda}_n$ as above, it is true that:

$$\widehat{\mathcal{S}}_n(t) = \prod_{T_{ni} \le t} \left(1 - \frac{A_r^{ni}}{c_n} \right), \quad 0 \le t \le T.$$

Since $D_{ni} \oplus r\check{B}$ is just dilation of D_{ni} by rB (see [8]), for computing A_r^{ni} we only need knowledge of A_{ni}, but the position of D_{ni} is not required.

3 Asymptotic Results

In this section we state and prove the Uniform Consistency and Asymptotic Gaussianity of the estimator $\widehat{\mathcal{S}}_n$.

Theorem 2 (Uniform consistency). *With the same definitions and notations as in the previous sections, the process $\widehat{\mathcal{S}}_n$ is a Uniform Consistent estimator of the fcsf ω_n, that is:*

$$\sup_{0 \leq t \leq T} |\widehat{\mathcal{S}}_n(t) - \omega_n(t)| \implies 0, \qquad as \ \ n \to \infty.$$

Proof. Note that

$$\sup_{0 \leq t \leq T} |\widehat{\mathcal{S}}_n(t) - \omega_n(t)| \leq$$

$$\leq \sup_{0 \leq t \leq T} |\widehat{\mathcal{S}}_n(t) - \mathcal{S}_n(t)| + \sup_{0 \leq t \leq T} |\mathcal{S}_n(t) - \mathcal{S}(t)| + \sup_{0 \leq t \leq T} |\omega_n(t) - \mathcal{S}(t)|.$$

Because of statement *b)* in Theorem 1 and (3), we have only to prove that

$$\sup_{0 \leq t \leq T} |\widehat{\mathcal{S}}_n(t) - \mathcal{S}_n(t)| \implies 0, \qquad as \ \ n \to \infty. \tag{5}$$

Note that

$$\mathcal{S}_n(t) := \prod_{s \leq t} (1 - d\Lambda_n(s)), \qquad with \quad \Lambda_n(s) := \frac{\mu_A}{c_n} N_n(s).$$

In view of (4) and the continuity of the product-integrals (see [1, p. 114] or [5]), the convergence in (5) will follow if we prove that

$$\sup_{0 \leq t \leq T} |\widehat{\Lambda}_n(t) - \Lambda_n(t)| \implies 0, \qquad as \ \ n \to \infty. \tag{6}$$

Let's denote by σ_A^2 the variance of A_r^{ni}:

$$\sigma_A^2 := Var(A_r^{ni}).$$

For any $\varepsilon > 0$ and $m \geq 1$, by **(A3)**,

$$\mathbb{E}\left[I\left(\sup_{0 \leq t \leq T} |\widehat{\Lambda}_n(t) - \Lambda_n(t)| \geq \varepsilon \right) - \frac{N_n(T)\sigma_A^2}{c_n^2 \varepsilon^2} \,\middle|\, N_n(T) = m \right] =$$

$$= \mathbb{E}\left[I\left(\sup_{k \leq m} \left| \sum_{1 \leq i \leq k} (A_r^{ni} - \mu_A) \right| \geq c_n \varepsilon \right) - \frac{Var\left(\sum_{1 \leq k \leq m} (A_r^{ni} - \mu_A) \right)}{c_n^2 \varepsilon^2} \right] =$$

$$= \mathbb{P}\left[\sup_{k \leq m} \left| \sum_{1 \leq i \leq k} (A_r^{ni} - \mu_A) \right| \geq c_n \varepsilon \right] - \frac{Var\left(\sum_{1 \leq k \leq m} (A_r^{ni} - \mu_A) \right)}{c_n^2 \varepsilon^2}$$

and the last term is ≤ 0 by Kolmogorov inequality. It follows that

$$\mathbb{E}\left[I\left(\sup_{0\leq t\leq T}|\widehat{\Lambda}_n(t)-\Lambda_n(t)|\geq\varepsilon\right)-\frac{N_n(T)\sigma_A^2}{c_n^2\varepsilon^2}\,\bigg|\,N_n(T)\right]\leq 0,$$

and then

$$\mathbb{E}\left[I\left(\sup_{0\leq t\leq T}|\widehat{\Lambda}_n(t)-\Lambda_n(t)|\geq\varepsilon\right)-\frac{N_n(T)\sigma_A^2}{c_n^2\varepsilon^2}\right]=$$

$$=\mathbb{E}\left[\mathbb{E}\left[I\left(\sup_{0\leq t\leq T}|\widehat{\Lambda}_n(t)-\Lambda_n(t)|\geq\varepsilon\right)-\frac{N_n(T)\sigma_A^2}{c_n^2\varepsilon^2}\,\bigg|\,N_n(T)\right]\right]\leq 0.$$

So

$$\mathbb{P}\left[\sup_{0\leq t\leq T}|\widehat{\Lambda}_n(t)-\Lambda_n(t)|\geq\varepsilon\right]\leq\frac{\mathbb{E}[N_n(T)]\sigma_A^2}{c_n^2\varepsilon^2}$$

and (6) follows from (2). $\square$

Theorem 3 (Asymptotic Gaussianity). *The process* $\mathcal{M}_n^{\mathcal{S}}=\{\mathcal{M}_n^{\mathcal{S}}(t)\,:\,0\leq t\leq T\}$, *defined by*

$$\mathcal{M}_n^{\mathcal{S}}(t):=\sqrt{c_n}\left(\frac{\widehat{\mathcal{S}}_n(t)-\mathcal{S}_n(t)}{\mathcal{S}_n(t)}\right),\qquad 0\leq t\leq T,$$

converges to $W(v)$:

$$\mathcal{M}_n^{\mathcal{S}}\Longrightarrow W(v),\qquad as\ \ n\to\infty, \tag{7}$$

where W *is a Standard Brownian motion on* $[0,T]$, *and* $v=\{v(t)\,:\,t\geq 0\}$ *is defined by:*

$$v(t):=\sigma_A^2\cdot\frac{t}{\mu_U}.$$

Proof. Let's define the process $\mathcal{M}_n^{\Lambda}=\{\mathcal{M}_n^{\Lambda}(t)\,:\,0\leq t\leq T\}$ by

$$\mathcal{M}_n^{\Lambda}(t):=\sqrt{c_n}\left(\widehat{\Lambda}_n(t)-\Lambda_n(t)\right)=\frac{1}{\sqrt{c_n}}\sum_{i=1}^{N_n(t)}(A_r^{ni}-\mu_A),\qquad 0\leq t\leq T.$$

We first prove that

$$\mathcal{M}_n^{\Lambda}\Longrightarrow W(v),\qquad as\ \ n\to\infty. \tag{8}$$

First suppose $T/\mu_U<1$. Let us define, for any $t\in[0,T]$:

$$\Phi_n(t):=\begin{cases}N_n(t)/c_n, & \text{if}\ \ N_n(t)/c_n\leq 1,\\[2mm]\dfrac{t}{\mu_U}, & \text{otherwise}\ .\end{cases}$$

Note that, because of (1):

$$\sup_{0 \le t \le T} \left| \Phi_n(t) - \frac{t}{\mu_U} \right| \le \sup_{0 \le t \le T} \left| \frac{N_n(t)}{c_n} - \frac{t}{\mu_U} \right| \implies 0, \qquad \text{as } n \to \infty.$$

So:

$$\Phi_n \implies \phi, \qquad \text{as } n \to \infty. \tag{9}$$

where

$$\phi(t) := \frac{t}{\mu_U}, \quad 0 \le t \le T.$$

By Donsker's Theorem (see [2, Th. 14.1]), the process $X_{c_n} = \{X_{c_n}(t) : 0 \le t \le T\}$ defined by

$$X_{c_n}(t) := \frac{1}{\sqrt{c_n}} \sum_{i=1}^{\lfloor c_n t \rfloor} (A_r^{ni} - \mu_A), \qquad 0 \le t \le T,$$

converges to $\sigma_A \cdot W$:

$$X_{c_n} \implies \sigma_A \cdot W, \qquad \text{as } n \to \infty. \tag{10}$$

By (9) and (10) it follows (see [2, Th. 3.9]) that:

$$(X_{c_n}, \Phi_n) \implies (\sigma_A \cdot W, \phi), \qquad \text{as } n \to \infty,$$

and, since W is a.s. continuous (see [2, Lemma p. 151]), then

$$(X_{c_n} \circ \Phi_n) \implies \sigma_A \cdot (W \circ \phi), \qquad \text{as } n \to \infty.$$

Fix now $\varepsilon > 0$ and put $\delta := 1 - T/\mu_U$. We have:

$$\mathbb{P}\left[\sup_{0 \le t \le T} |\mathcal{M}_n^A(t) - (X_{c_n} \circ \Phi_n)(t)| > \varepsilon \right] \le \mathbb{P}\left[\sup_{0 \le t \le T} \frac{N_n(t)}{c_n} > 1 \right] \le$$

$$\le \mathbb{P}\left[\sup_{0 \le t \le T} \left| \frac{N_n(t)}{c_n} - \frac{t}{\mu_U} \right| > \delta \right],$$

and, because of (1), the last probability goes to 0, as $n \to \infty$. So

$$\mathcal{M}_n^A \implies \sigma_A \cdot (W \circ \phi), \qquad \text{as } n \to \infty,$$

and hence (8) follows because $\sigma_A \cdot (W \circ \phi)$ and $W(v)$ have the same distribution.

If $T/\mu_U \ge 1$ and $a > 0$ is such that $T/a\mu_U < 1$, the proof of (8) can be arranged as before, by substituting c_n with ac_n.

Now, after having established (8), we note that, by Duhamel's Equation (see [1, eq. (2.6.5)]):

$$\mathcal{M}_n^S(t) = - \int_0^t \frac{\widehat{S}_n(s^-)}{S_n(s)} \, d\mathcal{M}_n^A(s),$$

so that

$$\sup_{0\leq t\leq T}\left|\mathcal{M}_n^{\mathcal{S}}(t)-\left(-\mathcal{M}_n^{\Lambda}(t)\right)\right| = \sup_{0\leq t\leq T}\left|\int_0^t\left(\frac{\widehat{\mathcal{S}}_n(s^-)}{\mathcal{S}_n(s)}-1\right)d\mathcal{M}_n^{\Lambda}(s)\right| \leq$$

$$\leq \sup_{0\leq t\leq T}\left|\frac{\widehat{\mathcal{S}}_n(t^-)}{\mathcal{S}_n(t)}-1\right|\cdot\sup_{0\leq t\leq T}\mathcal{M}_n^{\Lambda}(t).$$

Moreover,

$$\sup_{0\leq t\leq T}\left|\frac{\widehat{\mathcal{S}}_n(t^-)}{\mathcal{S}_n(t)}-1\right| \leq \frac{1}{\mathcal{S}_n(T)}\cdot\sup_{0\leq t\leq T}\left|\widehat{\mathcal{S}}_n(t^-)-\mathcal{S}_n(t)\right|,$$

and because of (3), (5) and the continuity of $\mathcal{S}$, we have:

$$\sup_{0\leq t\leq T}\left|\frac{\widehat{\mathcal{S}}_n(t^-)}{\mathcal{S}_n(t)}-1\right| \Longrightarrow 0, \quad \text{as } n\to\infty.$$

Furthermore, (8) implies that

$$\sup_{0\leq t\leq T}\mathcal{M}_n^{\Lambda}(t) \Longrightarrow \sup_{0\leq t\leq T}W(v(t)), \quad \text{as } n\to\infty.$$

Hence

$$\sup_{0\leq t\leq T}\left|\mathcal{M}_n^{\mathcal{S}}(t)-\left(-\mathcal{M}_n^{\Lambda}(t)\right)\right| \Longrightarrow 0, \quad \text{as } n\to\infty,$$

and, again because of (8), we arrive at the desired convergence (7). $\square$

The next step is to use Theorems 2 and 3 to derive confidence bands. First we have to find a good estimator for the variance function v. Let us define the process $\widehat{v}_n = \{\widehat{v}_n(t) \ : \ 0\leq t\leq T\}$ by

$$\widehat{v}_n(t) := \frac{1}{c_n}\sum_{i=1}^{N_n(t)}\left(A_r^{ni}-\frac{1}{N_n(t)}\sum_{j=1}^{N_n(t)}A_r^{nj}\right)^2, \quad 0\leq t\leq T.$$

Theorem 4. *The process $\widehat{v}_n$ is a Uniformly Consistent estimator of the variance function v, that is:*

$$\sup_{0\leq t\leq T}\left|\widehat{v}_n(t)-v(t)\right| \Longrightarrow 0, \quad \text{as } n\to\infty.$$

Proof. Note that, for any $t\in[0,T]$, we have

$$\widehat{v}_n(t) := \frac{1}{c_n}\sum_{i=1}^{N_n(t)}\left(A_r^{ni}-\mu_A\right)^2-\frac{1}{N_n(t)}\left(\mathcal{M}_n^{\Lambda}(t)\right)^2.$$

So

$$|\widehat{v}_n(t) - v(t)| \leq \mathcal{B}_n(t) + \sigma_A^2 \left| \frac{N_n(t)}{c_n} - \frac{t}{\mu_U} \right| + \frac{1}{N_n(t)} \left(\mathcal{M}_n^\Lambda(t) \right)^2, \qquad (11)$$

where, for notational convenience, we have put

$$\mathcal{B}_n(t) := \frac{1}{c_n} \left| \sum_{i=1}^{N_n(t)} \left((A_r^{ni} - \mu_A)^2 - \sigma_A^2 \right) \right|.$$

The last term in (11) goes uniformly to 0 in probability because of (1) and (8). The second term goes uniformly to 0 in probability because of (1). It follows that we have only to show that

$$\sup_{0 \leq t \leq T} \mathcal{B}_n(t) \Longrightarrow 0, \qquad \text{as } n \to \infty.$$

Let $\varepsilon > 0$. For any $m \geq 1$, by $(\mathbf{A3})$:

$$\mathbb{E}\left[I\left(\sup_{0 \leq t \leq T} \mathcal{B}_n(t) \geq \varepsilon \right) - \frac{N_n(T) Var((A_r^{ni} - \mu_A)^2)}{\varepsilon^2 c_n^2} \,\middle|\, N_n(T) = m \right] =$$

$$= \mathbb{E}\left[I\left(\sup_{k \leq m} \left| \sum_{1 \leq i \leq k} \left((A_r^{ni} - \mu_A)^2 - \sigma_A^2 \right) \right| \geq \varepsilon c_n \right) - \frac{m Var((A_r^{ni} - \mu_A)^2)}{\varepsilon^2 c_n^2} \right] =$$

$$= \mathbb{P}\left[\sup_{k \leq m} \left| \sum_{1 \leq i \leq k} \left((A_r^{ni} - \mu_A)^2 - \sigma_A^2 \right) \right| \geq \varepsilon c_n \right] - \frac{Var(\sum_{1 \leq i \leq m} (A_r^{ni} - \mu_A)^2)}{\varepsilon^2 c_n^2},$$

and the last term is ≤ 0 by Kolmogorov's inequality. It follows that

$$\mathbb{E}\left[I\left(\sup_{0 \leq t \leq T} \mathcal{B}_n(t) \geq \varepsilon \right) - \frac{N_n(T) Var((A_r^{ni} - \mu_A)^2)}{\varepsilon^2 c_n^2} \,\middle|\, N_n(T) \right] \leq 0,$$

so that

$$\mathbb{E}\left[I\left(\sup_{0 \leq t \leq T} \mathcal{B}_n(t) \geq \varepsilon \right) - \frac{N_n(T) Var((A_r^{ni} - \mu_A)^2)}{\varepsilon^2 c_n^2} \right] =$$

$$\mathbb{E}\left[\mathbb{E}\left[I\left(\sup_{0 \leq t \leq T} \mathcal{B}_n(t) \geq \varepsilon \right) - \frac{N_n(T) Var((A_r^{ni} - \mu_A)^2)}{\varepsilon^2 c_n^2} \,\middle|\, N_n(T) \right] \right] \leq 0.$$

Hence

$$\mathbb{P}\left[\sup_{0 \leq t \leq T} \mathcal{B}_n(t) \geq \varepsilon \right] \leq \frac{\mathbb{E}[N_n(T)]}{\varepsilon^2 c_n^2} Var\left[(A_r^{ni} - \mu_A)^2 \right]$$

and the conclusion follows from (2). $\square$

4 Confidence Bands

In order to find Confidence Bands, let us show that the following theorem holds.

Theorem 5. *Under the same notations and assumptions as in the previous sections, the following convergence result holds:*

$$\sup_{0 \le t \le T} \left| \frac{\sqrt{c_n}}{1 + \widehat{v}_n(t)} \frac{\widehat{\mathcal{S}}_n(t) - \mathcal{S}_n(t)}{\widehat{\mathcal{S}}_n(t)} \right| \Longrightarrow \sup_{0 \le x \le c} \left| W^0(x) \right|, \qquad as \ \ n \to \infty,$$

where W^0 is a standard Brownian bridge and $c := v(T)/(1 + v(T))$.

Proof. From (5), Theorem 3 and Theorem 4, it follows that

$$\frac{\sqrt{c_n}}{1 + \widehat{v}_n} \frac{\widehat{\mathcal{S}}_n - \mathcal{S}_n}{\widehat{\mathcal{S}}_n} = \frac{\mathcal{M}_n^{\mathcal{S}}}{(1 + \widehat{v}_n)} \cdot \frac{\mathcal{S}_n}{\widehat{\mathcal{S}}_n} \Longrightarrow \frac{W(v)}{1 + v}, \qquad as \ \ n \to \infty,$$

where W denotes standard Brownian motion on $[0, T]$. So, it is enough to see that $\dfrac{W(v)}{1 + v}$ and $W^0 \left(\dfrac{v}{1 + v} \right)$ have the same distribution. $\square$

From the previous result, it follows that, for any $y > 0$,

$$\mathbb{P} \left[\sup_{0 \le t \le T} \left| \frac{\sqrt{c_n}}{1 + \widehat{v}_n(t)} \frac{\widehat{\mathcal{S}}_n(t) - \mathcal{S}_n(t)}{\widehat{\mathcal{S}}_n(t)} \right| \le y \right] \xrightarrow[n \to \infty]{} \mathbb{P} \left[\sup_{0 \le x \le c} \left| W^0(x) \right| \le y \right].$$

Then, the asymptotic $100(1 - \alpha)\%$ Confidence Band for $\mathcal{S}_n$ in $[0, T]$ is:

$$\left[\widehat{\mathcal{S}}_n(t) \left(1 - \frac{1 + \widehat{v}_n(t)}{\sqrt{c_n}} e_\alpha(c) \right), \widehat{\mathcal{S}}_n(t) \left(1 + \frac{1 + \widehat{v}_n(t)}{\sqrt{c_n}} e_\alpha(c) \right) \right], \qquad 0 \le t \le T,$$

where $e_\alpha(c)$ denotes the upper α-quantile of the distribution of

$$\sup_{0 \le x \le c} \left| W^0(x) \right|.$$

References

1. Andersen, P.K., Borgan, O., Gill, R.D. and Keiding, N.: Statistical Models Based on Counting Processes. Springer, New York (1997)
2. Billingsley, P.: Convergence of Probability Measures. Wiley, New York (1999)
3. Daley, D.J. and Vere-Jones, D.: An Introduction to the Theory of Point Processes. Springer, New York (1988)
4. De Giosa, M.: Free area estimation in a dynamic germ-grain model with renewal dropping process. J. Appl. Math. Stoch. Anal. in press (2006)

5. Gill, R.D., Johansen, S.: A survey of product-integration with a view toward application in survival analysis. Ann. Statist. **18**, 1501–1555 (1990)
6. Hansen, M.B., Baddeley, A.J., Gill, R.D.: First contact distribution for spatial patterns: regularity and estimation. Adv. Appl. Prob. **31**, 15–33 (1999)
7. Karlin, S. and Taylor, H.M.: A First Course in Stochastic Processes. Academic Press, New York (1975)
8. Stoyan, D., Kendall, W.S., Mecke, J.: Stochastic Geometry and its Applications. Wiley, New York (1995)

An Extension of the Kolmogorov-Avrami Formula to Inhomogeneous Birth-and-Growth Processes

Martin Burger[1], Vincenzo Capasso[2], and Alessandra Micheletti[2]

[1] Institut für Industriemathematik, Johannes Kepler Universität, Altenbergerstr. 69, A 4040 Linz, Austria
   `martin.burger@jku.at`
[2] ADAMSS(Centre for Advanced Applied Mathematical and Statistical Sciences) & Department of Mathematics, Universitá degli Studi di Milano, via Saldini 50, 20133 Milano, Italy
   `{vincenzo.capasso,Alessandra.Micheletti}@unimi.it`

Summary. It has been shown by a substantial body of literature that the hazard function plays an important role in the derivation of evolution equations of volume and $n-$facet densities of Johnson-Mehl tessellations generated by germ-grain models associated with spatially homogeneous birth-and-growth processes.

In this paper, we analyze a more general class of space-time inhomogeneous birth-and-growth processes, emphasizing the role played by the hazard function. A special result is the extension of the well-known formula that Kolmogorov and Avrami had found in connection with problems of crystal growth. Recent literature shows the relevance of a theory for the hazard function in other important areas of application such as tumor growth and angiogenesis, crystallization of sea shells, etc. Moreover, a detailed analysis of the hazard function in terms of relevant volume and surface densities is carried out; its relationship with the local spherical contact distribution function is given, too.

1 Introduction

Many important real world phenomena, such as phase-change and crystallization processes (see [6, 9, 22]) or tumor growth and angiogenesis [20], can be modeled as heterogeneous birth and growth processes. After the random birth (nucleation) of germs, grains are formed, which usually grow in a strongly heterogeneous way. The birth-and-growth process finally forms a Johnson-Mehl tessellation of the space.

A Johnson-Mehl tessellation [15, 21] is generated by a spatially marked point process $N = \{(T_i, X_i)\}_{i \in \mathbb{N}}$, where T_i represents the random time of birth of the i-th germ and X_i its random spatial location. Once born, each germ generates a grain which grows at the surface (growth front), with a speed

$G(x, t) > 0$, which is, in general, assumed to be deterministic and space-time dependent.

When two growing cells meet, they stop growing at contact points, thus forming interfaces (n-facets) at various Hausdorff dimensions; this phenomenon is called *impingement*.

In many applications, the characterization of the final morphology of the tessellation is of interest, in particular geometric measures of n-facets [19]. As we shall see in this paper, it is of fundamental importance to understand the role of the hazard function for this process in order to obtain evolution equations for n-facet densities in a generalized and more realistic setup (allowing heterogeneous birth and growth). We are considering the *hazard function* associated with the survival function of a point with respect to its capture by growing grains (crystalline phase) [19].

In Section 2, we introduce basic ingredients of a birth-and-growth process, i.e. a space-time inhomogeneous Poisson process for the birth of germs, and a *normal growth* model for the growth of grains.

In Section 3, basic concepts regarding mean densities are introduced in the framework of stochastic geometry of birth-and-growth processes.

In Section 4, we introduce the hazard function associated with a stochastic birth-and-growth process, and relate it to mean volume and surface densities. Here, we derive a significant extension of the classical Kolmogorov-Avrami theory to the case of space-time inhomogeneous processes.

Section 4.1 relates the hazard function to another classical concept of stochastic geometry, the spherical contact distribution function.

2 Stochastic Birth-and-growth Processes

2.1 Random Closed Sets

Consider the measure space $(\mathbb{R}^d, \mathcal{B}_{\mathbb{R}^d}, \nu^d)$ endowed with the usual Lebesgue measure ν^d, and the measurable space $(\mathcal{F}, \sigma_{\mathcal{F}})$ where $\mathcal{F}$ is the family of closed subsets of $\mathbb{R}^d$, and $\sigma_{\mathcal{F}}$ is the $\sigma-$algebra on $\mathcal{F}$ generated by the hit-or-miss topology [18], which coincides with the $\sigma-$ algebra generated by the family

$$F_K = \{C \in \mathcal{F} | C \cap K \neq \emptyset\}, \quad K \in \{\text{compact subsets of } \mathbb{R}^d\}$$

The following definition introduces the key ingredient of stochastic geometry.

Definition 1. *Let* $(\Omega, \mathcal{A}, \mathbb{P})$ *be a probability space. A random closed set* (RACS) Θ *is a measurable function*

$$\Theta : (\Omega, \mathcal{A}) \longrightarrow (\mathcal{F}, \sigma_{\mathcal{F}}).$$

In order to define the probability law induced on $(\mathcal{F}, \sigma_{\mathcal{F}})$ by Θ, we follow the well-known theory of Choquet-Matheron [18], according to which it is possible to assign a unique probability law $\mathbb{P}_\Theta$ associated with the *RACS* Θ by assigning its *hitting functional* T_Θ.

If we denote by $\mathcal{K}$ the family of compact sets in $\mathbb{R}^d$, then the hitting functional of Θ is defined as

$$T_\Theta : K \in \mathcal{K} \longmapsto \mathbb{P}(\Theta \cap K \neq \emptyset).$$

Actually, it is sufficient to assign the restriction of T_Θ to the family of closed balls $\{B_\varepsilon(x); x \in \mathbb{R}^d, \varepsilon \in \mathbb{R}_+ - \{0\}\}$.

2.2 A Birth-and-Growth Model

A birth-and-growth process is a dynamic germ-grain model whose birth process is modelled as a marked point process (MPP). For the model presented here we refer to [6, 8, 11].

Consider a Borel set $E \subset \mathbb{R}^d$ endowed with its Borel σ-algebra $\mathcal{E}$. A marked point process (MPP) N on $E \times \mathbb{R}_+$ is defined as a random measure given by

$$N = \sum_{j=1}^{\infty} \epsilon_{X_j, T_j}$$

where

- T_j is an $\mathbb{R}_+$-valued random variable representing the time of birth of the $j-$th nucleus,
- X_j is an E-valued random variable representing the spatial location of the nucleus born at time T_j,
- $\epsilon_{x,t}$ is the Dirac measure on $\mathcal{E} \times \mathcal{B}_{\mathbb{R}_+}$ such that for any $B \in \mathcal{E}$ and $t_1 < t_2$,

$$\epsilon_{x,t}(B \times [t_1, t_2]) = \begin{cases} 1 & \text{if } x \in B, t \in [t_1, t_2], \\ 0 & \text{otherwise.} \end{cases}$$

Thus we have that

$$N(A \times B) = \sharp\{X_j \in A, T_j \in B\}, \qquad A \in \mathcal{E}, B \in \mathcal{B}_{\mathbb{R}_+}$$

is the (random) number of germs born in the region A, during B.

Let $\Theta^j(t)$ be the RACS obtained as the evolution up to time $t > T_j$ of the germ born at time T_j in X_j, according to some growth model; this will be the *grain* associated with the *germ* (X_j, T_j).

The family of RACS's given by

$$\Theta^t = \bigcup_{T_j < t} \Theta^j(t), \ \ t \in \mathbb{R}_+ \tag{1}$$

is called a *birth-and-growth process*.

The Birth Model

It is well known that, under general conditions [3, 17], a marked point process (MPP) is characterized by its compensator (or stochastic intensity). We assume that the MPP N is a space-time inhomogeneous Poisson process with a given (deterministic) intensity $\alpha(x,t), x \in E, t \geq 0$. It will be assumed that α is a real valued measurable function on $E \times \mathbb{R}_+$ such that $\alpha(\cdot, t) \in \mathcal{L}^1(E)$, for all $t > 0$ and such that

$$0 < \int_0^T \int_E \alpha(x,t)dx \, dt < \infty$$

for any $0 < T < \infty$, but $\int_0^{+\infty} \int_E \alpha(x,t)dx \, dt = +\infty$.

Whenever we want to exclude germs which are born within the region already occupied by Θ^t, we consider the *thinned stochastic intensity*

$$\nu(dx \times dt) = \alpha(x,t)(1 - I_{\Theta^{t-}}(x))dxdt.$$

In this respect we shall call

$$\nu_0(dx \times dt) = \alpha(x,t)dxdt$$

the *free space intensity* .

The Growth Model

In order to complete the definition of the birth-and-growth process we need to define a growth model for any grain associated with each individual germ.

We assume that the growth of a nucleus occurs with a nonnegative normal velocity $G(x,t)$, i.e., the velocity of boundary points is determined by

$$V = Gn, \qquad \text{on } \partial\left(\bigcup_j \Theta^j(t)\right),$$

where n is the unit outer normal. As usual, initial growth is considered from a spherical nucleus with an infinitesimal radius $R \to 0$.

Without further notice, we shall assume that G is bounded and continuous on $E \times [0,T]$ with

$$g_0 := \inf_{x \in E, t \in [0,T]} G(x,t) > 0, \qquad G_0 := \sup_{x \in E, t \in [0,T]} G(x,t).$$

Moreover, we assume that G is (globally) Lipschitz-continuous with respect to the space variable x.

As a consequence, given a nucleation event at time t_0 and location x_0, the corresponding grain $\Theta(t; x_0, t_0)$, freely grown up to time $t > t_0$, is given by [5]

$$\Theta(t; x_0, t_0) = \{x \in E | \exists \xi \in W^{1,\infty}([t_0, t]) : \xi(t_0) = x_0, \xi(t) = x,$$
$$|\dot{\xi}(s)| \leq G(\xi(s), s), s \in (t_0, t)\} \tag{2}$$

for $t \geq t_0$ and $\Theta(t; x_0, t_0) = \emptyset$ for $t < t_0$ (here, $W^{1,\infty}$ is the classical Sobolev space).

Note that in general the inclusion $\Theta^j(t) \subset \Theta(t; X_j, T_j)$ holds without equality. However, the total crystalline phase defined by (1) can be computed as

$$\Theta^t = \bigcup_{T_j < t} \Theta(t; X_j, T_j), \quad t \in \mathbb{R}_+. \tag{3}$$

2.3 The Causal Cone

So far, we have taken a Lagrangian approach and looked at the evolution of the grain starting from the location where it nucleated. Alternatively, we can adopt an Eulerian approach, i.e., fix a time t and a spatial location x, and investigate under which conditions the point x will be covered by the phase $\Theta(t)$ at time t. This investigation is simplified significantly by the results of the previous section, which allow to look at the freely grown grains.

For the birth-and-growth model defined above we may introduce a *causal cone* associated with a point $x \in E$, and a time $t > 0$. By looking at the possible nucleation events for which $x \in \Theta^t$, the *causal cone* is defined by

$$\mathcal{C}(x, t) := \{(y, s) \in E \times [0, t] | x \in \Theta(t; y, s)\}.$$

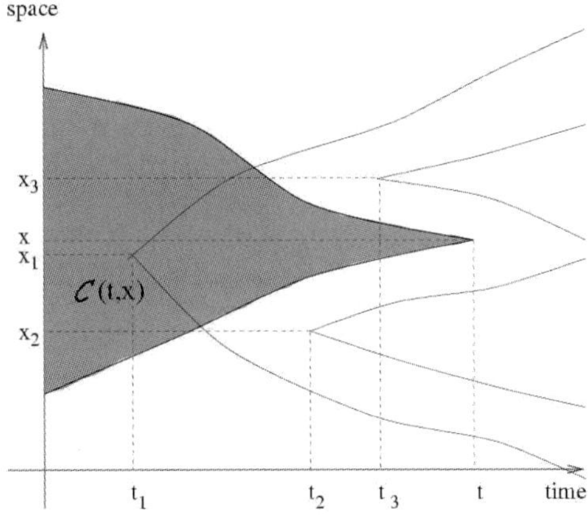

Fig. 1: The causal cone $\mathcal{C}(x, t)$ of point x at time t: it is the space-time region where a nucleation has to take place so that point x is reached by a growing grain by time t.

Some information on the properties of the boundaries in a sense of geometric measure theory has been obtained in [4] (see also [2]), for a freely grown crystal $\Theta(t; y, s)$,

Proposition 1. *For almost every $t > s$, the set $\Theta(t; y, s)$ has finite nontrivial Hausdorff-measure $\mathcal{H}^d$; its boundary $\partial\Theta(t; y, s)$ has finite nontrivial Hausdorff-measure $\mathcal{H}^{d-1}$.*

From the theory of Poisson processes, it is easily seen that

$$\mathbb{P}(N(\mathcal{C}(x, t)) = 0) = e^{-\nu_0(\mathcal{C}(x,t))},$$

where $\nu_0(\mathcal{C}(x, t))$ is the volume of the causal cone with respect to the intensity measure of the Poisson process

$$\nu_0(\mathcal{C}(x, t)) = \int_{\mathcal{C}(x,t)} \alpha(y, s) d(y, s).$$

The following result holds [5] for the time derivative of the measure $\nu_0(\mathcal{C}(x, t))$.

Proposition 2. *Let the standard assumptions on the nucleation and growth rates be satisfied. Then $\nu_0(\mathcal{C}(x, t))$ is continuously differentiable with respect to t and*

$$\frac{\partial}{\partial t}\nu_0(\mathcal{C}(x, t)) = G(x, t) \int_0^t dt_0 \int_{\mathbb{R}^d} dx_0 K(x_0, t_0; x, t)\alpha(x_0, t_0) \tag{4}$$

with

$$K(x_0, t_0; x, t) := \int_{\{z \in \mathbb{R}^d | \tau(x_0, t_0; z) = t\}} da(z)\delta(z - x).$$

Here δ is the Dirac function, $da(z)$ is a $(d-1)$-surface element, and $\tau(x_0, t_0; z)$ is the solution of the eikonal problem

$$|\frac{\partial \tau}{\partial x_0}(x_0, t_0, x)| = \frac{1}{G(x_0, t_0)}\frac{\partial \tau}{\partial t_0}(x_0, t_0, x)$$

$$|\frac{\partial \tau}{\partial x}(x_0, t_0, x)| = \frac{1}{G(x, \tau(x_0, t_0, x))},$$

subject to suitable initial and boundary conditions.

3 Mean Geometric Densities

Since the growth model generates sufficiently regular grains $\Theta(t; x_0, t_0)$, together with their boundaries $\partial\Theta(t; x_0, t_0)$, we may describe them in terms of generalized densities of Radon measures, with respect to the usual Lebesgue measure on $\mathbb{R}^d$.

Given an n-regular set Θ_n in $\mathbb{R}^d$ as defined in [13], consider the Radon measure on the Borel σ-algebra $\mathcal{B}_{\mathbb{R}^d}$

$$\mu_{\Theta_n}(\cdot) := \mathcal{H}^n(\Theta_n \cap \cdot);$$

we may then identify the set Θ_n by its generalized density (distribution)

$$\delta_{\Theta_n}(x) := \lim_{r \to 0} \frac{\mathcal{H}^n(\Theta_n \cap B_r(x))}{b_d r^d},$$

finite or not. From the results above, we may assume that a grain $\Theta(t; x_0, t_0)$ born at time t_0 at location x_0 is a d-regular set; we recognize that its density is the indicator function

$$\delta_{\Theta(t;x_0,t_0)}(x) = \begin{cases} 1 \text{ for } x \in \Theta(t; x_0, t_0) \\ 0 \text{ otherwise} \end{cases}.$$

Its boundary $\partial\Theta(t; x_0, t_0)$ is a $(d-1)$-regular set, so that its density is a geometric Dirac δ-distribution [23], $\delta_{\partial\Theta(t;x_0,t_0)}$ such that, for any $B \in \mathcal{B}_{\mathbb{R}^d}$,

$$\int_B \delta_{\partial\Theta(t;x_0,t_0)} \nu^d(dx) := \mathcal{H}^{d-1}(\partial\Theta(t; x_0, t_0) \cap B),$$

where ν^d is the classical Lebesgue measure in dimension d.

If the growth model is well posed (which is true under our regularity assumptions on the growth rate $G(x, t)$), it can be shown that a probability law of the birth-and-growth process can be defined [10]. From now on, this will be taken as an underlying assumption.

In the stochastic setting we assume that the model assumptions are such that if (Y, S) is a random point of birth in the space-time region $E \times \mathbb{R}_+ \subset \mathbb{R}^d \times \mathbb{R}_+$ the set $\Theta(t; Y, S)$, respectively $\partial\Theta(t; Y, S)$ are random d-regular, respectively $(d-1)$-regular sets; their geometric densities $\delta_{\Theta(t;Y,S)}(x)$ and $\delta_{\partial\Theta(t;Y,S)}$ are now random distributions.

Given a random n-regular set Θ_n, its mean geometric density $\mathbb{E}[\delta_{\Theta_n}]$ is defined as the generalized density of the measure

$$\mathbb{E}[\mu_{\Theta_n}](\cdot) := \mathbb{E}[\mathcal{H}^n(\Theta_n \cap \cdot)].$$

When $n = d$, both μ_{Θ_d} and $\mathbb{E}[\mu_{\Theta_d}]$ are absolutely continuous with respect to ν^d and $\delta_{\Theta_d}(x) = \mathbf{1}_{\Theta_d}(x)$, ν^d-a.s.

Moreover, due to the assumptions on the growth field $G(x, t)$, grains $\Theta(t; x_0, t_0)$ are a.s. uniformly bounded at any time $t > 0$. This implies the existence of uniformly bounded volume densities $v_{\Theta(t;Y,S)}(x)$ for all individual random grains; they are such that

$$v_{\Theta(t;Y,S)}(x) = \mathbb{E}_{(Y,S)}(\delta_{\Theta(t;Y,S)}(x)) = \mathbb{P}(x \in \Theta(t; Y, S)).$$

Under our modelling assumptions, the expected value of the measure associated with the boundary $\partial\Theta(t; Y, S)$ can also be assumed to be absolutely continuous with respect to ν^d [12], so that a mean geometric density is obtained as a classical function, the surface density of the individual random grain,

$$s_{\Theta(t;Y,S)}(x) := \mathbb{E}[\partial\delta_{\Theta(t;Y,S)}](x).$$

All these densities are themselves uniformly bounded.

Consider now the *extended* birth-and-growth process which evolves in such a way that germs are born with birth rate $\alpha(x,t)$ and grains grow with growth rate $G(x,t)$, independently of each other, i.e. ignoring overlapping of germs and grains; under the mentioned above regularity assumptions, the following quantities are well defined a.e.

Definition 2. *We call* mean extended volume density *at point x and time t the quantity $V_{ex}(x,t)$ such that, for any $B \in \mathcal{B}_{\mathbb{R}_+}$,*

$$\mathbb{E}[\sum_{T_j<t} \nu^d(\Theta(t; X_j, T_j) \cap B)] = \int_B V_{ex}(x,t)\nu^d(dx).$$

It represents the mean of the sum of the volume densities of the grains freely born and grown, up to time t [8].

Correspondingly, we can define an extended surface density:

Definition 3. *We call* mean local extended surface density *at point x and time t the function $S_{ex}(x,t)$ such that, for any $B \in \mathcal{B}_{\mathbb{R}^d}$,*

$$\mathbb{E}[\sum_{T_j<t} \nu^{d-1}(\partial\Theta(t; X_j, T_j) \cap B)] = \int_B S_{ex}(x,t)\nu^d(dx).$$

It represents the mean of the sum of the surface densities of the grains freely born and grown, up to time t.

We show now that the volume of the causal cone can be expressed in terms of the extended volume density.

Theorem 1. *Under the previous modelling assumptions on birth and on growth, if the growth field G makes (2) well defined, the following equality holds for $\nu^d \times \nu^1$-almost all (x,t)*

$$\nu_0(\mathcal{C}(x,t)) = V_{ex}(x,t),$$

Proof. We will prove the theorem by showing that for any $B \in \mathcal{B}_{\mathbb{R}^d}$, we have

$$\int_B V_{ex}(x,t)\nu^d(dx) = \int_B \nu_0(\mathcal{C}(x,t))\nu^d(dx).$$

Let $B \in \mathcal{B}_{\mathbb{R}^d}$. By definition of the extended volume density, we have

$$\int_B V_{ex}(x,t)\nu^d(dx)$$

$$= \mathbb{E}\left[\sum_{T_j < t} \nu^d(\Theta(t; X_j, T_j) \cap B)\right]$$

$$= \sum_{n=1}^{\infty} \mathbb{E}\left[\sum_{j=1}^{n} \nu^d(\Theta(t; X_j, T_j) \cap B)\bigg| N_0(t) = n\right] \mathbb{P}[N_0(t) = n]$$

$$= \sum_{n=1}^{\infty} \sum_{j=1}^{n} \mathbb{E}\left[\nu^d(\Theta(t; X_j, T_j) \cap B)|N_0(t) = n\right] \mathbb{P}[N_0(t) = n].$$

Here N_0 is the *free* birth process, having intensity $\alpha(x,t)$. Given $\{N_0(t) = n\}$, from the general theory of Poisson processes we know that all $(X_j, T_j)_{j=1,\dots,n}$ are jointly distributed as n i.i.d. (Y,S) random vectors, having probability density function

$$f_{(Y,S)}(y,s) = \frac{\alpha(y,s)}{\int_{E \times [0,t]} \alpha(y,s)dyds}.$$

The last identity becomes

$$\mathbb{E}\left[\sum_{T_j < t} \nu^d(\Theta(t; X_j, T_j) \cap B)\right] =$$

$$= \sum_{n=1}^{\infty} n\mathbb{E}_{(Y,S)}[\nu^d(\Theta(t; Y, S) \cap B)]\mathbb{P}[N_0(t) = n]$$

$$= \mathbb{E}_{(Y,S)}[\nu_d(\Theta(t; Y, S) \cap B)] \sum_{n=1}^{\infty} n\mathbb{P}[N_0(t) = n]$$

$$= \mathbb{E}_{(Y,S)}[\nu_d(\Theta(t; Y, S) \cap B)]\mathbb{E}[N_0(t)]$$

$$= \mathbb{E}_{(Y,S)}\left(\int_B I_{\Theta(t;Y,S)}(x)\nu^d(dx)\right)\mathbb{E}[N_0(t)], \tag{5}$$

where we have denoted by $\mathbb{E}_{(Y,S)}$ the expectation with respect to the probability law of the birth marked point process.

Under our regularity assumptions, it can be shown [13] that Fubini's theorem applies, so that we have

$$\mathbb{E}_{(Y,S)}\Big(\int_B I_{\Theta(t;Y,S)}(x)\nu^d(dx)\Big) = \int_\Omega d\mathbb{P}(\omega)\int_B I_{\Theta(t;Y(\omega),S(\omega))}(x)\nu^d(dx)$$

$$= \int_B \nu^d(dx)\int_\Omega d\mathbb{P}(\omega)I_{\Theta(t;Y(\omega),S(\omega))}(x)$$

$$= \int_B \nu^d(dx)\int_{E\times[0,t]} P(dy\times ds)I_{\mathcal{C}(x,t)}(y,s)$$

$$= \int_B \nu^d(dx)\frac{\int_{\mathcal{C}(x,t)}\alpha(y,s)dyds}{\int_{E\times[0,t]}\alpha(y,s)dyds}$$

Now, since $\int_0^t[\int_E \alpha(x,s)dy]ds = \mathbb{E}(N_0(t))$ and $\nu_0(\mathcal{C}(x,t)) = \int_{\mathcal{C}(x,t)}\alpha(y,s)$ $dyds$, (5) leads to

$$\int_B V_{ex}(x,t)\nu^d(dx) = \int_B \nu_0(\mathcal{C}(x,t))\nu^d(dx).$$

$\square$

4 The Hazard Function

In a birth-and-growth process the RACS Θ^t evolves with time, so that the question arises about *when* a point $x \in E$ is reached (*captured*) by this growing RACS ; or viceversa up to when a point $x \in E$ survives capture?

In this respect the *degree of crystallinity* or *mean volume density*, defined by

$$V_V(x,t): \ = \mathbb{P}(x \in \Theta^t),$$

may be seen as the probability of capture of point $x \in E$, by time $t > 0$. In this sense the complement to 1 of the crystallinity, also known as *porosity*

$$p_x(t) = 1 - V_V(x,t) = \mathbb{P}(x \notin \Theta^t)$$

represents the *survival function* of the point x at time t, i.e. the probability that the point x is not yet covered by the random set Θ^t.

With reference to the growing RACS Θ^t we may introduce the (random) time $\tau(x)$ of survival of a point $x \in E$ with respect to its capture by Θ^t , such that

$$p_x(t) = \mathbb{P}(\tau(x) > t).$$

Correspondingly, a *hazard function* $h(x,t)$ can be defined (a.e. with respect to x) as the rate of capture by the process Θ^t , i.e.

$$h(x,t) = \lim_{\Delta t \to 0}\frac{\mathbb{P}(x \in \Theta^{t+\Delta t}|x \notin \Theta^t)}{\Delta t}.$$

Under our modelling assumptions,

$$p_x(t) = \mathbb{P}(x \notin \Theta^t) = \mathbb{P}(N(\mathcal{C}(x,t)) = 0) = e^{-\nu_0(\mathcal{C}(x,t))}.$$

Thanks to Proposition 2, $\nu_0(\mathcal{C}(x,t))$ is continuously differentiable with respect to t, so that the hazard function

$$h(x,t) = -\frac{\partial}{\partial t} \ln p_x(t) = \frac{\partial}{\partial t} \nu_0(\mathcal{C}(x,t)),$$

is well defined; hence the time of capture $\tau(x)$ is an absolutely continuous random variable, having probability density function

$$f_x(t) = p_x(t) h(x,t).$$

Since

$$f_x(t) = \frac{d}{dt}(1 - p_x(t)) = \frac{\partial V_V(x,t)}{\partial t}$$

we immediately obtain

$$\frac{\partial V_V(x,t)}{\partial t} = (1 - V_V(x,t)) h(x,t).$$

This is an extension of the well known Avrami-Kolmogorov formula [16, 1],

$$\frac{dV_V}{dt}(t) = (1 - V_V(t)) \frac{dV_{ex}}{dt}(t)$$

proven for a very specific space and time homogeneous birth and growth process; instead our expression holds whenever a mean volume density and an hazard function are well defined. The remaining problem is to relate the hazard function $h(x,t)$ to the defining parameters of the process; we follow here Kolmogorov [16], using the previous analysis on the causal cone.

Because of Theorem 3,

$$h(x,t) = -\frac{\partial}{\partial t} \ln p_x(t) = \frac{\partial}{\partial t} \nu_0(\mathcal{C}(x,t)) = \frac{\partial}{\partial t} V_{ex}(x,t)$$

so that we also have

$$\frac{\partial}{\partial t} V_V(x,t) = (1 - V_V(x,t)) \frac{\partial}{\partial t} V_{ex}(x,t). \tag{6}$$

By Proposition 2

$$\frac{\partial}{\partial t} \nu_0(\mathcal{C}(x,t)) = G(x,t) \int_0^t dt_0 \int_{\mathbb{R}^d} dx_0 K(x_0,t_0;x,t) \alpha(x_0,t_0).$$

Consequently

$$\frac{\partial}{\partial t} V_{ex}(x,t) = G(x,t) \int_0^t dt_0 \int_{\mathbb{R}^d} dx_0 K(x_0,t_0;x,t) \alpha(x_0,t_0), \tag{7}$$

and

$$h(x,t) = G(x,t) \int_0^t dt_0 \int_{\mathbb{R}^d} dx_0 K(x_0,t_0;x,t)\alpha(x_0,t_0).$$

On the other hand, from the results in [13] we may claim that, for any individual crystal $\Theta_j{}^t := \Theta(t; X_j, T_j)$, the following evolution equation holds relating its mean volume and surface densities

$$\frac{\partial}{\partial t}\mathbb{E}[\delta_{\Theta_j{}^t}](x) = G(t,x)\mathbb{E}[\delta_{\partial\Theta_j{}^t}](x).$$

By linearity arguments, by considering all crystals individually born, and grown independently of each other, we get

$$\frac{\partial}{\partial t}V_{ex}(x,t) = G(x,t)S_{ex}(x,t). \tag{8}$$

A comparison of equations (7) and (8) yields the interesting expression

$$S_{ex}(x,t) = \int_0^t dt_0 \int_{\mathbb{R}^d} dx_0 K(x_0,t_0;x,t)\alpha(x_0,t_0) = \frac{h(x,t)}{G(x,t)},$$

i.e. the available free surface can be described directly in terms of the hazard function and the growth rate (and vice versa). Using (6) and (8) we finally have

$$\frac{\partial}{\partial t}V_V(x,t) = (1 - V_V(x,t))\frac{\partial}{\partial t}V_{ex}(x,t)) = (1 - V_V(x,t))G(x,t)S_{ex}(x,t).$$

4.1 Hazard Function and Spherical Contact Distribution Function

Let us recall the definition of the *local spherical contact distribution function* H_S of a random set Ξ [7, 21]

$$H_S(x,r): = \mathbb{P}(x \in \Xi \oplus B_r(0)|x \notin \Xi),$$

where $\oplus$ is Minkowski addition and $B_r(0)$ is a d-dimensional ball of radius r centered at the origin. This function has a strong connection with the surface density of a random closed set, but H_S is more easily computable from digitised images of the studied objects than the surface density itself (see e.g. [7, 14]).

We may generalise the concept of spherical contact distribution function to our birth-and-growth process in the following way [7]. Consider the set

$$\Theta^{t,\Delta t}: = \Theta^t \cup \bigcup_{x \in \Theta^t} B_{G(x,t)\Delta t}(x)$$

where $G(x,t)$ is the (strictly positive) growth rate at point x and time t, and Δt is a sufficiently small time increment. We may call the set $\Theta^{t,\Delta t}$ *inhomogeneous parallel set* of Θ^t; it represents (up to first order in Δt) the growth of the union of the grains up to time $t + \Delta t$.

Definition 4. *We call the quantity*

$$H_S(x,t,\tau) = \mathbb{P}(x \in \Theta^{t+\tau} | x \notin \Theta^t),$$

generalised local spherical contact distribution function *of the random set Θ^t,* *where $\tau \geq 0, t \geq 0, x \in \mathbb{R}^d$.*

By comparing their definitions we may relate the generalised spherical contact distribution function to the hazard function by

$$\frac{\partial H_S(x,t,\tau)}{\partial \tau}\bigg|_{\tau=0} = h(x,t).$$

As a particular consequence we may rewrite the generalized Kolmogorov-Avrami equation in the form

$$\frac{\partial V_V(x,t)}{\partial t} = (1 - V_V(x,t))\frac{\partial H_S(x,t,\tau)}{\partial \tau}\bigg|_{\tau=0}.$$

The formula (9) is benefitial for the computational prediction of the evolution of V_V, since the first-order asymptotic of the spherical contact distribution can be rather easily numerically computed.

Acknowledgements

It is a pleasure to acknowledge the significant contribution of E. Villa of the University of Milan, in the development of joint research projects relevant for this presentation. The authors gratefully acknowledge relevant contributions by G. Aletti during the final revision of the paper.

The work of MB has been supported by the Austrian Science Foundation FWF through project SFB F 013 / 08 and the Johann Radon Institute for Computational and Applied Mathematics (Austrian Academy of Sciences). The work of AM, and VC has been partially supported by the Italian PRIN/COFIN programme "Multiple scale stochastic modelling of biomineral interfaces".

VC acknowledges the warm hospitality of the Austrian Academy of Sciences at RICAM (Radon Institute for Computational and Applied Mathematics) in Linz, chaired by Prof. H. Engl.

References

1. A. Avrami, Kinetic of phase change. Part I, *J. Chem. Phys.*, **7**(1939), 1103–112.
2. G. Barles, H.M. Soner, P.E. Souganidis, Front propagation and phase-field theory, *SIAM J. Contr.Optim.*, **31**(1993), 439–469.
3. P. Brémaud, *Point Processes and Queues, Martingale Dynamics*, Springer-Verlag, New York, 1981.

4. M. Burger, Growth fronts of first-order Hamilton-Jacobi equations. SFB Report 02–8, J. Kepler University, Linz (2002).

5. M. Burger, V. Capasso, L. Pizzocchero, Mesoscale averaging of nucleation and growth models. SIAM J. Multiscale Modeling and Simulation, (2006). In press.

6. V. Capasso, Ed., *Mathematical Modelling for Polymer Processing. Polymerization, Crystallization, Manufacturing*, Springer-Verlag, Heidelberg, 2003.

7. V. Capasso, A. Micheletti, Local spherical contact distribution function and local mean densities for inhomogeneous random sets, *Stochastics and Stoch. Rep.*, **71** (2000), 51–67.

8. V. Capasso, A. Micheletti, Stochastic geometry of spatially structured birth-and-growth processes. Application to crystallization processes. In *Topics in Spatial Stochastic Processes* (E. Merzbach, Ed.). Lecture Notes in Mathematics, Vol. 1802 - CIME Subseries, Springer-Verlag, Heidelberg, 2002, 1–39.

9. V. Capasso, A. Micheletti, Stochastic geometry and related statistical problems in Biomedicine In "Complex Systems in Biomedicine" (A. Quarteroni et al, Eds.) Springer, Milano, 2006.

10. V. Capasso, C. Salani, Stochastic-birth-and-growth processes modelling crystallization of polymers with spatially heterogeneous parameters, *Nonlinear Analysis: Real World Application*, **1** (2000), 485–498.

11. V. Capasso, E. Villa, On the evolution equations of mean geometric densities for a class of space and time inhomogeneous stochastic birth-and-growth processes In "Stochastic Geometry" (W. Weil, Editor) Lecture Notes in Mathematics - CIME subseries - Springer, Heidelberg, 2005.

12. V. Capasso, E. Villa, Continuous and absolutely continuous random sets. Stoch. Anal. Appl., **24** (2006), 381–397.

13. V. Capasso, E. Villa, On the geometric densities of random closed sets, 2005. RICAM Report 13/2006, Linz, Austria.

14. U. Hahn, A. Micheletti, R. Pohlink, D. Stoyan, H. Wendrock, Stereological Analysis and Modeling of Gradient Structures, *J. of Microscopy*, **195** (1999), 113–124.

15. W.A. Johnson, R.F. Mehl, Reaction kinetics in processes of nucleation and growth, *Trans. A.I.M.M.E.*, **135** (1939), 416–458.

16. A.N. Kolmogorov, On the statistical theory of the crystallization of metals, *Bull. Acad. Sci. USSR, Math. Ser.*,**1** (1937), 355–359.

17. G. Last, A. Brandt, *Marked Point Processes on the Real Line. The Dynamic Approach*, Springer, New York, 1995.

18. G. Matheron, *Random Sets and Integral Geometry*, Wiley, New York, 1975.

19. J. Møller, Random Johnson-Mehl tessellations, *Adv. Appl. Prob.*, **24** (1992), 814–844.

20. G. Serini, D. Ambrosi, E. Giraudo, A. Gamba, L. Preziosi, F. Bussolino, Modeling the early stages of vascular network assembly, *EMBO J.*, **22** (2003), 1771–1779.

21. D. Stoyan, W.S. Kendall, J. Mecke, *Stochastic Geometry and its Application*, John Wiley & Sons, New York, 1995.

22. T. Ubukata, Computer modelling of microscopic features of molluscan shells. In *Morphogenesis and Pattern Formation in Biological Systems* (T. Sekimura et al. eds.), Springer-Verlag, Tokyo, 2003, 355–368.

23. V.S. Vladimirov, *Generalized Functions in Mathematical Physics*, Mir Publishers, Moscow, 1979.

On the Generalized Geometric Densities of Random Closed Sets. An Application to Growth Processes

Vincenzo Capasso and Elena Villa

ADAMSS (Advanced Applied Mathematical and Statistical Sciences) & Dept. of Mathematics, University of Milan, via Saldini 50, 20133 Milano, Italy
`vincenzo.capasso@unimi.it,villa@mat.unimi.it`

Summary. In recent literature the authors have introduced a *Delta formalism*, á la Dirac, for the description of random closed sets of lower dimension with respect to the environment space $\mathbb{R}^d$. Mean densities can be introduced for expected measures associated with such sets, with respect to the usual Lebesgue measure. In this paper we offer a review of the main results; in particular approximating sequences for the quoted mean densities are provided, that are of interest in the concrete estimation of mean densities of fibre processes, surface processes, etc. For time dependent random closed sets, as the ones describing the evolution of birth-and-growth processes (of interest for many models in material science and in biomedicine), the Delta formalism provides a natural framework for deriving evolution equations for mean densities at any (integer) Hausdorff dimension, in terms of the relevant kinetic parameters. In this context connections with the concepts of hazard functions, and spherical contact functions are presented.

1 Introduction

Many real phenomena may be modelled as random closed sets in $\mathbb{R}^d$, and in several situations as evolving random closed sets (see for example [10, 11]).

We remind that a *random closed set* Ξ in $\mathbb{R}^d$ is a measurable map

$$\Xi : (\Omega, \mathcal{F}, \mathbb{P}) \longrightarrow (\mathbb{F}, \sigma_{\mathbb{F}}),$$

where $\mathbb{F}$ denotes the class of the closed subsets in $\mathbb{R}^d$, and $\sigma_{\mathbb{F}}$ is the so called *hit-or-miss topology* (see [22]).

Let us consider a random closed set Θ_n with Hausdorff dimension $\dim_{\mathcal{H}}(\Theta_n) = n$ such that $\mathbb{E}[\mathcal{H}^n(\Theta_n \cap B_r(0))] < \infty$ for all $r > 0$, where $\mathcal{H}^n$ is the n-dimensional Hausdorff measure and $B_r(0)$ is the closed ball with radius r and center 0. (For a discussion about measurability of $\mathcal{H}^n(\Theta_n)$ we refer to [5, 26].) A random measure μ_{Θ_n} is induced by the random set Θ_n, defined by:

$$\mu_{\Theta_n}(A) := \mathcal{H}^n(\Theta_n \cap A), \qquad A \in \mathcal{B}_{\mathbb{R}^d}; \tag{1}$$

it is clear that, if $n < d$, for a.e. $\omega \in \Omega$ the measure $\mu_{\Theta_n(\omega)}$ is singular with respect to the d-dimensional Lebesgue measure ν^d, and so its Radon-Nikodym derivative is zero almost everywhere. On the other hand, in dependence of the probability law of Θ_n, the expected measure

$$\mathbb{E}[\mu_{\Theta_n}](A) := \mathbb{E}[\mathcal{H}^n(\Theta_n \cap A)], \qquad A \in \mathcal{B}_{\mathbb{R}^d}$$

may be either singular or absolutely continuous with respect to ν^d; in this second case its Radon-Nikodym derivative may be a non trivial classical function. If Θ_n is sufficiently regular, even though $\mathbb{E}[\mu_{\Theta_n}]$ is singular, we may introduce a *generalized Radon-Nikodym derivative*, say $\mathbb{E}[\delta_{\Theta_n}](x)$ (see Section 2), i.e. a generalized function (a continuous linear functional on a suitable test space), in a similar way as the usual Dirac delta δ_{x_0} of a point x_0. That is, formally, we may write $\int f(x)\mathbb{E}[\delta_{\Theta_n}](x)\mathrm{d}x := \int f(x)\mathbb{E}[\mu_{\Theta_n}](\mathrm{d}x)$ for any test function f.

By introducing the generalized density $\mathbb{E}[\delta_{\Theta_n}]$, we may formally deal with it as a classical function; it will be clear by the context, i.e. by the underlying assumptions, whether $\mathbb{E}[\mu_{\Theta_n}]$ is an absolutely continuous measure with respect to ν^d or not; consequently whether $\mathbb{E}[\delta_{\Theta_n}](x)$ has to be considered a generalized function, or a classical function (the usual Radon-Nikodym derivative) associated with the measure $\mathbb{E}[\mu_{\Theta_n}]$.

As the well known Dirac delta $\delta_{x_0}(x)$, associated with a point x_0, allows for example the localization of a mass at point x_0, the *delta function* $\delta_{\Theta_n}(x)$ allows the "localization" of any relevant quantity along points x belonging to an *n-regular* closed set Θ_n.

On the other hand, again as for the usual Dirac delta (generalized) function we may express it in terms of a suitable approximating sequence of classical functions, it can be shown that it is possible to approximate δ_{Θ_n} and $\mathbb{E}[\delta_{\Theta_n}]$ by sequences of classical functions (see Section 3). This turns out of great importance in several real applications, whenever we wish to estimate the density of the mean measure $\mathbb{E}[\mu_{\Theta_n}]$. For example, when $n = 1$ in the case of a fibre process, or a line process, or when $n = d - 1$ in the case of a surface process (see also [1]).

Further, in case the random closed set depends upon time as, for example, when it models the evolution of a growth process (see Section 5), in which case the associated delta function will also be a function of time, we take advantage of the "localizing" action of the Delta formalism for writing evolution equations in terms of the relevant local (in time and space) kinetic parameters of the system.

In particular, for a wide class of growth processes, which satisfy a *mean first order Steiner formula* (Section 4), we may write an evolution equation of the *mean volume density* $\mathbb{E}[\delta_{\Theta^t}]$ of Θ^t, and relate it to relevant quantities describing the process, such as, for example, the hazard function associated with the random time of capture of a point $x \in \mathbb{R}^d$.

2 Generalized Densities

For any lower dimensional random closed set Θ_n in $\mathbb{R}^d$, it is clear that $\mu_{\Theta_n(\omega)}$ defined in (1) is a singular measure, but in general, when we consider the expected measure $\mathbb{E}[\mu_{\Theta_n}]$, it may be absolutely continuous with respect to ν^d, and so it may have density, say $\mathbb{E}[\delta_{\Theta_n}](x)$, that is a real-valued integrable function on $\mathbb{R}^d$. In such case we say that the random closed set Θ_n is *absolutely continuous in mean* [25].

We are going to introduce a *generalized Radon-Nikodym derivative* of the measure $\mu_{\Theta_n(\omega)}$, say $\delta_{\Theta_n(\omega)}(x)$, in order to take formally its expected value and obtain $\mathbb{E}[\delta_{\Theta_n}](x)$.

To this end, as the Dirac delta function δ_{x_0} associated to a point $x_0 \in \mathbb{R}^d$ may be seen as the density of the singular measure $\mathcal{H}^0(x_0 \cap \cdot)$, and, mathematically, it has to be considered a continuous linear functional on a suitable test space (e.g. [19]), we define $\delta_{\Theta_n(\omega)}$ and $\mathbb{E}[\delta_{\Theta_n}]$ as linear functionals (generalized functions), so that, when Θ_n is absolutely continuous, $\mathbb{E}[\delta_{\Theta_n}]$ turns to be a regular generalized function, i.e. a classical integrable function. (See [13].)

Definition 1 (*n*-regular sets). *Given an integer* $n \in [0, d]$, *we say that a closed subset S of $\mathbb{R}^d$ is n-regular, if it satisfies the following conditions:*

(i) $\mathcal{H}^n(S \cap B_R(0)) < \infty$ *for any* $R > 0$;

(ii) $\displaystyle\lim_{r \to 0} \frac{\mathcal{H}^n(S \cap B_r(x))}{b_n r^n} = 1$ *for* $\mathcal{H}^n$*-a.e.* $x \in S$.

Here b_n is the volume of the unit ball in $\mathbb{R}^n$.

Remark 1. Note that condition (ii) is related to a characterization of the countable $\mathcal{H}^n$-rectifiability of the set S ([14], p.256,267, [3], p.83).

Definition 2 (Random *n*-regular sets). *Given an integer n, with $0 \leq n \leq d$, we say that a random closed set Θ_n in $\mathbb{R}^d$ is n-regular, if it satisfies the following conditions:*

(i) for almost all $\omega \in \Omega$, $\Theta_n(\omega)$ *is an n-regular closed set in* $\mathbb{R}^d$;
(ii) $\mathbb{E}[\mathcal{H}^n(\Theta_n \cap B_R(0))] < \infty$ *for any* $R > 0$.

As a consequence (by assuming $0 \cdot \infty = 0$), for any $0 \leq n < d$ we have:

$$\lim_{r \to 0} \frac{\mathcal{H}^n(\Theta_n(\omega) \cap B_r(x))}{b_d r^d} = \lim_{r \to 0} \frac{\mathcal{H}^n(\Theta_n(\omega) \cap B_r(x))}{b_n r^n} \frac{b_n r^n}{b_d r^d}$$

$$= \begin{cases} \infty & \mathcal{H}^n\text{-a.e. } x \in \Theta_n(\omega), \\ 0 & \forall x \notin \Theta_n(\omega). \end{cases}$$

Note that in the particular case $n = 0$, with $\Theta_0 = X_0$ random point in $\mathbb{R}^d$ (X_0 is indeed a 0-regular random closed set),

$$\lim_{r \to 0} \frac{\mathcal{H}^0(X_0(\omega) \cap B_r(x))}{b_d r^d} = \begin{cases} \infty & \text{if } x = X_0(\omega), \\ 0 & \text{if } x \neq X_0(\omega); \end{cases}$$

In analogy with the Dirac delta function $\delta_{x_0}(x)$ associated with a point $x_0 \in \mathbb{R}^d$, we may introduce the following definition:

Definition 3. *We call $\delta_{\Theta_n(\omega)}$, the* generalized density *(or, briefly, the density) associated with $\Theta_n(\omega)$, the quantity*

$$\delta_{\Theta_n(\omega)}(x) := \lim_{r \to 0} \frac{\mathcal{H}^n(\Theta_n(\omega) \cap B_r(x))}{b_d r^d},$$

finite or not.

In this way $\delta_{\Theta_n(\omega)}(x)$ can be considered as the *generalized density* (or the *generalized Radon-Nikodym derivative*) of the measure $\mu_{\Theta_n(\omega)}$ with respect to the d-dimensional Lebesgue measure ν^d.

Now we are ready to introduce the delta function of the set $\Theta_n(\omega)$ as the linear functional (the generalized function) $\delta_{\Theta_n(\omega)}(x)$ in a similar way as for the usual Delta dirac associated to a point.

Define the function

$$\delta^{(r)}_{\Theta_n(\omega)}(x) := \frac{\mathcal{H}^n(\Theta_n(\omega) \cap B_r(x))}{b_d r^d},$$

and correspondingly the associated Radon measure

$$\mu^{(r)}_{\Theta_n(\omega)}(A) := \int_A \delta^{(r)}_{\Theta_n(\omega)}(x)\mathrm{d}x, \qquad A \in \mathcal{B}_{\mathbb{R}^d}.$$

We recall that, according to Riesz theorem, Radon measures in $\mathbb{R}^d$ (i.e. non-negative and σ-additive set functions defined on the Borel σ-algebra $\mathcal{B}_{\mathbb{R}^d}$ which are finite on bounded sets) can be canonically identified with linear and order preserving functionals on $C_c(\mathbb{R}^d, \mathbb{R})$, the space of continuous functions with compact support in $\mathbb{R}^d$. The identification is provided by the integral operator, i.e.

$$(\mu, f) = \int_{\mathbb{R}^d} f \, d\mu \qquad \forall f \in C_c(\mathbb{R}^d, \mathbb{R}).$$

If $\mu \ll \nu^d$, it admits, as Radon-Nikodym density, a classical function δ_μ defined almost everywhere in $\mathbb{R}^d$, so that

$$(\mu, f) = \int_{\mathbb{R}^d} f(x)\delta_\mu(x)\mathrm{d}x \qquad \forall f \in C_c(\mathbb{R}^d, \mathbb{R})$$

in the usual sense of Lebesgue integral.

If $\mu \perp \nu^d$, we may speak of a density δ_μ only in the sense of distributions (it is almost everywhere trivial, but it is ∞ on a set of ν^d-measure zero). In this case the symbol

$$\int_{\mathbb{R}^d} f(x)\delta_\mu(x)\mathrm{d}x := (\mu, f)$$

can still be adopted, provided the integral on the left hand side is understood in a generalized sense, and not as a Lebesgue integral.

In either cases, from now on, we will denote by (δ_μ, f) the quantity (μ, f).

With an abuse of notations, we may introduce the linear functionals $\delta^{(r)}_{\Theta_n(\omega)}$ and $\delta_{\Theta_n(\omega)}$ associated with the measure $\mu^{(r)}_{\Theta_n(\omega)}$ and $\mu_{\Theta_n(\omega)}$, respectively, as follows:

$$(\delta^{(r)}_{\Theta_n(\omega)}, f) := \int_{\mathbb{R}^d} f(x)\mu^{(r)}_{\Theta_n(\omega)}\mathrm{d}x,$$

$$(\delta_{\Theta_n(\omega)}, f) := \int_{\mathbb{R}^d} f(x)\mu_{\Theta_n(\omega)}\mathrm{d}x,$$

for any $f \in C_c(\mathbb{R}^d, \mathbb{R})$.

Proposition 1. *[13] The sequence of measures* $\mu^{(r)}_{\Theta_n(\omega)}$ *weakly* converges to the measure* $\mu_{\Theta_n(\omega)}$, *i.e.*

$$\lim_{r \to 0} \int_{\mathbb{R}^d} f(x)\mu^{(r)}_{\Theta_n}\mathrm{d}x = \int_{\mathbb{R}^d} f(x)\mu_{\Theta_n}\mathrm{d}x \qquad \forall f \in C_c(\mathbb{R}^d, \mathbb{R}).$$

In other words, the sequence of linear functionals $\delta^{(r)}_{\Theta_n(\omega)}$ weakly* converges to the linear functional $\delta_{\Theta_n(\omega)}$.

Remark 2. In analogy with the classical Dirac delta, we may regard the continuous linear functional δ_{Θ_n} as a generalized function on the usual test space $C_c(\mathbb{R}^d, \mathbb{R})$, and, in accordance with the usual representation of distributions in the theory of generalized functions, we formally write

$$\int_{\mathbb{R}^d} f(x)\delta_{\Theta_n(\omega)}(x)\mathrm{d}x := (\delta_{\Theta_n(\omega)}, f).$$

Since $\delta_{\Theta_n}(x)$ is a random quantity, δ_{Θ_n} is a *random linear functional* (i.e. (δ_{Θ_n}, f) is a real random variable for any test function f).

Definition 4. *By extending the definition of expected value of a random operator à la Pettis (or Gelfand-Pettis, [4, 7]), we may define the* expected linear functional $\mathbb{E}[\delta_{\Theta_n}]$ *associated with* δ_{Θ_n} *as follows:*

$$(\mathbb{E}[\delta_{\Theta_n}], f) := \mathbb{E}[(\delta_{\Theta_n}, f)], \quad \forall f \in C_c(\mathbb{R}^d\mathbb{R}) \tag{2}$$

and the mean generalized density $\mathbb{E}[\delta_{\Theta_n}](x)$ *of* $\mathbb{E}[\mu_{\Theta_n}]$ *by the formal integral representation:*

$$\int_{\mathbb{R}^d} f(x)\mathbb{E}[\delta_{\Theta_n}](x)\mathrm{d}x := \int_{\mathbb{R}^d} f(x)\mathbb{E}[\mu_{\Theta_n}](\mathrm{d}x), \quad \forall f \in C_c(\mathbb{R}^d\mathbb{R})$$

with

$$\mathbb{E}[\delta_{\Theta_n}](x) := \lim_{r \to 0} \frac{\mathbb{E}[\mathcal{H}^n(\Theta_n \cap B_r(x))]}{b_d r^d}.$$

An equivalent definition of (2) can be given in terms of the expected measure $\mathbb{E}[\mu_{\Theta_n}]$ by

$$(\mathbb{E}[\delta_{\Theta_n}], f) := \int_{\mathbb{R}^d} f(x)\mathbb{E}[\mu_{\Theta_n}](dx), \qquad (3)$$

for any test function f. In fact, by condition (ii) in Definition 2, the expected measure $\mathbb{E}[\mu_{\Theta_n}]$ is a Radon measure in $\mathbb{R}^d$; as usual, we may consider the associated linear functional as follows:

$$(\tilde{\delta}_{\Theta_n}, f) := \int_{\mathbb{R}^d} f(x)\mathbb{E}[\mu_{\Theta_n}](dx), \qquad f \in C_c(\mathbb{R}^d, \mathbb{R}). \qquad (4)$$

Proposition 2. *[13] The linear functionals $\mathbb{E}[\delta_{\Theta_n}]$ and $\tilde{\delta}_{\Theta_n}$ defined in (3) and (4), respectively, are equivalent.*

By using the integral representation of (δ_{Θ_n}, f) and $(\mathbb{E}[\delta_{\Theta_n}], f)$, Eq. (2) becomes

$$\int_{\mathbb{R}^d} f(x)\mathbb{E}[\delta_{\Theta_n}](x)dx = \mathbb{E}\left[\int_{\mathbb{R}^d} f(x)\delta_{\Theta_n}(x)dx\right];$$

so that, formally, we may exchange integral and expectation.

Remark 3. When $n = d$, integral and expectation can be really exchanged by Fubini's theorem. Since in this case $\delta_{\Theta_d}(x) = \mathbf{1}_{\Theta_d}(x)$, ν^d-a.s., it follows that $\mathbb{E}[\delta_{\Theta_d}](x) = \mathbb{P}(x \in \Theta_d)$. In particular, in material science, the density $\rho(x) := \mathbb{P}(x \in \Theta_d)$ is known as the *(degree of) crystallinity.*

If $n = 0$ and $\Theta_0 = X_0$ is a continuous random point with pdf p_{X_0}, then $\mathbb{E}[\mathcal{H}^0(X_0 \cap \cdot)] = \mathbb{P}(X_0 \in A)$ is absolutely continuous and, in this case, $\mathbb{E}[\delta_{X_0}](x)$ is just the probability density function $p_{X_0}(x)$.

3 Approximation of the Mean Densities

In many real applications, several problems are related to the estimation of the local mean density $\mathbb{E}[\delta_{\Theta_n}]$ of a lower dimensional random closed set such as a fiber process of dimension $n = 1$ in a space of dimension $d > 1$.

As for the estimation of probability densities of real random variables we refer to the histogram, or more generally to kernel estimators for facing the problem of the measure ν^1 zero for points in $\mathbb{R}$, we need to introduce some sort of spatial histogram for facing the problem that lines in $\mathbb{R}^2$ have measure ν^2 zero. Histograms provide a natural 1D box approximation of points in $\mathbb{R}$; we may provide a 2D box approximation of lines in $\mathbb{R}^2$. As a matter of fact, a computer graphic representation is anyway provided in terms of pixels, which can only offer a 2D box approximation of points in $\mathbb{R}^2$ (for a useful introduction to the subject we refer to [24]).

We denote by $A_{\oplus r}$ the Minkowski addition of A with the ball $B_r(0)$, i.e.

$$A_{\oplus r} := A \oplus B_r(0) = \{x \in \mathbb{R}^d : \mathrm{dist}(x, A) \leq r\}.$$

The following is proved in [1].

Proposition 3. *Let Θ_n be a random n-regular set, and let $A \in \mathcal{B}_{\mathbb{R}^d}$. If*

$$\lim_{r \to 0} \frac{\mathbb{E}[\nu^d(\Theta_{n \oplus r} \cap A)]}{b_{d-n} r^{d-n}} = \mathbb{E}[\mathcal{H}^n(\Theta_n \cap A)], \tag{5}$$

then

$$\lim_{r \to 0} \int_A \frac{\mathbb{P}(x \in \Theta_{n \oplus r})}{b_{d-n} r^{d-n}} \, \mathrm{d}x = \mathbb{E}[\mathcal{H}^n(\Theta_n \cap A)].$$

As a consequence of the proposition above, if we denote by $\mu^{\oplus r}$ the measure on $\mathcal{B}_{\mathbb{R}^d}$ so defined

$$\mu^{\oplus r}(A) := \int_A \frac{\mathbb{P}(x \in \Theta_{n \oplus r})}{b_{d-n} r^{d-n}} \, \mathrm{d}x,$$

then it follows that $\mu^{\oplus r}$ weakly* converges to $\mathbb{E}[\mu_{\Theta_n}]$.

For every fixed $r > 0$, the measure $\mu^{\oplus r}$ is absolutely continuous with respect to the d-dimensional Lebesgue measure with density

$$\delta_n^{\oplus r}(x) := \frac{\mathbb{P}(x \in \Theta_{n \oplus r})}{b_{d-n} r^{d-n}}. \tag{6}$$

Such a function defines a linear functional, say $\delta_n^{\oplus r}$, associated with the measure $\mu^{\oplus r}$ as follows

$$(\delta_n^{\oplus r}, f) := \int_{\mathbb{R}^d} f(x) \mu^{\oplus r}(\mathrm{d}x), \qquad f \in C_c(\mathbb{R}^d, \mathbb{R}).$$

A sufficient condition for (5) is given by the following result, proved in [1].

Theorem 1. *Let Θ_n be a countably $\mathcal{H}^n$-rectifiable random closed set in $\mathbb{R}^d$ (i.e., for $\mathbb{P}$-a.e. $\omega \in \Omega$, $\Theta_n(\omega) \subseteq \mathbb{R}^d$ is a countably $\mathcal{H}^n$-rectifiable closed set), such that $\mathbb{E}[\mu_{\Theta_n}]$ is a Radon measure. Let $W \subset \mathbb{R}^d$ be a compact set and let $\Gamma_W : \Omega \longrightarrow \mathbb{R}$ be the function so defined:*

$$\Gamma_W(\omega) := \max\{\gamma \geq 0 : \exists \ a \ probability \ measure \ \eta \ll \mathcal{H}^n \ such \ that$$

$$\eta(B_r(x)) \geq \gamma r^n \quad \forall x \in \Theta_n(\omega) \cap W_{\oplus 1}, \ r \in (0,1)\}.$$

If there exists a random variable Y with $\mathbb{E}[Y] < \infty$, such that $1/\Gamma_W(\omega) \leq Y(\omega)$ for $\mathbb{P}$-a.e. $\omega \in \Omega$, then, for all $A \in \mathcal{B}_{\mathbb{R}^d}$ such that

$$A \subset \mathrm{int}\, W_{\oplus 1} \quad and \quad \mathbb{E}[\mathcal{H}^n(\Theta_n \cap \partial A)] = 0,$$

we have

$$\lim_{r \to 0} \frac{\mathbb{E}[\nu^d(\Theta_{n \oplus r} \cap A)]}{b_{d-n} r^{d-n}} = \mathbb{E}[\mathcal{H}^n(\Theta_n \cap A)]. \tag{7}$$

Note that many kinds of random closed sets satisfy the proposition above, as fibre processes, line and segment processes, Boolean models,... (see [1]). As a consequence, by estimating the probability that a point x belongs to the enlarged set Θ_n in (6), we might give an estimation of $\mathbb{E}[\mu_{\Theta_n}]$, and so of the mean density $\mathbb{E}[\delta_{\Theta_n}]$.

Remark 4. In the case $n = 0$ and $\Theta_0 = X$ is a real random variable, $\delta_0^{\oplus r}(x)$ leads to the usual estimation of the density of X by histograms.

4 Mean First Order Steiner Formulas

If we consider a d-dimensional random closed set Θ with $\dim_{\mathcal{H}}(\partial\Theta) = d - 1$, sufficiently regular such that $\partial\Theta$ satisfies the conditions of Theorem 1, then we may rephrase (7) as

$$\lim_{r \to 0} \frac{\mathbb{E}[\nu^d(\partial\Theta_{\oplus r} \cap A)]}{r} = 2\mathbb{E}[\mathcal{H}^{d-1}(\partial\Theta \cap A)]. \tag{8}$$

Note that $\mathbb{E}[\nu^d(\partial\Theta)] = 0$, so that, roughly speaking, we may regard (8) as the derivative in $r = 0$ of the expected Hausdorff measure of $\partial\Theta$ with respect to the Minkowski enlargement.

If we enlarge $\partial\Theta$ only in the complement of Θ (i.e. we consider $\Theta_{\oplus r} \setminus \Theta$), we ask if Θ satisfies a *local mean first order Steiner formula*, i.e:

$$\lim_{r \to 0} \frac{\mathbb{E}[\nu^d(\Theta_{\oplus r} \setminus \Theta \cap A)]}{r} = \mathbb{E}[\mathcal{H}^{d-1}(\partial\Theta \cap A)].$$

By a *Steiner formula*, we mean a polynomial expansion of the volume of the enlarged set of a given subset of the Euclidean space $\mathbb{R}^d$. Namely, let $A \subset \mathbb{R}^d$; A is said to satisfy a Steiner formula if there exist numbers $\Phi_m(A)$, $m = 1, \ldots, d$, such that, for every (sufficiently small) $r > 0$ (e.g., see [15, 17])

$$\mathcal{H}^d(A_{\oplus r}) = \sum_{m=0}^{d} r^{d-m} b_{d-m} \Phi_m(A).$$

Definition 5. *We say that a random closed set Θ satisfies a* first order Steiner formula *almost surely if*

$$\lim_{r \to 0} \frac{\mathcal{H}^d(\Theta(\omega)_{\oplus r} \setminus \Theta(\omega))}{r} = \mathcal{H}^{d-1}(\partial\Theta(\omega)), \qquad \text{for } \mathbb{P}\text{-}a.e.\ \omega \in \Omega.$$

In [2] it has been shown that the following two classes of sets admit a first order Steiner formula

(i) sets which are union of finitely many sets with positive reach, such that each possible intersection has still positive reach (see also [23]);
(ii) sets with Lipschitz boundary.

It is well known that almost sure convergence does not imply L^1-convergence; on the other hand, if either the family of random variables $\left\{\frac{\mathcal{H}^d(\Theta_{\oplus r} \setminus \Theta)}{r}\right\}_r$ is uniformly integrable, or we may directly apply the Dominated Convergence Theorem, we obtain that the so called *mean first order Steiner formula* is also satisfied by the random closed set Θ, i.e.

$$\lim_{r \to 0} \frac{\mathbb{E}[\mathcal{H}^d(\Theta_{\oplus r} \setminus \Theta)]}{r} = \mathbb{E}[\mathcal{H}^{d-1}(\partial\Theta)].$$

In particular, in [2] the following is proved:

Theorem 2. *Let Θ^t be a random closed set in $\mathbb{R}^d$ with boundary $\partial\Theta^t$ countably $\mathcal{H}^{d-1}$-rectifiable and compact, and let $A \in \mathcal{B}_{\mathbb{R}^d}$ be such that*

$$\lim_{r \to 0} \frac{\mathcal{H}^d((\Theta(\omega)_{\oplus r} \setminus \Theta(\omega)) \cap A)}{r} = \mathcal{H}^{d-1}(\partial\Theta(\omega) \cap A), \qquad \text{for } \mathbb{P}\text{-a.e. } \omega \in \Omega.$$

Let $\Gamma : \Omega \longrightarrow \mathbb{R}$ be the function so defined:

$$\Gamma(\omega) := \max\{\gamma \geq 0 : \exists \text{ a probability measure } \eta \ll \mathcal{H}^{d-1} \text{ such that}$$
$$\eta(B_r(x)) \geq \gamma r^{d-1} \quad \forall x \in \partial\Theta^t(\omega), \ r \in (0,1)\}.$$

If there exists a random variable Y with $\mathbb{E}[Y] < \infty$, such that $\frac{1}{\Gamma(\omega)} \leq Y(\omega)$ for $\mathbb{P}$-a.e. $\omega \in \Omega$, then

$$\lim_{r \to 0} \frac{\mathbb{E}[\mathcal{H}^d(\Theta^t_{\oplus r} \setminus \Theta^t \cap A)]}{r} = \mathbb{E}[\mathcal{H}^{d-1}(\partial\Theta^t \cap A)],$$

for any $A \in \mathcal{B}_{\mathbb{R}^d}$ such that $\mathbb{P}(\mathcal{H}^{d-1}(\partial\Theta^t \cap \partial A) > 0) = 0$.

First order Steiner formulas play important rules in various applications (see also [18]). For instance, *birth-and-growth stochastic processes* are described by random closed sets in $\mathbb{R}^d$ which evolve in time accordingly to a given growth model, so that evolution equations of their mean geometric densities are of great interest in applications (see e.g. [13] and references therein). To this end, a mean first order Steiner formula is required for the relevant random closed set, as we shall see in the next section.

5 Time Dependent Random Closed Sets

In this section we wish to analyze the case in which a random closed set Θ may depend upon time as, for example, when it models the evolution due to a growth process, so that we have a geometric random process $\{\Theta^t, \ t \in \mathbb{R}_+\}$, such that for any $t \in \mathbb{R}_+$, the random set Θ^t satisfies all the relevant assumptions required in the previous sections. Correspondingly the associated linear functional δ_{Θ^t} will also be a functional depending on time, and so we need to define partial derivatives of linear functionals depending on more than one variable.

Consider a linear functional L acting on the test space $\mathcal{S}_k$ of functions s in k variables; we formally represent it as

$$(L, s) =: \int_{\mathbb{R}^k} \phi(x_1, \ldots, x_k) s(x_1, \ldots, x_k) \mathrm{d}(x_1, \ldots, x_k).$$

Let us denote by L_i^h the linear functional defined by

$$(L_i^h, s) =: \int_{\mathbb{R}^k} \phi(x_1, \ldots, x_i + h, \ldots, x_k) s(x_1, \ldots, x_k) \mathrm{d}(x_1, \ldots, x_k).$$

We define the *weak partial derivative* of the functional L with respect to the variable x_i as follows (see also [16], p. 20).

Definition 6. *We say that a linear functional L on the space $\mathcal{S}_k$, admits a weak partial derivative with respect to x_i, denoted by $\frac{\partial}{\partial x_i} L$, if and only if $\frac{\partial}{\partial x_i} L$ is a linear functional on the same space $\mathcal{S}_k$ and $\left\{ \frac{L_i^h - L}{h} \right\}$ weakly* converges to $\frac{\partial}{\partial x_i} L$, i.e.*

$$\lim_{h \to 0} \left(\frac{L_i^h - L}{h}, s \right) = \left(\frac{\partial}{\partial x_i} L, s \right) \qquad \text{for all } s \in \mathcal{S}_k.$$

Let us consider, as an example, the case in which $\{\Theta^t\}_t$ is given by a *birth-and-growth process*, that is a dynamic germ-grain model whose birth process is modelled as a marked point process. Thus δ_{Θ^t} depends now on $d+1$ variables, and $\mathcal{S}_{d+1} = C_c(\mathbb{R}_+ \times \mathbb{R}^d, \mathbb{R})$.

Consider a Borel set $E \subset \mathbb{R}^d$, $d \geq 2$, endowed with its Borel σ-algebra $\mathcal{E}$. A marked point process N on $\mathbb{R}_+$, with marks in E, is a point process on $\mathbb{R}_+ \times E$ with the property that the marginal process $\{N(B \times E) : B \in \mathcal{B}_{\mathbb{R}_+}\}$ is itself a point process. So, it is defined as a random measure given by

$$N = \sum_{j=1}^{\infty} \varepsilon_{T_j, X_j},$$

where

- T_j is an $\mathbb{R}_+$-valued random variable representing the time of birth of the n-th nucleus,
- X_j is an E-valued random variable representing the spatial location of the nucleus born at time T_j,
- $\varepsilon_{t,x}$ is the Dirac measure on $\mathcal{B}_{\mathbb{R}_+} \times \mathcal{E}$ such that for any $t_1 < t_2$ and $A \in \mathcal{E}$,

$$\varepsilon_{t,x}([t_1, t_2] \times A) = \begin{cases} 1 & \text{if } t \in [t_1, t_2], \ x \in A, \\ 0 & \text{otherwise.} \end{cases}$$

Hence, in particular, for any $B \in \mathcal{B}_{\mathbb{R}_+}$ and $A \in \mathcal{E}$ bounded, we have

$$N(B \times A) = \#\{T_j \in B, \ X_j \in A\} < \infty,$$

i.e. it is the (random) number of germs born in the region A, during time B. It is well known (see e.g. [20]) that the *intensity measure* of the process:

$$\Lambda(\mathrm{d}t \times \mathrm{d}x) := \mathbb{E}(\nu(\mathrm{d}t \times \mathrm{d}x)) = \mathbb{E}[\mathbb{E}(N(\mathrm{d}t \times \mathrm{d}x) \mid \mathcal{F}_{t-})] = \mathbb{E}[N(\mathrm{d}t \times \mathrm{d}x)]$$

can be factorized in the following way:

$$\Lambda(\mathrm{d}t \times \mathrm{d}x) = \tilde{\Lambda}(\mathrm{d}t) Q(t, \mathrm{d}x),$$

where $\tilde{\Lambda}$ is the intensity measure of the marginal process and, $\forall t \in \mathbb{R}_+$, $Q(t, \cdot)$ is a probability measure on E, called the *mark distribution* at time t.

We assume that the nucleation process N is such that the marginal process is *simple* (i.e. $N(\mathrm{d}t \times E) \leq 1$ for every infinitesimal time interval $\mathrm{d}t$), and so the mark distribution $Q(t, A)$ represents the probability that a nucleus belongs to A, given that it is born during $[t, t + \mathrm{d}t)$.

As far as the growth is concerned, we assume that the growth of each grain is given by a normal growth model with space and time dependent growth rate $G(t, x)$, i.e. we assume that almost every point of $\partial\Theta^t$ admits a unit outer normal, and that the growth of Θ^t occurs with nonnegative normal velocity $G(t, x)$ [9].

Denoted by $\Theta_s^t(y)$ the grain born at time s at point y and grown up to time t, then, for any fixed $t \in \mathbb{R}_+$, Θ^t is the random closed set given by

$$\Theta^t = \bigcup_{T_j \leq t} \Theta_{T_j}^t(X_j).$$

With reference to our birth-and-growth process $\{\Theta^t\}_t$, we may introduce the random variable $\tau(x)$, representing the *time of capture* of a given point $x \in E$, i.e.

$$\{x \in \Theta^t\} = \{\tau(x) \leq t\},$$

and the well known *hazard function* $h(\cdot, x)$ associated with point x so defined:

$$h(t, x) := \lim_{\Delta t \downarrow 0} \frac{\mathbb{P}(x \in \Theta^{t+\Delta t} \mid x \notin \Theta^t)}{\Delta t}.$$

Depending upon the regularity of the birth-and-growth parameters, we may assume that the process $\{\Theta^t\}_t$ is such that:

1. for any $t \in \mathbb{R}_+$, and any $s > 0$, Θ^t is well contained in Θ^{t+s}, i.e. $\partial\Theta^t \subset \mathrm{int}\Theta^{t+s}$;
2. for any $t \in \mathbb{R}_+$, Θ^t is a d-regular random closed set in $\mathbb{R}^d$, and $\partial\Theta^t$ is a $(d-1)$-regular random closed set;
3. $\tau(x)$ is a continuous random variable with probability density function $p_{\tau(x)}(t)$.

For the assumptions 1. and 2. see for example [8]; while assumption 3. strongly depends on the intensity of the marked point process of birth-and-growth (see e.g. [12, 25]).

In particular, the absolute continuity of the intensity of the birth process with respect to both time and space, together with sufficient regularity of the growth rate may guarantee the absolute continuity of $\mathbb{E}[\mu_{\partial\Theta^t}]$, so that $\mathbb{E}[\delta_{\partial\Theta^t}](x)$ is a real integrable function and it is usually called *mean free surface density* and denoted by $S_V(t, x)$.

Remark 5. In the simple case in which each grain grows with constant rate G, for any fixed $t \in \mathbb{R}_+$, we have a random collection of balls with random centers and radii, and we may show [1] that $\partial\Theta^t$ and $\bigcup_{T_j\leq t}\partial\Theta^t_{T_j}(X_j)$ satisfy to the hypotheses of Proposition 3, so that an estimation of $\mathring{S}_V$ might be given. Further, it is clear that

$$\lim_{\Delta t\to 0}\frac{\mathcal{H}^d(\Theta^{t+\Delta t}(\omega)\setminus\Theta^t(\omega))}{\Delta t} = \lim_{\Delta t\to 0}\frac{\mathcal{H}^d(\Theta^t_{\oplus G\Delta t}(\omega)\setminus\Theta^t(\omega))}{\Delta t}$$
$$= G\lim_{r\to 0}\frac{\mathcal{H}^d(\Theta^t_{\oplus r}(\omega)\setminus\Theta^t(\omega))}{r},$$

and, for any $t\in\mathbb{R}_+$, $\Theta^t(\omega)$ satisfies a first order Steiner formula, so that we have

$$\lim_{\Delta t\to 0}\frac{\mathcal{H}^d(\Theta^{t+\Delta t}(\omega))-\mathcal{H}^d(\Theta^t(\omega)))}{\Delta t} = G\mathcal{H}^{d-1}(\partial\Theta^t(\omega)).$$

In particular Theorem 2 applies, so Θ^t satisfies a mean first order Steiner formula:

$$\lim_{\Delta t\to 0}\frac{\mathbb{E}[\mathcal{H}^d(\Theta^{t+\Delta t})]-\mathbb{E}[\mathcal{H}^d(\Theta^t)]}{\Delta t} = G\mathbb{E}[\mathcal{H}^{d-1}(\partial\Theta^t)].$$

As a consequence of assumptions 1. and 2. we have that [13]

$$\frac{\partial}{\partial t}\delta_{\Theta^t}(x) = \delta_{\tau(x)}(t)$$

as functional on $C_c(\mathbb{R}_+\times\mathbb{R}^d,\mathbb{R})$, i.e.

$$\int_{\mathbb{R}_+\times\mathbb{R}^d}f(t,x)\frac{\partial}{\partial t}\delta_{\Theta^t}(x)\,\mathrm{d}x\mathrm{d}t = \int_{\mathbb{R}_+\times\mathbb{R}^d}f(t,x)\delta_{\tau(x)}(t)\,\mathrm{d}x\mathrm{d}t$$
$$= \int_{\mathbb{R}^d}f(\tau(x),x)\,\mathrm{d}x$$

for any test function $f\in C_c(\mathbb{R}_+\times\mathbb{R}^d,\mathbb{R})$.

By the assumption 3. and Remark 3, it follows

$$\mathbb{E}\left[\frac{\partial}{\partial t}\delta_{\Theta^t}\right](x) = p_{\tau(x)}(t) = \frac{\partial}{\partial t}\mathbb{P}(x\in\Theta^t) = \frac{\partial}{\partial t}\mathbb{E}[\delta_{\Theta^t}](x).$$

In [13] an evolution equation for the mean density $\mathbb{E}[\delta_{\Theta^t}](x)$ has been obtained in terms of $G(t,x)$ and the mean density of the boundary of Θ^t, as follows.

Proposition 4. *Under the above assumption on the growth model, let G be sufficiently regular so that, for any $t\in\mathbb{R}_+$,*

$$\lim_{r\to 0}\frac{\mathbb{E}[\mathcal{H}^d(\Theta^t_{\oplus r}\setminus\Theta^t\cap A)]}{r} = \mathbb{E}[\mathcal{H}^{d-1}(\partial\Theta^t\cap A)],$$

for any $A\in\mathcal{B}_{\mathbb{R}^d}$ such that $\mathbb{E}[\mathcal{H}^{d-1}(\partial\Theta^t\cap\partial A)] = 0$.

If the time of capture $\tau(x)$ is a continuous random variable with density $p_{\tau(x)}$, the following evolution equation holds for the mean density $\mathbb{E}[\delta_{\Theta^t}](x)$:

$$\frac{\partial}{\partial t}\mathbb{E}[\delta_{\Theta^t}](x) = G(t,x)\mathbb{E}[\delta_{\partial\Theta^t}](x), \tag{9}$$

to be taken, as usual, in weak form.

Note that, whenever for a.e. $\omega \in \Omega$ the evolution of the realization $\Theta^t(\omega)$ can be described by the following (weak) equation (e.g. [6, 8]):

$$\frac{\partial}{\partial t}\delta_{\Theta^t}(x) = G(t,x)\delta_{\partial\Theta^t}(x), \tag{10}$$

then equation (9) can be formally obtained by taking the expected value in (10), by the linearity properties of the expectation and since G is a deterministic function.

We remind the definition of the spherical contact distribution function associated to a random closed set.

Definition 7. *The* local spherical contact distribution function $H_{S,\Xi}$ *of an inhomogeneous random set Ξ is defined as*

$$H_{S,\Xi}(r,x) := \mathbb{P}(x \in \Xi_{\oplus r} \mid x \notin \Xi).$$

Denote by $H_{S,\Theta^t}(\cdot,x)$ the spherical contact distribution of Θ^t associated to a point x. In the proof of the above proposition the following relation between $H_{S,\Theta^t}(\cdot,x)$ with the hazard function (see [12])

$$h(t,x) = G(t,x)\frac{\partial}{\partial r}H_{S,\Theta^t}(r,x)_{|_{r=0}}$$

plays a crucial rule.

As a corollary, it follows that

$$\mathbb{E}[\delta_{\partial\Theta^t}](x) = \mathbb{P}(x \notin \Theta^t)\frac{\partial}{\partial r}H_{S,\Theta^t}(r,x)_{|_{r=0}},$$

which leads to the following interesting interpretation (see [13])

$$\frac{\partial}{\partial r}H_{S,\Theta^t}(r,x)_{|_{r=0}} = \mathbb{E}[\delta_{\partial\Theta^t}(x) \mid x \notin \mathrm{int}\Theta^t].$$

Acknowledgements

It is a pleasure to acknowledge fruitful discussions with L. Ambrosio, of the Scuola Normale Superiore in Pisa, M. Burger of the J.Kepler University in Linz, A. Colesanti, of the University of Florence, and A. Micheletti, of the Milan University. A special thank is due to D. Jeulin for having attracted the attention of the authors on the contribution of Matheron [21] to the theory of random distributions in Geostatistics.

VC acknowledges the warm hospitality of the Austrian Academy of Sciences at RICAM (Radon Institute for Computational and Applied Mathematics) in Linz, chaired by Prof. H. Engl.

References

1. Ambrosio, L., Capasso, V., Villa, E.: On the approximation of geometric densities of random closed sets. RICAM Report 14/2006, Linz. *Available at:* http://www.ricam.oeaw.ac.at/publications/reports.
2. Ambrosio, L., Colesanti, A., Villa, E.: First order Steiner formulas for some classes of closed sets. An application to stochastic geometry. In preparation.
3. Ambrosio, L., Fusco, N., Pallara, D.: Functions of Bounded Variation and Free Discontinuity Problems. Clarendon Press, Oxford, (2000)
4. Araujo, A., Giné, E.: The Central Limit Theorem for Real and Banach Valued Random Variables. John Wiley & Sons, New York, (1980)
5. Baddeley, A.J., Molchanov, I.S.: On the expected measure of a random set. In: Proceedings of the International Symposium on Advances in Theory and Applications of Random Sets (Fontainebleau, 1996). World Sci. Publishing, River Edge, NJ, 3–20, (1997)
6. Barles, G., Soner, H.M., Souganidis, P.E.: Front propagation and phase-field theory. SIAM J. Contr.Optim., **31**, 439–469 (1993)
7. Bosq, D.: Linear Processes in Function Spaces. Theory and Applications. Lecture Notes in Statistics **149**, Springer-Verlag, New York, (2000)
8. Burger, M.: Growth fronts of first-order Hamilton-Jacobi equations. SFB Report 02-8, J. Kepler University, Linz (2002)
9. Burger, M., Capasso, V., Salani, C.: Modelling multi-dimensional crystallization of polymers in interaction with heat transfer. Nonlinear Analysis: Real World Application, **3**, 139–160 (2002)
10. Mathematical Modelling for Polymer Processing. Polymerization, Crystallization, Manufacturing (V. Capasso, Editor) Mathematics in Industry Vol 2, Springer Verlag, Heidelberg (2003)
11. Capasso, V., Micheletti, A.: Stochastic geometry and related statistical problems in biomedicine. In: Complex Systems in Biomedicine (Quarteroni, A. et al., Eds.) Springer, Milano (2006)
12. Capasso, V., Villa, E.: Survival functions and contact distribution functions for inhomogeneous, stochastic geometric marked point processes. Stoch. An. Appl., **23**, 79–96 (2005)
13. Capasso, V., Villa, E.: On the geometric densities of random closed sets. RICAM Report 13/2006, Linz. *Available at:* http://www.ricam.oeaw.ac.at/publications/reports.
14. Falconer, K.J.: The Geometry of Fractal Sets. Cambridge University press, Cambridge, (1985)
15. Federer, H.: Curvature Measures, *Trans. Amer. Math. Soc.*, **93**, 418–491 (1959)
16. Gelfand I.M., Shilov G.E.: Generalized Functions. Properties and operations. Academic Press, New York, (1964)
17. Hug, D., Last, G., Weil, W.: A local Steiner-type formula for general closed sets and applications. Math. Z. **246**, no. 1-2, 237–272 (2004)
18. Kiderlen, M., Rataj, J.: On infinitesimal increase of volumes of morphological transforms. Thiele Research Report 14/2005, Aarhus. *Available at:* http://www.imf.au.dk/cgi-bin/dlf/viewpublications.cgi?id=580
19. Kolmogorov, A.N., Fomin S.V.: Introductory Real Analysis. Prentice-Hall, Englewood Cliffs (N.J.), (1970)
20. Last, G., Brandt, A.: Marked Point Processes on the Real Line. The Dynamic Approach. Springer, New York (1995)

21. Matheron, G.: Les Variables Regionalisées et leur Estimation, Masson et Cie, Paris, (1965)
22. Matheron, G.: Random Sets and Integral Geometry. John Wiley & Sons, New York, (1975)
23. Rataj, J.: On boundaries of unions of sets with positive reach. Beiträge Algebra Geom. **46**, 397–404 (2005)
24. Serra, J.: Image Analysis and Mathematical Morphology. Academic Press, London, (1984)
25. Villa, E.: Methods of Geometric Measure Theory in Stochastic Geometry. PhD thesis, University of Milan, Milan (2006)
26. Zähle M.; Random processes of Hausdorff rectifiable closed sets. Math. Nachr., **108**, 49–72 (1982)

The Multiparameter Fractional Brownian Motion

Erick Herbin[1] and Ely Merzbach[2]

[1] Dassault Aviation, 78 quai Marcel Dassault, 92552 Saint-Cloud Cedex, France
`erick.herbin@dassault-aviation.fr`
[2] Dept. of Mathematics, Bar Ilan University, 52900 Ramat-Gan, Israel
`merzbach@macs.biu.ac.il`

Summary. We define and study the multiparameter fractional Brownian motion. This process is a generalization of both the classical fractional Brownian motion and the multiparameter Brownian motion, when the condition of independence is relaxed. Relations with the Lévy fractional Brownian motion and with the fractional Brownian sheet are discussed. Different notions of stationarity of the increments for a multiparameter process are studied and applied to the fractional property. Using self-similarity we present a characterization for such processes. Finally, behavior of the multiparameter fractional Brownian motion along increasing paths is analysed.

1 Introduction

The aim of this paper is to give a satisfactory definition of the concept of Multiparameter Fractional Brownian Motion (MpfBm). The definition given here is a particular case of the Set-indexed Fractional Brownian Motion studied in [2], but in the multiparameter case, the various stationarity properties can be compared.

In the last decade, two other definitions for the MpfBm appeared in the literature (see [1] for a review of their properties). Both are problematic as extensions of the classical fractional Brownian motion. In this work, we hope to persuade the reader that our definition is natural, is the "right" generalization of the fractional Brownian motion (fBm) and can be applied directly to real applied problems.

2 Definition of the MpfBm

In [2], a set-indexed extension of fractional Brownian motion was defined and some extensions of fractal properties were established. Let $\mathcal{A}$ be an indexing collection of compact subsets of a metric measure space (metric d and measure

m) satisfying certain assumptions, the *Set-indexed fractional Brownian motion (SifBm)* was defined as the centered Gaussian process $\mathbf{B}^H = \{\mathbf{B}_U^H;\ U \in \mathcal{A}\}$ such that

$$\forall\ U, V \in \mathcal{A};\ E\left[\mathbf{B}_U^H \mathbf{B}_V^H\right] = \frac{1}{2}\left[m(U)^{2H} + m(V)^{2H} - m(U \triangle V)^{2H}\right], \qquad (1)$$

where $0 < H \leq \frac{1}{2}$ and m is a measure defined on the σ-algebra generated by $\mathcal{A}$.

As the collection $\mathcal{A} = \{[0, t];\ t \in \mathbb{R}_+^N\} \cup \{\emptyset\}$ is a particular indexing collection, definition (1) provides a multiparameter process which can be seen as a multiparameter extension of fractional Brownian motion. We get the following definition.

Definition 1. *The* Multiparameter Fractional Brownian Motion (MpfBm) *is defined as the centered Gaussian process* $\mathbf{B}^H = \{\mathbf{B}_t^H;\ t \in \mathbb{R}_+^N\}$ *such that*

$$\forall\ s, t \in \mathbb{R}_+^N;\ E\left[\mathbf{B}_s^H \mathbf{B}_t^H\right] = \frac{1}{2}\left[m([0, s])^{2H} + m([0, t])^{2H} - m([0, s] \triangle [0, t])^{2H}\right]$$

where m is a measure on $\mathbb{R}^N$ and $H \in (0, 1/2]$ is called the index of similarity.

This definition looks very natural since it relies on a set-indexed process and thus, structure of the space $\mathbb{R}^N$ is only present in indices and not in the shape of the covariance function.

Notice that the definition of the MpfBm depends on the measure m.

In the particular case of $\mathbb{R}_+^2$ with the Lebesgue measure m, we can explicitly give the covariance between $s = (s_1, s_2)$ and $t = (t_1, t_2)$

$$E\left[\mathbf{B}_s^H \mathbf{B}_t^H\right] = \frac{1}{2}\left[(s_1 s_2)^{2H} + (t_1 t_2)^{2H}\right.$$
$$\left. - (s_1 s_2 + t_1 t_2 - 2(s_1 \wedge t_1)(s_2 \wedge t_2))^{2H}\right].$$

Let us notice that parameter H is restricted to be in $(0, 1/2]$, on the contrary to standard fractional Brownian motion, in which H is in $(0, 1)$.

Remark 1. If the measure m is absolutely continuous with respect to the Lebesgue measure, the process $\mathbf{B}^H$ is almost surely null on the axis.

Self-similarity is the first property of MpfBm. As a particular case of the set-indexed fractional Brownian motion, the multiparameter process inherits its properties. It is self-similar of index $N.H$: for all $a \in \mathbb{R}_+$,

$$\{\mathbf{B}_{at}^H;\ t \in \mathbb{R}_+^N\} \overset{(d)}{=} \{a^{NH}\mathbf{B}_t^H;\ t \in \mathbb{R}_+^N\}.$$

where $\overset{(d)}{=}$ denotes equality of finite dimensional distributions.

3 Comparisons with Other Multiparameter Extensions of fBm

The following two multiparameter extensions of fractional Brownian motions are classical. Their definitions rely on a generalization of covariance structure of fBm based on euclidian structure of $\mathbb{R}^N$. The first definition uses the euclidian norm and the second one uses the canonical basis of $\mathbb{R}^N$.

3.1 The Lévy fractional Brownian motion

The Lévy fractional Brownian motion (Lévy fBm) is defined as the mean-zero Gaussian process $\mathscr{B}^H = \left\{ \mathscr{B}^H_t ; \ t \in \mathbb{R}^N_+ \right\}$ such that

$$\forall s,t \in \mathbb{R}^N_+; \quad E\left[\mathscr{B}^H_s \ \mathscr{B}^H_t \right] = \frac{1}{2} \left[\|s\|^{2H} + \|t\|^{2H} - \|t - s\|^{2H} \right]$$

where $H \in (0,1)$.

The structure of the covariance function of $\mathscr{B}^H$ provides an extension of fractional Brownian motion where the absolute value in $\mathbb{R}_+$ is substituted with the euclidian norm of the space $\mathbb{R}^N_+$. From this point of view, the Lévy fBm is usually called an isotropic extension of fBm. However, with this simple generalization, the process does not seem to be really a multiparameter process.

This simple definition allows to state directly the self-similarity property. For all $a \in \mathbb{R}_+$,

$$\left\{ \mathscr{B}^H_{at} ; \ t \in \mathbb{R}^N_+ \right\} \overset{(d)}{=} \left\{ a^H \mathscr{B}^H_t ; \ t \in \mathbb{R}^N_+ \right\}.$$

3.2 The fractional Brownian sheet

The fractional Brownian sheet is defined as the mean-zero Gaussian process $\mathbb{B}^H = \left\{ \mathbb{B}^H_t ; \ t \in \mathbb{R}^N_+ \right\}$ such that

$$\forall s,t \in \mathbb{R}^N_+; \quad E\left[\mathbb{B}^H_s \ \mathbb{B}^H_t \right] = \frac{1}{2} \prod_{i=1}^{N} \left[s_i^{2H_i} + t_i^{2H_i} - |t_i - s_i|^{2H_i} \right]$$

where $H = (H_1, \dots, H_N) \in (0,1)^N$.

In this definition, the euclidian structure of the space $\mathbb{R}^N$ is strongly present in the shape of the covariance function of the fractional Brownian sheet. Particularly, this kind of tensor product of standard fractional Brownian motions along each direction of the canonical basis of $\mathbb{R}^N$ seems quite artificial and lacks generality to be really efficient in concrete applications.

From the covariance structure of fractional Brownian sheet, the self-similarity property can be easily established. For all $a \in \mathbb{R}_+$,

$$\left\{ \mathbb{B}^H_{at} ; \ t \in \mathbb{R}^N_+ \right\} \overset{(d)}{=} \left\{ a^{\sum_j H_j} \mathbb{B}^H_t ; \ t \in \mathbb{R}^N_+ \right\}$$

4 Different Notions of Stationarity

Stationarity of increments is one of the two characteristic properties of the classical fractional Brownian motion. In the framework of multiparameter processes, the notion of stationarity can take different forms:

- Stationarity against translation

$$\forall h \in \mathbb{R}_+^N; \quad \{X_t - X_0;\ t \in \mathbb{R}_+^N\} \overset{(d)}{=} \{X_{t+h} - X_h;\ t \in \mathbb{R}_+^N\} \tag{2}$$

- Stationarity in the strong sense

$$\forall g \in \mathcal{G}\left(\mathbb{R}^N\right); \quad \{X_t - X_0;\ t \in \mathbb{R}_+^N\} \overset{(d)}{=} \{X_{g(t)} - X_{g(0)};\ t \in \mathbb{R}_+^N\} \tag{3}$$

where $\mathcal{G}\left(\mathbb{R}^N\right)$ is the set of rigid motions on $\mathbb{R}^N$; see [6, p. 392].

For the next definitions, one needs the notion of the increment of a process X on a rectangle $D = [s,t]$, $s = (s_1, \ldots, s_N)$ and $t = (t_1, \ldots, t_N)$ where $s \prec t$ $(s_i \le t_i,\ i = 1, \ldots, N)$

$$\Delta X(D) = \sum_{r \in \{0,1\}^N} (-1)^{N - \sum_i r_i} X_{[s_i + r_i(t_i - s_i)]_i}.$$

This definition can be extended to finite unions of rectangles of $\mathbb{R}_+^N$. For $C = \bigcup_{i=1}^n D_i$, where the D_i' are rectangles such that

$$\forall i, j \in \{1, \ldots, n\} \quad D_i \cap D_j \neq \emptyset \Rightarrow i = j,$$

the increment $\Delta X(C)$ is defined by

$$\Delta X(C) = \sum_{i=1}^n \Delta X(D_i).$$

This definition is consistent as the previous expression is independent of the representation of C.

- Increment stationarity against translation

$$\forall h \in \mathbb{R}_+^N; \quad \{\Delta X_{[0,t]};\ t \in \mathbb{R}_+^N\} \overset{(d)}{=} \{\Delta X_{[h,t+h]};\ t \in \mathbb{R}_+^N\} \tag{4}$$

- Increment stationarity in the strong sense

$$\forall g \in \mathcal{G}\left(\mathbb{R}^N\right); \quad \{\Delta X_{[0,t]};\ t \in \mathbb{R}_+^N\} \overset{(d)}{=} \{\Delta X_{[g(0),g(t)]};\ t \in \mathbb{R}_+^N\} \tag{5}$$

- Measure stationarity (also called $\mathcal{C}_0$-increment stationarity)

$$\forall\, t,\ \forall \tau \succ \tau' \in \mathbb{R}_+^N;$$

$$m([0,\tau]) - m([0,\tau']) = m([0,t]) \Rightarrow X_t - X_0 \overset{(d)}{=} X_\tau - X_{\tau'} \tag{6}$$

- Increment measure stationarity
  For all finite unions of rectangles C and C',

$$m(C) = m(C') \Rightarrow \Delta X_C \overset{(d)}{=} \Delta X_{C'}. \tag{7}$$

Notice that, among these 6 properties of stationarity, the first 4 are process properties, but the last 2 properties are pointwise properties and depend of the chosen measure m.

The following result summarizes the connections between these different stationarity properties:

Proposition 1. *The following implications hold:*

$$(3) \Rightarrow (2) \Rightarrow (4);$$
$$(3) \Rightarrow (5) \Rightarrow (4);$$
$$(7) \Rightarrow (6).$$

From proposition 3.6 and theorem 4.4 in [2], the following can be stated:

Proposition 2. *The MpfBm is C_0-increment stationary, but not increment measure stationary if $H \neq \frac{1}{2}$.*

Let $\mathbf{B}^H$ be a MpfBm. The increment covariance between two rectangles D and D', $E[\Delta \mathbf{B}^H(D) \cdot \Delta \mathbf{B}^H(D')]$ can be computed, but the formula is quite complicated.

In the particular case of $\mathbb{R}^2_+$, with the Lebesgue measure and $D = D' = (s, t]$, we get:

$$E[\Delta \mathbf{B}^H(D)]^2 = (t_1 t_2 - s_1 t_2)^{2H} + (t_1 t_2 - t_1 s_2)^{2H} - (t_1 t_2 - s_1 s_2)^{2H}$$
$$- (s_1 t_2 + t_1 s_2 - 2 s_1 s_2)^{2H} + (s_1 t_2 - s_1 s_2)^{2H} + (t_1 s_2 - s_1 s_2)^{2H}.$$

We summarize stationarity properties for other definitions of multiparameter fractional Brownian motion (see [1], [6] and [2]).

Proposition 3. *The Lévy fractional Brownian motion $\mathscr{B}^H$ ($H \in (0, 1)$) satisfies (2), (3), (4), (5), and the fractional Brownian sheet $\mathbb{B}^H$ ($H \in (0, 1)^N$) satisfies (4). Moreover, if $\mathbb{B}^H$ has constant parameter H in every axis, then it satisfies (6).*

5 Characterization

In Sections 2 and 4, the multiparameter fractional Brownian motion was shown to be self-similar and C_0-increment stationary. As standard fractional Brownian motion is characterized by its two fractal properties, self-similarity and stationarity, it is natural to wonder what are the multiparameter processes satisfying the two properties.

As a particular case of set-indexed fractional Brownian motion, the multiparameter fractional Brownian motion satisfies a pseudo-characterization property.

Proposition 4. *Let $X = \left\{ X_t;\ t \in \mathbb{R}_+^N \right\}$ be a multiparameter process satisfying the following two properties:*

1. self-similarity of index $\alpha \in (0, N/2)$,
2. $\mathcal{C}_0$-increment stationarity, for Lebesgue measure m.

Then, the covariance function between s and t such that $s \prec t$ is

$$E\left[X_s . X_t\right] = K \left[m([0, s])^{2\alpha/N} + m([0, t])^{2\alpha/N} - m([0, t] \setminus [0, s])^{2\alpha/N} \right].$$

Proof. The result simply relies on Proposition 4.1 of [2], where we consider the operation of $\mathbb{R}_+$ on $\left\{ [0, t];\ t \in \mathbb{R}_+^N \right\}$ such that

$$\forall a > 0, \forall t \in \mathbb{R}_+^N; \quad a.[0, t] = [0, at].$$

In that framework, we have

$$\forall a > 0, \forall t \in \mathbb{R}_+^N; \quad m(a.[0, t]) = a^N m([0, t])$$

and then, μ is the function $a \mapsto a^N$, which is surjective. $\square$

A consequence of Proposition 4 is that the fractal properties of self-similarity and $\mathcal{C}_0$-increments stationarity prescribe the covariance between points s and t that are comparable for the partial order $\prec$ of $\mathbb{R}^N$. Since there are non ordered points, we cannot get a complete characterization of the MpfBm by the two properties of self-similarity and stationarity.

A natural question is then, what are the self-similar processes which are stationary in the different definitions of Section 4? The following result shows that for some choice of stationarity definition, we obtain characterization of the Lévy fBm.

Proposition 5. *Let $H \in (0, 1)$. The Lévy fBm is the only Gaussian process which is self-similar of index H and stationary in the strong sense (property (3)).*

Proof. (cf. [6, p. 393])

It is known (Sections 3 and 4) that the Lévy fBm is self-similar and has stationary increments in the strong sense.

Conversely, let $X = \left\{ X_t;\ t \in \mathbb{R}_+^N \right\}$ be a Gaussian process such that

$$\forall a \in \mathbb{R}_+; \quad \left\{ X_{at};\ t \in \mathbb{R}_+^N \right\} \overset{(d)}{=} \left\{ a^H X_t;\ t \in \mathbb{R}_+^N \right\}$$

and

$$\forall g \in \mathcal{G}\left(\mathbb{R}^N\right); \quad \left\{X_t - X_0;\ t \in \mathbb{R}_+^N\right\} \stackrel{(d)}{=} \left\{X_{g(t)} - X_{g(0)};\ t \in \mathbb{R}_+^N\right\}$$

First of all, considering the canonical basis $(\epsilon_i)_{1 \leq i \leq N}$ of $\mathbb{R}^N$, and the rotation g_u that maps ϵ_1 onto any unit vector u, the stationarity property leads to

$$E\left[X_u\right] = E\left[X_{g_u(\epsilon_1)} - X_0\right] = E\left[X_{\epsilon_1}\right]$$

For any s and t in $\mathbb{R}_+^N$, the self-similarity property leads to

$$E\left[X_t - X_s\right] = E\left[X_{t-s}\right] - E\left[X_0\right] = \|t - s\|^H E\left[X_{\epsilon_1}\right].$$

As we also have

$$E\left[X_t - X_s\right] = \left(\|t\|^H - \|s\|^H\right) E\left[X_{\epsilon_0}\right],$$

we get $E\left[X_t\right] = 0$ for all $t \in \mathbb{R}_+^N$.

In the same way, we prove that for any s and t in $\mathbb{R}_+^N$,

$$E\left[(X_t - X_s)^2\right] = E\left[(X_{t-s} - X_0)^2\right] = \|t - s\|^{2H} E\left[X_{\epsilon_1}^2\right].$$

The result follows. $\square$

In the fractional Brownian sheet case, several supplementary assumptions are needed to obtain a characterization of the process. Particularly, a null value of the process on each axis must be imposed as well as a condition of self-similarity for each parameter, when the $N-1$ other ones are fixed (see [5]). From that point of view, the fractional Brownian sheet has no real motivation to be considered, although it satisfies the two properties of stationarity and self-similarity.

6 Projection on Flows and Regularity

The notion of flow is the key to reduce the proof of many theorems. It was extensively studied in [3] and [4].

Definition 2. *Let $S = [a, b] \subseteq R$. An increasing function $f : S \to \mathbb{R}_+^N$ $(x < y \Rightarrow f(x) \prec f(y))$ is called a* flow.

The following results, proved in [2], give a good justification of the definition of the MpfBm.

Proposition 6. *Let $\mathbf{B}^H$ be a MpfBm and f be a flow. Then the process $(\mathbf{B}^H)^f = \{\mathbf{B}^H_{f(t)},\ t \in [a, b]\}$ is a time changed fractional Brownian motion.*

However, in general, the projection of a multiparameter process does not inherit its different properties.

Proposition 7. *Let f be a flow, and X be a multiparameter process.*

1. *If X is a Lévy fBm, then $(X)^f$ is a classical fractional Brownian motion iff $f(t) = \alpha t$ where $\alpha \in \mathbb{R}_+^N$.*
2. *If X is a fractional Brownian sheet, then $(X)^f$ is a classical fractional Brownian motion iff f is a line parallel to one axis of $\mathbb{R}_+^N$.*

We conclude this section by giving an interpretation of H parameter.

Let us recall the definition of the two classical Hölder exponents of a stochastic process X at $t_0 \in \mathbb{R}_+$:

- the pointwise Hölder exponent

$$
\boldsymbol{\alpha}_X(t_0) = \sup \left\{ \alpha : \limsup_{\rho \to 0} \ \sup_{s,t \in \mathcal{B}(t_0,\rho)} \frac{|X_t - X_s|}{\rho^\alpha} < \infty \right\}
$$

- the local Hölder exponent

$$
\widetilde{\boldsymbol{\alpha}}_X(t_0) = \sup \left\{ \alpha : \limsup_{\rho \to 0} \ \sup_{s,t \in \mathcal{B}(t_0,\rho)} \frac{|X_t - X_s|}{|t - s|^\alpha} < \infty \right\}
$$

Corollary 1. *Let $\mathbf{B}^H$ be a multiparameter fractional Brownian motion with self-similarity index H. The pointwise and local Hölder exponents of the projection $(\mathbf{B}^H)^f$ along any flows f at $t_0 \in [0,1]$, satisfy almost surely*

$$
\boldsymbol{\alpha}_{(\mathbf{B}^H)^f}(t_0) = \begin{cases} \alpha_\theta(t_0).H & \text{if } \alpha_\theta(t_0) < 1 \\ H & \text{otherwise} \end{cases}
$$

$$
\widetilde{\boldsymbol{\alpha}}_{(\mathbf{B}^H)^f}(t_0) = \begin{cases} \widetilde{\alpha}_\theta(t_0).H & \text{if } \widetilde{\alpha}_\theta(t_0) < 1 \\ H & \text{otherwise} \end{cases}
$$

where θ is the real function such that $\theta(t) = m\,[f(t)]$ ($\forall t \in [0,1]$), and $\alpha_\theta(t_0)$ (resp. $\widetilde{\alpha}_\theta(t_0)$) is the pointwise (resp. local) Hölder exponent of θ at t_0.

Consequently, the H parameter of the MpfBm $\mathbf{B}^H$ represents the regularity of the projection on any regular flow. This fact gives a way to estimate H from real data, in the frame of applications.

Acknowledgement

The authors wish to thank Prof. M. Dozzi for his helpful comments and suggestions.

References

1. Herbin, E.: From N-parameter fractional Brownian motions to N-parameter multifractional Brownian motions. Rocky Mountain J. Math. (2006)
2. Herbin, E., Merzbach, E.: A set-indexed fractional Brownian motion. J. Theoret. Probab., to appear (2006)
3. Ivanoff, G.: Set-indexed processes: distributions and weak convergence. In: Topics in Spatial Stochastic Processes, Lecture Notes in Mathematics, 1802, 85-126, Springer (2003)
4. Ivanoff, G., Merzbach, E.: Set-Indexed Martingales, Chapman & Hall/CRC, 2000.
5. Leger, S., Pontier, M.: Drap brownien fractionnaire. CRAS 329 série I, 893-898 (1999)
6. Samorodnitsky, G., Taqqu, M.S.: Stable Non-Gaussian Random Processes. Chapman & Hall (1994)

Filtering of Multiparameter Processes: Theory and Applications

Alberto Carabarín-Aguirre, B. Gail Ivanoff, and Adriana Jordan

Department of Mathematics and Statistics, University of Ottawa, Ottawa K1N
6N5, Canada
`acara553@science.uottawa.ca`, `givanoff@uottawa.ca`,
`ajord687@science.uottawa.ca`

*Dedicated to Professor Vincenzo Capasso on the occasion of his sixtieth birth-
day.*

1 Introduction

Stopping times and related random sets play a fundamental role in the analysis
of stochastic processes on $\mathbb{R}_+$. In particular, a stochastic process $(X(t) : t \in
\mathbb{R}_+)$ on a complete probability space $(\Omega, \mathcal{F}, P)$ adapted to a filtration $(\mathcal{F}_t \subseteq
\mathcal{F} : t \in \mathbb{R}_+)$ is said to be *filtered* by a random set ξ if one can only observe
$X(t)$ when $t \in \xi$. It is generally assumed that ξ can be expressed as a disjoint
union of random intervals:

$$\xi = \cup_{i=1}^{r}(\tau_1^{(i)}, \tau_2^{(i)}]\tag{1}$$

where the endpoints $\tau_j^{(i)}$ are stopping times, $j = 1, 2, i = 1, ..., r$. This ensures
that the filtered process X^ξ defined by

$$X^\xi(t) := \int_0^t I\{s \in \xi\}dX(s)$$

remains adapted and is a martingale whenever X is a martingale.

The concept of filtering by a random set has been extended in [5] and [6]
to processes indexed by $\mathbb{R}_+^d$ (or more generally, by a class of sets). The goal
of this article is to review and extend this generalized version of filtering. We
will be focussing on two main applications: precedence tests and estimation
in survival analysis. These examples will demonstrate the importance of the
type of information available to the practitioner, and how it affects the filtering problem in higher dimensions. In both cases, we develop techniques that
illustrate how to deal with the more complex multidimensional structure.

We begin with a brief description of the one-dimensional versions of our
examples.

Example 1 (Precedence tests on $\mathbb{R}_+$). Given two continuous distributions F and G on $\mathbb{R}_+$, we want to test $H_0 : F = G$ vs. $H_1 : F \leq G$ (i.e. $F(t) \leq G(t)\ \forall t \in \mathbb{R}_+$ and $\exists t'$ such that $F(t') < G(t')$). If $X_1, ..., X_n$ are i.i.d. F and $Y_1, ..., Y_m$ are i.i.d. G, a precedence test tells us to reject H_0 if the test statistic

$$G_m(X_{(k)}) = G_m([0, X_{(k)}])$$

$$= \frac{1}{m} \sum_{i=1}^{m} I\{Y_i \in [0, X_{(k)}]\}$$

is too large, where $X_{(k)}$ is the kth order statistic of the sample $(X_1, ..., X_n)$. Precedence tests are not only distribution free (see [2]), but they allow us to reach a conclusion without having to observe all the data points. This can be reformulated in terms of stopping times: the order statistic $X_{(k)}$ can be viewed as a stopping time with respect to the minimal filtration $(\mathcal{F}_t)$ generated by the empirical distributions F_n and G_m:

$$\mathcal{F}_t := \sigma\{F_n(u), G_m(v) : 0 \leq u, v \leq t\}, \tag{2}$$

and so in fact the observations $Y_1, ..., Y_m$ have been filtered by $(0, X_{(k)}]$. As a result, given the available information at any time t, we know whether or not we need to observe more data points: i.e. the experiment is over by time t if and only if $t \geq X_{(k)}$, and this is an $\mathcal{F}_t$-measurable event. This observation, while trivial in one dimension, is less so in higher dimensions and will motivate the general definition of a precedence test in $\mathbb{R}_+^2$, given in Section 3.

Example 2 (Survival Analysis on $\mathbb{R}_+$ and the Nelson-Aalen Estimator). The integrated hazard function H plays an important role in survival analysis. In particular, if F is a continuous distribution on $\mathbb{R}_+$ with density f and survival function $\overline{F} := 1 - F$, we have $H(t) := \int_0^t \frac{f(s)}{\overline{F}(s)} ds$. Given a sample $X_1, ..., X_n$ from F, define the associated counting process $N_n(t) := \sum_{i=1}^{n} I\{X_i \in [0, t]\}$. The Nelson-Aalen estimator of H is based on a martingale estimating equation, and is defined by

$$\hat{H}_n(t) := \int_0^t \frac{N_n(du)}{Z_n(u)}, \tag{3}$$

where $Z_n(t) := \sum_{i=1}^{n} I\{X_i \geq t\}$. Letting $\tilde{H}_n(t) = \int_0^t I\{Z_n(u) > 0\}dH(u)$, the crucial fact is that $\hat{H}_n - \tilde{H}_n$ is a martingale, and this is still the case if each of the observations X_i is filtered by a set ξ_i of the form (1). Since the martingale in the estimating equation remains a martingale under filtering, (3) remains the appropriate estimator with N_n replaced by $N_n^\xi(t) := \sum_{i=1}^{n} I\{X_i \in [0, t] \cap \xi_i\}$ and Z_n redefined as $Z_n(t) := \sum_{i=1}^{n} I\{X_i \geq t\}I\{t \in \xi_i\}$ (cf. [1]). (Note that here we do not use the notation Z_n^ξ, since the redefined process is not the filtered version of the process Z_n.)

In Section 2 we present the framework and definitions for a dynamical theory of stochastic processes indexed by $\mathbb{R}_+^2$, and we introduce *anti-clouds,* the multidimensional analogue of the random set ξ in (1). (The term anti-cloud is suggested by the idea that the process cannot be observed when obscured by the cloud ξ^c.) In Section 3 we introduce the general concept of a precedence test on $\mathbb{R}_+^2$. Two different scenarios will be considered, depending on the information structure of the data set in question. The asymptotics of one precedence test statistic will be discussed. In Section 4 we review the extension of the Nelson-Aalen estimator to filtered data on $\mathbb{R}_+^2$ as developed in [5] and [6]. It will be seen that there is a fundamental problem with observability of the estimator under the usual sort of data structure. We propose a solution via filtering by a more general type of anti-cloud (a $*$-anti-cloud). The asymptotic distribution of the Nelson-Aalen estimator will be given. Sketches of proofs will be given in Sections 3 and 4; a more complete development of both examples will be published elsewhere.

2 Framework and Definitions

Although the framework used in both [5] and [6] was based on the general theory of set-indexed martingales as developed in [4], for clarity here we will focus on processes indexed by $\mathbb{R}_+^2$ and consequently we specialize and simplify the notation and assumptions of [4]. The usual partial order on $\mathbb{R}_+^2$ is denoted by "$\leq$". We write $(z_1, z_2) = z << z' = (z_1', z_2')$ if and only if $z_i < z_i', i = 1, 2$.

Given a complete probability space $(\Omega, \mathcal{F}, P)$, the information structure is defined by a filtration $(\mathcal{F}_z : z \in \mathbb{R}_+^2)$ satisfying

- $\mathcal{F}_z$ contains all the P-null sets, $\forall z$;
- $z \leq z' \Rightarrow \mathcal{F}_z \subseteq \mathcal{F}_{z'}$;
- $\mathcal{F}_z = \cap_{z' >> z} \mathcal{F}_{z'}$.

The σ-algebra $\mathcal{F}_z$ represents the information in the past of the point z. In addition, we define

$$\mathcal{F}_z^* = \vee_{z' \not\gg z} \mathcal{F}_{z'};$$

this is the σ-algebra of all the information not strictly in the future of z. A stochastic process $W = (W(z) : z \in \mathbb{R}_+^2)$ is

- adapted if $W(z)$ is $\mathcal{F}_z$-measurable $\forall z \in \mathbb{R}_+^2$;
- a pseudo-strong martingale if $W(z)$ is integrable $\forall z \in \mathbb{R}_+^2$ and for all $z \leq z' \in \mathbb{R}_+^2$, $E(W(z, z']|\mathcal{F}_z^*) = 0$ where $W(z, z'] := W(z') - W(z_1', z_2) - W(z_1, z_2') + W(z)$;
- a strong martingale if W is an adapted pseudo-strong martingale.

A process W is filtered by a random Borel set $\xi \subseteq \mathbb{R}_+^2$ if we observe

$$W^\xi(z) = \int_{(0,z]} I\{u \in \xi\} dW(u) = \int_{(0,z] \cap \xi} dW. \tag{4}$$

In order for the filtered process W^ξ to be well-defined and adapted, further assumptions are required: in particular that ξ is an anti-cloud. The definition below of an anti-cloud is motivated by the observation that for ξ as in (1), $\{t \in \xi\} \in \mathcal{F}_t \; \forall t$. This is a result of the fact that the endpoints of the intervals are stopping times.

We denote by $\mathcal{K}$ the class of *domains* in $\mathbb{R}_+^2$: D is a domain if $D = \overline{D^o}$, where "$\overline{(\cdot)}$" and "$(\cdot)^o$" denote respectively the closure and interior of a set.

Definition 1. *A random set* $\xi : \Omega \to \mathcal{K}$ *is an anti-cloud if* $\{z \in \xi\} \in \mathcal{F}_z \; \forall z \in \mathbb{R}_+^2$.

The measurability properties of anti-clouds are developed in [6]. In particular, we have the following stopping theorem which is key to our applications:

Theorem 1 ([6], Theorem 3.12). *Let ξ be an anti-cloud and W a process of bounded variation such that $W_{\partial\xi} = 0$ a.s. ("$\partial(\cdot)$" denotes the boundary of a set).*

- *If W is adapted, then so is W^ξ.*
- *If W is a (pseudo-)strong martingale, then so is W^ξ.*

In the next two sections, we will make use of the following spaces. For $T \subseteq [0, \infty)^2$, the Banach space $l^\infty(T)$ is the set of all functions $f : T \to \mathbb{R}$ that are bounded uniformly equipped with the norm $\|f\| = \sup_x |f(x)|$. As usual, $C(T)$ is the space of continuous functions $f : T \to \mathbb{R}$ equipped with the uniform norm. Furthermore, $D([0, \infty)^2)$ is the Banach space of all functions $f : [0, \infty)^2 \to \mathbb{R}$ continuous at each point from the upper right quadrant and with limits from the other quadrants, also equipped with the uniform norm; for $\eta \in \mathbb{R}_+^2$, $D([0, \eta]) = D([0, \eta_1] \times [0, \eta_2])$ is defined similarly. Finally, $BV_M([0, \infty)^2)$ denotes the space of all functions in $D([0, \infty)^2)$ with total variation bounded by M. Products of any of these spaces will always be equipped with a product norm.

The proofs of the limit theorems in the following sections will be based on the delta-method, which in turn is based on the concept of Hadamard differentiability tangentially to a set. This definition, as well as an excellent description of the delta-method, can be found in [8].

3 Precedence Tests on the Plane

The set-up on $\mathbb{R}_+^2$ is similar to that described in Example 1. We have continuous distributions F and G on $\mathbb{R}_+^2$ which are null on the axes, and we want to test $H_0 : F = G$ versus $H_1 : F <_{st} G$, where "$<_{st}$" denotes a particular stochastic order. (There are many such orders on $\mathbb{R}_+^2$; see, for example, [7].) If $X_1, ..., X_n$ are i.i.d. F and $Y_1, ..., Y_m$ are i.i.d. G, we reject H_0 if the test statistic

$$G_m(\xi_n) := \frac{1}{m} \sum_{i=1}^{m} I\{Y_i \in \xi_n\}$$

is too large, where ξ_n is an appropriately chosen random set depending on $(X_1, ..., X_n)$. This test will be called a precedence test on $\mathbb{R}_+^2$ provided that ξ_n is an anti-cloud, since in this case we do not have to observe all of the data points in order to calculate the test statistic. This fact will have important implications in practice, and in particular for clinical trials.

The choice of ξ_n depends both on the stochastic order in the alternative and on the structure of the data available to us. We will describe two typical scenarios in detail.

3.1 Data Filtered by an $(\mathcal{F}_z)$-anti-Cloud

We first deal with the case in which the underlying filtration is the minimal. In analogy to (2), we define the minimal filtration in $\mathbb{R}_+^2$ to be the σ-field generated by the bivariate empirical distributions F_n and G_m generated, respectively, by $(X_1, \ldots, X_n)$ and $(Y_1, \ldots, Y_m)$: for all $z \in \mathbb{R}_+^2$,

$$\mathcal{F}_z := \sigma\{F_n(u), G_m(v) : 0 \le u, v \le z\}.$$

It is easy to see that given $(\mathcal{F}_z)$, the only information available to us is the number of observations from each sample that lie in $[0, z]$, their exact locations, and the number of observations outside $[0, z]$. This kind of filtration is appropriate for geographical data, for example, where any additional information such as the identity of the individual at a particular location is either unavailable or not required.

The simple structure of the minimal filtration gives rise to anti-clouds that are defined by the contours of the empirical distribution F_n.

Lemma 1. *The random set* $\xi_k := \{u \in \mathbb{R}_+^2 : F_n(u-) := F_n([0, u)) \le \frac{k-1}{n}\}$ *is an anti-cloud with respect to* $(\mathcal{F}_z)$.

Proof. It is easily seen that ξ_k is a domain since F is null on the axes. The measurability criterion of Definition 1 is satisfied since $\{z \in \xi_k\} = \{F_n(z-) \le \frac{k-1}{n}\} \in \mathcal{F}_z, \ \forall z \in \mathbb{R}_+^2$. $\qquad\square$

3.2 Data Filtered by an $(\mathcal{F}_z^p)$-anti-Cloud

We now turn to the definition of a larger filtration that is appropriate for clinical trials. Given the samples $(X_1, \ldots, X_n)$ and $(Y_1, \ldots, Y_m)$ $(X_i = (X_i^1, X_i^2), Y_j = (Y_j^1, Y_j^2))$, the product filtration $(\mathcal{F}_z^p)$ is defined by

$$\mathcal{F}_z^p := \sigma\{I\{X_i^1 \le u_1\}, I\{X_i^2 \le u_2\}, I\{Y_j^1 \le v_1\}, I\{Y_j^2 \le v_2\} :$$
$$0 \le u_1, v_1 \le z_1, 0 \le u_2, v_2 \le z_2, i = 1, 2, \ldots, n, j = 1, 2, \ldots, m\}$$

for all $z = (z_1, z_2) \in \mathbb{R}^2_+$. This filtration is much larger than the minimal, since not only do we have additional information about the locations of observations that lie outside $[0, z]$, but we can distinguish one test subject from another. In particular, we know the exact location of the observations in $[0, z]$, the first component of those in $[0, z_1] \times (z_2, \infty)$, as well as the second component of the ones lying in $(z_1, \infty) \times [0, z_2]$. Generally, this sort of information structure would be observed in data arising from medical studies where, for example, X^1 and X^2, denote respectively the age of onset of two different diseases in an individual test subject exposed to a risk factor common to the two diseases. Y^1 and Y^2 are the corresponding ages in a control population. (A classic example would be the ages of onset of heart disease (X_i^1) and lung cancer (X_i^2) for a sample of smokers compared with the corresponding ages of onset $(Y_j^1$ and $Y_j^2)$ in a sample of non-smokers.) For every $z = (z_1, z_2) \in \mathbb{R}^2_+$, the σ-field $\mathcal{F}_z^p$ identifies the test subjects who developed the first disease by age z_1 and/or the second disease by age z_2, and the exact age of onset in each of these subjects.

When using $(\mathcal{F}_z^p)$ as the underlying filtration, there are several interesting anti-clouds to consider in addition to those defined in Lemma 1. For notational purposes let $X_{(i)}^1$ be the ith order statistic of $(X_1^1, ..., X_n^1)$ and $X_{(j)}^2$ be the jth order statistic of $(X_1^2, ..., X_n^2)$.

Lemma 2. *Let $\tau = (\tau_1, \tau_2) = (X_{(i)}^1, X_{(j)}^2)$. The set $[0, \tau]$ is an anti-cloud with respect to $(\mathcal{F}_z^p)$.*

Proof. Clearly the set $[0, \tau]$ is a domain since F is null on the axes. Next, we have that

$$\{z \in [0, \tau]\} = \{z_1 \le X_{(i)}^1\} \cap \{z_2 \le X_{(j)}^2\}$$

$$= \{(\sum_{k=1}^n I\{X_k^1 < z_1\}) \le i - 1\} \cap \{(\sum_{l=1}^n I\{X_l^2 < z_2\}) \le j - 1\}$$

$$= \{\sum_{k=1}^n I\{\cup_{r \in \mathbf{Q}, r < z_1}\{X_k^1 \le r\}\} \le i - 1\}$$

$$\cap \{\sum_{l=1}^n I\{\cup_{s \in \mathbf{Q}, s < z_2}\{X_l^2 \le s\}\} \le j - 1\}$$

$$\in \mathcal{F}_z^p.$$

Therefore, $[0, \tau]$ is an anti-cloud. $\qquad\square$

Similarly, we can prove that the sets $\{[0, \tau_1] \times [0, \infty)\} \cup \{[0, \infty) \times [0, \tau_2]\}$ and $\{[0, \tau_1] \times (\tau_2, \infty)\} \cup \{(\tau_1, \infty) \times [0, \tau_2]\}$ are anti-clouds with respect to $(\mathcal{F}_z^p)$ as well. However, it should be noted that none of these sets are anti-clouds with respect to the minimal filtration $(\mathcal{F}_z)$.

3.3 Limiting Distribution of a Precedence Test Statistic

We now discuss the asymptotics of a specific precedence test statistic in $\mathbb{R}_+^2$. We assume that the filtration is $(\mathcal{F}_z^p)$, and as in Example 1 we want to test $H_0 : F = G$ versus $H_1 : F \leq G$ (i.e. $F(z) \leq G(z)\ \forall z \in \mathbb{R}_+^2$ and $\exists z'$ such that $F(z') < G(z')$). This corresponds to the lower orthant stochastic order. The appropriate precedence test statistic is of the form $G_m([0, \tau])$ where $\tau = (X_{(i)}^1, X_{(j)}^2)$, as defined in Lemma 2. In fact, we are able to identify the asymptotic behaviour of a functional form of the test statistic, which includes all possible pairs $(X_{(i)}^1, X_{(j)}^2)$, $i = 1, ..., n$, $j = 1, ..., m$.

In what follows, let F and G have marginal distribution functions F_1, F_2 and G_1, G_2. The copulas associated with F and G are denoted by C^F and C^G respectively. For a distribution H on $[0, 1]^2$, U^H will denote the Brownian bridge on $[0, 1]^2$ with covariance

$$E(U^H(s_1, s_2)U^H(t_1, t_2)) = H(\min\{(s_1, s_2), (t_1, t_2)\}) - H(s_1, s_2)H(t_1, t_2).$$

For any distribution function J on $\mathbb{R}_+$, let J^- denote the left continuous inverse of J: for $0 \leq p \leq 1$,

$$J^-(p) := \inf\{x \geq 0 : J(x) \geq p\}.$$

In particular, we note that if F_n^1 and F_n^2 are the marginals of the empirical distribution F_n, then for $0 < p, q \leq 1$,

$$F_n^{1-}(p) = X_{(\lceil np \rceil)}^1, F_n^{2-}(q) = X_{(\lceil nq \rceil)}^2,$$

where "$\lceil r \rceil$" denotes the smallest integer greater than or equal to r. We now see that $G_m \circ (F_n^{1-}, F_n^{2-})$ defines a process on $[0, 1]^2$:

$$G_m \circ (F_n^{1-}, F_n^{2-})(p, q) := G_m([0, F_n^{1-}(p)] \times [0, F_n^{2-}(q)]).$$

The process $G_m \circ (F_n^{1-}, F_n^{2-})$ may be regarded as a functional version of the precedence test statistic.

Theorem 2. *Suppose F and G are continuous and differentiable distribution functions on $\mathbb{R}_+^2$ with marginal distributions F_1, F_2, G_1, G_2 that have continuous positive derivatives f_1, f_2, g_1, g_2 on their open support. Furthermore, assume that C^G is continuously differentiable on $[0, 1]^2$. Let $v_p^{F_1} = F_1^-(p)$ and $v_q^{F_2} = F_2^-(q)$. If $\frac{m}{n} \to \lambda$ as $n, m \to \infty$, then $\sqrt{m}[G_m \circ (F_n^{1-}, F_n^{2-}) - G \circ (F_1^-, F_2^-)]$ converges weakly to a Gaussian process in $\ell^\infty([0, 1]^2)$ which is equal in distribution to*

$$W(p, q) = U^{C^G}(G_1(v_p^{F_1}), G_2(v_q^{F_2}))$$
$$- \sqrt{\lambda}\frac{\partial C^G(G_1(v_p^{F_1}), G_2(v_q^{F_2}))}{\partial G_1(v_p^{F_1})} \frac{g_1(v_p^{F_1})}{f_1(v_p^{F_1})} U^{C^F}(p, 1)$$
$$- \sqrt{\lambda}\frac{\partial C^G(G_1(v_p^{F_1}), G_2(v_q^{F_2}))}{\partial G_2(v_q^{F_2})} \frac{g_2(v_q^{F_2})}{f_2(v_q^{F_2})} U^{C^F}(1, q),$$

where U^{C^F} and U^{C^G} are independent bridges.

Proof (Sketch). Following the procedure of [3], we define the pseudo-variables $(X_1^*, X_2^*) = (F_1(X_1), F_2(X_2))$ and $(Y_1^*, Y_2^*) = (F_1(Y_1), F_2(Y_2))$, the corresponding distributions F^* and G^*, and empirical distributions F_n^* and G_m^*. In what follows, we shall see that this allows us to restrict our attention to distributions on $[0,1]^2$ and therefore, as in [3], yields functional convergence on the entire unit square. We have that $\sqrt{m}[(F_n^*, G_m^*) - (F^*, G^*)] \to_D (\sqrt{\lambda} U^{F^*}, U^{G^*})$, where U^{F^*} and U^{G^*} are independent Brownian bridges. It can be shown that $G^*(F_1^{*-}(x_1), F_2^{*-}(x_2)) = G(F_1^-(x_1), F_2^-(x_2))$ and that $G_m^* \circ (F_n^{*1-}, F_n^{*2-}) = G_m \circ (F_n^{1-}, F_n^{2-})$. The last assertion, along with the fact that for all $x, y \in [0,1]$ there exist i, j such that $G_m(F_n^{1-}(x), F_n^{2-}(y)) = G_m(F_n^{1-}(\frac{i}{n})), F_n^{2-}(\frac{j}{n}))$, implies that

$$\sqrt{m}[G_m \circ (F_n^{1-}, F_n^{2-}) - G \circ (F_1^-, F_2^-)](x, y)$$
$$= \sqrt{m}[G_m^* \circ (F_n^{*1-}, F_n^{*2-}) - G^* \circ (F_1^{*-}, F_2^{*-})](x, y), \quad \forall (x, y) \in [0,1]^2.$$

On the other hand, it can also be shown that the map

$$(F^*, G^*) \to (F_1^*, F_2^*, G^*) \to (F_1^{*-}, F_2^{*-}, G^*) \to G^* \circ (F_1^{*-}, F_2^{*-})$$

is Hadamard differentiable tangentially to $(C([0,1]^2))^2$. The result follows by applying the delta-method to $\sqrt{m}[(F_n^*, G_m^*) - (F^*, G^*)]$, noting that F_1^* and F_2^* are uniform distributions, and finally rewriting the result in terms of the original distributions F and G. $\square$

4 Survival Analysis on the Plane and the Nelson-Aalen Estimator

Let F be a continuous distribution on $\mathbb{R}_+^2$ with density f. Denote by $\overline{F}$ the corresponding survival function: if X has distribution F, $\overline{F}(z) = P(X \geq z)$, $z \in \mathbb{R}_+^2$. Analogously to the univariate case, the integrated hazard H is defined by $H(z) := \int_{(0,z]} h(u)du = \int_{(0,z]} \frac{f(u)}{\overline{F}(u)} du$ where for $z = (z_1, z_2)$, $(0, z] := (0, z_1] \times (0, z_2]$. We are given a sample $X_1, ..., X_n$ from F and a sequence of independent anti-clouds $\xi_1, ..., \xi_n$, such that X_i is filtered by $\xi_i, i = 1, ..., n$. We may again define $\hat{H}_n$, a Nelson-Aalen estimator of H, by

$$\hat{H}_n(z) = \int_{(0,z]} \frac{N_n^\xi(du)}{Z_n(u)}, \tag{5}$$

where $N_n^\xi(u) := \sum_{i=1}^n I\{X_i \in [0, u] \cap \xi_i\}$ and $Z_n(u) := \sum_{i=1}^n I\{X_i \geq u\} I\{u \in \xi_i\}$. Letting $\tilde{H}_n(z) ;= \int_{(0,z]} I\{Z_n(u) > 0\} dH(u)$, it follows from Theorem 1 that $\hat{H}_n - \tilde{H}_n$ is a pseudo-strong martingale (cf. [6]). If $I\{Z_n(u) > 0\} \to 1$ a.s. for all $u \leq z$, the pseudo-strong martingale property implies that $\hat{H}_n(z)$ is asymptotically unbiased for $H(z)$, and in [6] it is also shown that $\hat{H}_n(z)$ is consistent. However, there are two important issues still to be addressed.

4.1 Observability of the Estimator $\hat{H}_n$

Example 3. Ideally, when conducting an experiment, we would like to have all the information regarding the events in the σ-algebra $\mathcal{F}_z^*$, which can be seen as the "wide history" of the point z. Unfortunately this is generally not possible in practice, and so we have to settle for somewhat more limited information. More specifically, if ξ is an anti-cloud and $D_z := \{u : u \not\gg z\}$, instead of having the whole $\mathcal{F}_z^*$ we can usually observe the more restrictive σ-field

$$\mathcal{H}_z := \sigma\{I\{X_i \in A \cap \xi_i\}, I\{u \in \xi_i\}, A \subseteq D_z, u \in D_z, i = 1, \dots n\} \subseteq \mathcal{F}_z^*.$$

We need the event $I\{X_i \geq z\}I\{z \in \xi_i\}$ to be observable in order to calculate the value of the estimator for the integrated hazard function proposed in (5). The problem is that this event is not $\mathcal{H}_z$-measurable, and so we cannot construct $\hat{H}_n$ in this case.

To resolve this kind of observability problem, we introduce a more general type of filtering. We will relax the adaptedness requirement in our filtering mechanism with the objective of making the events of the form $I\{X_i \geq z\}I\{z \in \xi_i\}$ observable. With this in mind, we define a $*$-*anti-cloud* as follows:

Definition 2. *A random set* $\xi : \Omega \to \mathcal{K}$ *is a* $*$-*anti-cloud if* $\{z \in \xi\} \in \mathcal{F}_z^*$ $\forall z \in \mathbb{R}_+^2$.

It is natural to expect $*$-anti-clouds to be very similar to anti-clouds. Indeed, they share most of their properties, such as the measurability of events of the type $\{\omega : B \subseteq \xi(\omega)\}$, $\{\omega : \xi(\omega) \subseteq B\}$ and $\{\omega : \xi(\omega) = B\}$ whenever $B \in \mathcal{K}$, as well as the measurability of the filtered process W^ξ defined as in (4). On the other hand, we will pay a small price for our modifications in the $*$-anti-cloud version of Theorem 1, which will differ from its anti-cloud counterpart in that the filtered process is not necessarily adapted. This is a consequence of the weaker requirement that $\{z \in \xi\} \in \mathcal{F}_z^*$.

Theorem 3. *Let* ξ *be a* $*$-*anti-cloud and* $X = Y - W$, *where* Y *and* W *are increasing processes such that* $Y_{\partial\xi} = W_{\partial\xi} = 0$ *a.s.*

1. *If* X *is a (pseudo-) strong martingale, then* X^ξ *is a pseudo-strong martingale.*
2. X^ξ *will not generally be adapted, even if* X *is.*

Now, with our new filtering mechanism in place, we turn to the Nelson-Aalen estimator. Again, suppose we have a sequence of i.i.d. random variables $X_1, \dots, X_n$ with distribution F, but now they are filtered by a sequence of independent $*$-anti-clouds $\xi_1, \dots, \xi_n$. Define the processes N_n^ξ and Z_n as in the beginning of this section, replacing anti-clouds with $*$-anti-clouds. Our new Nelson-Aalen estimator is

$$\hat{H}_n(z) = \int_{(0,z]} \frac{N_n^\xi(du)}{Z_n(u)}.$$

It can be shown that, if we let $\tilde{H}_n(z) = \int_{(0,z]} I\{Z_n(u) > 0\}dH(u)$, the difference $\hat{H}_n - \tilde{H}_n$ is still a pseudo-strong martingale. As in the case of filtering by anti-clouds, $\hat{H}_n(z)$ is a consistent and asymptotically unbiased estimator for $H(z)$ under the conditions outlined in [6]. The proofs of these properties are exactly the same as in the anti-cloud case.

In order to better illustrate the benefits of the switch from the anti-cloud model to the $*$-anti-cloud one, we go back to Example 3 and recall that the main issue was that $I\{X_i \geq z\}I\{z \in \xi_i\} \notin \mathcal{H}_z$. To correct this, define $\xi_i^*(\omega) = \{z : D_z \cap \xi_i^c(\omega) = \emptyset\}$. ξ_i^* is a $*$-anti-cloud, since

$$\{z \in \xi_i^*\} = \{D_z \cap \xi_i^c = \emptyset\} = \{D_z \subseteq \xi_i\} = \bigcap_{u \in D_z} \{u \in \xi_i\}$$

$$= \bigcap_{u \in T_{D_z}} \{u \in \xi_i\} \in \bigvee_{u \in T_{D_z}} \mathcal{F}_u \subseteq \bigvee_{u:u \not\gg z} \mathcal{F}_u = \mathcal{F}_z^*,$$

where T_{D_z} stands for a countable dense subset of D_z.

Now consider $I\{X_i \geq z\}I\{z \in \xi_i^*\}$. We have that if $z \in \xi_i^*$, then $D_z \subseteq \xi_i$ and so

$$\{X_i \geq z\} \cap \{z \in \xi_i^*\} = \{X_i \in D_z^o\}^c \cap \{z \in \xi_i^*\}$$

$$= \{X_i \in D_z^o \cap \xi_i\}^c \cap \{z \in \xi_i^*\} \in \mathcal{H}_z.$$

Therefore, $I\{X_i \geq z\}I\{z \in \xi_i^*\}$ is observable and we are able to construct a Nelson-Aalen estimator.

4.2 A Functional Central Limit Theorem for the Estimator $\hat{H}_n$

The other point that we would like to address is the existence of a functional central limit theorem for the process $U_n(z) := \sqrt{n}(\hat{H}_n(z) - H(z))$. The convergence in finite-dimensional distribution of the slightly different (but asymptotically equivalent) process $\sqrt{n}(\hat{H}_n(z) - \tilde{H}_n(z))$ to a mean-zero Gaussian process was proven in [5] in the case of filtering by a stopping set, a type of anti-cloud with a particular geometric structure. The proof in [5] exploited the fact that if ξ is a stopping set, then the sample paths of the process $I\{z \in \xi\}$ have certain regularity properties. These properties are lost when we filter by an anti-cloud or a $*$-anti-cloud, and so here we take a different approach. In what follows ξ may represent either an anti-cloud or a $*$-anti-cloud.

Before the statement of the functional central limit theorem, we have to make some assumptions.

Assumption 1 *For all $z, z' \in \mathbb{R}_+^2$, $P(z \in \xi) - P(z, z' \in \xi) \leq K |z - z'|$, where K is a constant and $|\cdot|$ denotes the Euclidean norm.*

Assumption 2 *$P(z \in \xi)$ is continuous in $z \in \mathbb{R}_+^2$ and there exists $\epsilon > 0$ such that $P(z \in \xi) > \epsilon$ for every $z \in \mathbb{R}_+^2$.*

Assumption 3 *The survival function $\overline{F}$ satisfies a Lipschitz condition of order 1.*

Theorem 4. *Under Assumptions 1, 2 and 3, $U_n \Rightarrow G$ in $D([0, \eta])$ for every $\eta \in \mathbb{R}_+^2$ such that $\overline{F}(\eta) > 0$, where G is a mean-zero Gaussian process with*

$$\mathrm{Cov}(G(z), G(z'))$$
$$= \int_{[0, z \wedge z']} \left(\overline{F}(t) P(t \in \xi) \right)^{-1} h(t) dt$$
$$+ \int \int_{([0,z] \setminus [0,z']) \cup ([0,z'] \setminus [0,z])} \frac{\overline{F}(s \vee t) P(s, t \in \xi)}{\overline{F}(s) \overline{F}(t) P(s \in \xi) P(t \in \xi)} h(s) h(t) ds dt.$$

Our approach to the proof of this Theorem is very similar to Example 3.9.19 in [8]. An obvious difference is that we are working on two dimensions instead of one. Another resides in our filtering mechanism and the information we are provided with; a consequence of this is that Z_n, the survivor function process, will not necessarily be in $D([0, \infty)^2)$.

Proof (Sketch). Once again we employ the delta-method.

We start with Assumption 1. This, together with Assumption 3 and using a very similar argument to that in Example 2.11.14 in [8], gives the convergence in distribution of the sequence of processes $\frac{1}{\sqrt{n}}[Z_n(\cdot) - E(Z_n(\cdot))]$ to a tight Gaussian process G_1, which can be proven to be continuous a.s. Moreover, since the ξ_i's are i.i.d., we also have that the sequence of processes $\frac{1}{\sqrt{n}}[N_n^\xi(\cdot) - E(N_n^\xi(\cdot))]$ converges in distribution to another tight Gaussian process G_2 on $D([0, \infty)^2)$. This follows from the CLT for empirical processes, since we are working with a subdistribution. This means that

$$\frac{1}{\sqrt{n}}[(Z_n(z), N_n^\xi(z)) - (E(Z_n(z)), E(N_n^\xi(z)))] \Rightarrow \tilde{G} = (G_1, G_2),$$

where $\tilde{G}$ is a Gaussian process on $C([0, \infty)^2) \times D([0, \infty)^2)$.

At this point, we note that the estimator depends on the pair $(\frac{Z_n}{n}, \frac{N_n^\xi}{n})$ through the maps

$$(A, B) \to (\frac{1}{A}, B) \to \int \frac{1}{A} dB.$$

We can show that the composition map is Hadamard-differentiable tangentially to $C([0, \infty)^2) \times BV_M([0, \infty)^2)$ on a certain domain, and that whenever z is restricted to a rectangle $[0, \eta]$ such that $\overline{F}(\eta) > 0$, the pair $(\frac{Z_n}{n}, \frac{N_n^\xi}{n})$ is contained in this domain with probability tending to 1 for $M \geq 1$ and ϵ sufficiently small. Now apply the delta-method to conclude that

$$U_n(\cdot) := \sqrt{n}(\hat{H}_n(\cdot) - H(\cdot)) \Rightarrow G(\cdot),$$

where G is again Gaussian.

The covariance structure of the limiting process is determined as in [5], Theorem 5.1, using Proposition 4.6 of [6]. $\Box$

Acknowledgments

The research of Alberto Carabarín-Aguirre is supported by Consejo Nacional de Ciencia y Tecnología, Mexico. The research of B. Gail Ivanoff is supported by a grant from the Natural Sciences and Engineering Research Council of Canada. The research of Adriana Jordan is supported by Consejo Nacional de Ciencia y Tecnología, Mexico.

References

1. Andersen, P.K., Borgan, O., Gill, R.D. and Keiding, N., *Statistical Models Based on Counting Processes*, Springer Series in Statistics, Springer-Verlag, New York, 1993.
2. Chakraborti, S. and Van der Laan, P., Precedence tests and confidence bounds for complete data: An overview and some results. *The Statistician* **45**, 1996, 351–369.
3. Fermanian, J.-D., Radulović, D. and Wegkamp, M., Weak convergence of empirical copula processes, *Bernoulli* **10**, 2004, 847–860
4. Ivanoff, B.G. and Merzbach, E., *Set-Indexed Martingales*, Chapman and Hall/CRC Press, Boca Raton, 2000.
5. Ivanoff, B.G. and Merzbach, E., Random censoring in set-indexed survival analysis, *The Annals of Applied Probability* **12**, 2002, 944–971.
6. Ivanoff, B.G. and Merzbach, E., Random clouds and an application to censoring in survival analysis, *Stochastic Processes and Their Applications* **111**, 2004, 259–279.
7. Shaked, M. and Shanthikumar, J.G., *Stochastic Orders and Their Applications*, Academic Press, San Diego, 1994.
8. van der Vaart, A.W. and Wellner, J.A., *Weak Convergence and Empirical Processes*, Springer Series in Statistics, Springer-Verlag, New York, 1996.

IFSM Representation of Brownian Motion with Applications to Simulation

Stefano Maria Iacus and Davide La Torre

Department of Economics, Business and Statistics, University of Milan, Via Conservatorio, 7, I-20122 Milan, Italy
{stefano.iacus,davide.latorre}@unimi.it

Summary. Several methods are currently available to simulate paths of the Brownian motion. In particular, paths of the BM can be simulated using the properties of the increments of the process like in the Euler scheme, or as the limit of a random walk or via L^2 decomposition like the Kac-Siegert/Karnounen-Loeve series. In this paper we first propose a IFSM (Iterated Function Systems with Maps) operator whose fixed point is the trajectory of the BM. We then use this representation of the process to simulate its trajectories. The resulting simulated trajectories are self-affine, continuous and fractal by construction. This fact produces more realistic trajectories than other schemes in the sense that their geometry is closer to the one of the true BM's trajectories. The IFSM trajectory of the BM can then be used to generate more realistic solutions of stochastic differential equations.

1 Introduction

In this paper we show how to solve the inverse problem for IFSM in the case of trajectories of stochastic processes in L^2. The method is based on the solution of the inverse problem for IFSM due to Forte and Vrscay [2]. This is an extension of classical IFS methods which can be used for approximating a given element of L^2 thus in particular trajectories of stochastic processes on this space. The final goal of this approach is simulation. Indeed, several methods are currently available to simulate paths of stochastic processes and in particular of the Brownian motion. Paths of the BM can be simulated using the properties of the increments of the process like in the Euler scheme [3], or as the limit of a random walk or via L^2 decomposition like the Kac-Siegert/Karnounen-Loeve series [4]. In this paper we first propose a IFSM (Iterated Function Systems with Maps) operator whose fixed point is the trajectory of the BM. We then use this representation of the process to simulate its trajectories. The resulting simulated trajectories are self-affine, continuous and fractal by construction. This fact produces more realistic trajectories than other schemes in the sense that their geometry is closer to the one of the true BM's trajectories. The IFSM trajectory of the BM can then be used to generate more realistic solutions of stochastic differential equations. The paper is organized as follows: Section 2 recalls the theory of IFSM on L^2, Section 3 recalls some details for stochastic processes with trajectories in L^2 and the link with the IFSM theory. Section 4 presents the application of the IFSM theory to the problem of simulation with particular attention to the case of the Brownian motion.

2 IFS with Maps (IFSM) on $L^2([0,1])$

The basic idea of Iterated Function Systems (IFS) can be traced back to some historical papers but the use of such systems to construct fractals and other similar sets was first described by Hutchinson (1981). The fundamental result on which the IFS method is based is Banach theorem. The mathematical context is the following: given y in a complete metric space (Y, d_Y), find a contractive operator $T : Y \to Y$ that admits a unique fixed point $y^* \in Y$ such that $d_Y(y, y^*)$ is small enough. In fact if one is able to solve *the inverse problem* with arbitrary precision, it is possible to identify y with the operator T which has it as fixed point. The fundamental theorems on which the IFS method is based on are the following:

Theorem 1. *(Banach Theorem) Let (Y, d_Y) be a complete metric space; suppose there exists a mapping $T : Y \to Y$ such that*

$$d_Y(T(x), T(y)) \leq c d_Y(x, y)$$

for all $x, y \in Y$ and some $c \in [0, 1)$. c is said to be the contractivity factor of T. Then there exits a unique $y^* \in Y$ such that $T(y^*) = y^*$ and for any $y \in Y$ we have $d_Y(T^n(y), y^*) \to 0$ when $n \to +\infty$.

Theorem 2. *(Collage Theorem) Let (Y, d_Y) be a complete metric space. Given $y \in Y$ suppose that there exists a contractive map T with contractivity factor $c \in [0, 1)$ such that $d_Y(y, T(y)) < \epsilon$. If y^* is the fixed point of T then $d_Y(y, y^*) \leq \frac{\epsilon}{1-c}$.*

Theorem 3. *Let (Y, d_Y) be a complete metric space and T_1, T_2 be two contractive mappings with fixed points y_1^* and y_2^*. Then*

$$d_Y(y_1^*, y_2^*) \leq \frac{1}{1 - c_1} d_{Y,\mathrm{sup}}(T_1, T_2)$$

where

$$d_{Y,\mathrm{sup}}(T_1, T_2) = \sup_{x \in Y} d_Y(T_1(x), T_2(x))$$

and c_1 is the contractivity factor of T_1.

We are going to use a particular class of IFS operators, known as IFSM (IFS with Maps), introduced by Forte and Vrscay in 1994. Let μ be the Lebesgue measure on $\mathcal{B}([0,1])$ (the Borel σ-algebra) and for any integer $p \geq 1$ let $L^p([0,1])$ denote the linear space of all real valued functions u such that u^p is integrable on $(\mathcal{B}([0,1]), \mu)$. To build a contraction map T on $L^2([0,1])$ we need N-map contractive IFS i.e. a set of maps $w = \{w_1, w_2, \ldots, w_N\}$ and a set of functions (grey level maps) $\phi = \{\phi_1, \phi_2, \ldots, \phi_N\}$ with $\phi_i : \mathbb{R} \to \mathbb{R}$. The operator T corresponding to the N map IFSM(w, ϕ) is

$$(Tu)(x) = \sum_{k=1}^{N}{}' \phi_k(u(w_k^{-1}(x))) \tag{1}$$

where the prime means that the sum operates on all those terms for which w_k^{-1} (the inverse function of w_k) is defined. Let us define the following two sets

$$\mathcal{S}im([0,1]) = \{w : [0,1] \to [0,1] : \exists c \in [0,1),$$
$$|w(x) - w(y)| = c|x - y|, \forall x, y \in [0,1]\}$$
$$\mathcal{L}ip(\mathbb{R}) = \{\phi : \mathbb{R} \to \mathbb{R} : \exists K \in [0, \infty),$$
$$|\phi(t_1) - \phi(t_2)| \leq K|t_1 - t_2|, \forall t_1, t_2 \in \mathbb{R}\}$$

Theorem 4. *[2] Let (w, ϕ) be an IFSM such that $w_k \in \mathcal{S}im([0,1])$ and $\phi_k \in \mathcal{L}ip(\mathbb{R})$ for $1 \leq k \leq N$. Then $T : L^2([0,1]) \to L^2([0,1])$ and for any $u, v \in L^2([0,1])$ we have*

$$||Tu - Tv||_2 \leq C||u - v||_2$$

where

$$C = \sum_{k=1}^{N} c_k^{\frac{1}{2}} K_k$$

Given $u \in L^2([0,1])$ the inverse problem consists of finding the operator T such that

$$u(x) = (Tu)(x) = \sum_{k=1}^{N}{}' \phi_k(u(w_k^{-1}(x))).$$

In the special case when

- $\bigcup_{k=1}^{N} H_k = \bigcup_{k=1}^{N} w_i([0,1]) = [0,1]$ i.e. the sets H_k "tile" $[0,1]$
- $\mu(w_i([0,1]) \cap w_j([0,1])) = 0$ for $i \neq j$

we say that the maps w_k are nonoverlapping. In [2] it is proved that in the non overlapping case the problem can be reduced to the determination of grey level maps ϕ_k which minimize the collage distance Δ^2

$$\Delta^2 = ||v - Tv||_2^2 = \int_0^1 \sum_{k=1}^{N}{}' ||\phi_k(v(w_k^{-1}(x))) - v(x)|| d\mu.$$

Later, in the applications, we will assume that, for $1 \leq k \leq N$,

- $w_k(x) = s_k x + a_k$
- $0 < c_k = |s_k| < 1$
- $\phi_k(t) = \alpha_k t + \beta_k$, $K_k = |\alpha_k|$

The collage distance becomes

$$\Delta^2 = <v - Tv, v - Tv> =$$

$$\sum_{k=1}^{N}\sum_{l=1}^{N} <\psi_k, \psi_l> \alpha_k \alpha_l + 2 <\psi_k, \xi_l> \alpha_k \beta_l + <\xi_k, \xi_l> \beta_k \beta_l$$

$$-2N \sum_{k=1}^{N} <v, \psi_k> \alpha_k + <v, \xi_k> \beta_k + <v, v>$$

where

$$\psi_k(x) = v(w_k^{-1}(x)), \qquad \xi_k(x) = I_{w_k([0,1])}(x)$$

Δ^2 is a quadratic form in α_i and β_i, that is

$$\Delta^2 = x^T A x + b^T x + c \tag{2}$$

where $x = (\alpha_1, \dots \alpha_k, \beta_1, \dots, \beta_k)$. The matrix A is symmetric and

$$a_{i,j} = <\psi_i, \psi_j>, a_{N+i,N+j} = <\xi_i, \xi_j>$$

$$a_{i,N+j} = <\psi_i, \xi_j>, b_i = -2 <v, \psi_i>, b_{N+i} = -2 <v, \xi_i>$$

and $c = \|v\|_2^2$. As in [2] we add an additional constraint in order to guarantee that the minimum of this quadratic form exists on a compact subset of feasible parameters α_i and β_i. The additional constraint is

$$\sum_{k=1}^{N} c_k(\alpha_k\|v\|_1 + \beta_k) - \|v\|_1 \le 0.$$

The maps w_k are choosen in an infinite set $\mathcal{W}$ of fixed affine contraction maps on $[0,1]$ which has the μ-dense and nonoverlapping property (in the sense of the following definition); When $(\alpha_k, \beta_k) = (0,0)$ the corresponding w_k is superfluous and the k-th term can be dropped from (1).

Definition 1. *We say that $\mathcal{W}$ generates a μ-dense and nonoverlapping family $\mathcal{F}$ of subsets of $[0,1]$ if for every $\epsilon > 0$ and every $B \subset [0,1]$ there exists a finite set of integers i_k, $i_k \ge 1$, $1 \le k \le N$, such that*

- $A = \cup_{k=1}^{N} w_{i_k}([0,1]) \subset B$
- $\mu(B \backslash A) < \epsilon$
- $\mu(w_{i_k}([0,1]) \cap w_{i_l}([0,1])) = 0$ *if* $k \ne l$

Let

$$\mathcal{W}^N = \{w_1, \dots w_N\}$$

be the N truncations of $\mathcal{W}$. Let $\Phi^N = \{\phi_1, \dots, \phi_N\}$ the N vector of affine grey level maps. Let x^N be the solution of the previous quadratic optimization problem (2) and $\Delta^2_{N,min} = \Delta^2_N(x^N)$. It can be shown that $\Delta^2_{N,min}$ may be arbitrarly small when $N \to \infty$ (see [2]).

3 IFSM for Stochastic Processes on $L^2([0,1])$

Let $(\Omega, \mathcal{F}, P)$ be a probability space and $\{\mathcal{F}_t, t \in [0,1]\}$ be a sequence of σ-algebras such that $\mathcal{F}_t \subset \mathcal{F}$. Let $X(\omega, t) : \Omega \times [0,1] \to \mathbb{R}$ be a stochastic process in $L^2([0,1])$, that is a sequence of random variables $\mathcal{F}_t$-adapted (that is each variable $X(\omega, t)$ is $\mathcal{F}_t$-measurable). Given $\omega \in \Omega$ a trajectory of the process is the function $X(\omega, t) : [0,1] \to \mathbb{R}$ belonging to $L^2([0,1])$. For a given $X(\omega, t)$, the trajectory of the stochastic process, the aim of the inverse problem consists in finding the parameters of the IFSM such that $X(\omega, t)$ is the solution of the equation

$$X(\omega, t) = TX(\omega, t) \quad \text{for a.a.} \quad \omega \in \Omega$$

In this case the coefficients of the matrix A and the vector b of the previous section become

$$a_{i,j}(\omega) = \int_0^1 X(\omega, w_i^{-1}(t))X(\omega, w_j^{-1}(t))dt$$

$$= \int_{w_i([0,1]) \cap w_j([0,1])} X(\omega, w_i^{-1}(t))X(\omega, w_j^{-1}(t))dt$$

and if $i = j$ it becomes

$$a_{i,i}(\omega) = c_i \int_0^1 X^2(\omega, t)dt$$

The other elements in the matrix A can be calculated as

$$a_{N+i,N+j} = <\xi_i, \xi_j> = \int_0^1 I_{w_i([0,1])}(t)I_{w_j([0,1])}(t)dt$$

$$= \mu(w_i([0,1]) \cap w_j([0,1]))$$

and

$$a_{i,N+j}(\omega) = <\psi_i, \xi_j> = \int_{w_i([0,1]) \cap w_j([0,1])} X(\omega, w_i^{-1}(t))dt$$

For the vector b

$$b_i(\omega) = -2 <X, \psi_i> = -2 \int_0^1 X(\omega, t)X(\omega, w_i^{-1}(t))dt$$

and

$$b_{N+i}(\omega) = -2 <X, \xi_i> = -2 \int_{w_i([0,1])} X(\omega, t)dt$$

In the nonoverlapping case, we have

- $a_{i,j} = 0$, $i \neq j$, and $a_{i,i}(\omega) = c_i \int_0^1 X^2(\omega, t)dt$, $1 \leq i, j \leq N$

- $a_{N+i,N+j} = 0$, $1 \leq i,j \leq N$, $i \neq j$ and $a_{N+i,N+i} = \mu(w_i([0,1]))$
- $a_{i,N+j} = 0$, $1 \leq i,j \leq N$, $i \neq j$ and $a_{i,N+i}(\omega) = c_i \int_0^1 X(\omega,t)dt$

It also holds this self-similarity property.

Theorem 5. *Let (α_k, β_k) be the solution of the inverse problem with a set of nonverlapping maps w_k and suppose that $X(\omega,t) = T\tilde{X}(\omega,t)$. Then*

$$\tilde{X}(\omega, w_i(t+h)) - \tilde{X}(\omega, w_i(t)) = \alpha_i(\tilde{X}(\omega, t+h) - \tilde{X}(\omega, t)).$$

for all $1 \leq i \leq N$.

Proof. In fact we have

$$\tilde{X}(\omega, w_i(t+h)) - \tilde{X}(\omega, w_i(t)) = T\tilde{X}(\omega, w_i(t+h)) - T\tilde{X}(\omega, w_i(t))$$

$$= \sum_{k=1}^{N} \alpha_k(\tilde{X}(\omega, w_k^{-1}(w_i(t+h)))) + \beta_k - \sum_{k=1}^{N} \alpha_k(\tilde{X}(\omega, w_k^{-1}(w_i(t)))) + \beta_k$$

$$= \alpha_i(\tilde{X}(\omega, w_i^{-1}(w_i(t+h)))) + \beta_i - \alpha_i(\tilde{X}(\omega, w_i^{-1}(w_i(t)))) + \beta_i$$

$$= \alpha_i(\tilde{X}(\omega, t+h) - \tilde{X}(\omega, t)). \qquad \square$$

3.1 The Kac-Siegert Decomposition of $L^2([0,1])$ Stochastic Processes

We suppose that a.e. $X(\omega,t)$ is an element of a subspace S of $L^2([0,1[)$ and that $X(\omega,t)$ is a zero-mean process. Let K be the covariance function of this process that is

$$K(s,t) = \text{Cov}\left[X(\omega,s), X(\omega,t)\right].$$

and assume

$$\int_0^1 K(t,t)dt < \infty.$$

If $\lambda_1 \geq \lambda_2 \geq \ldots > 0$ comprises the entire spectrum of eigenvalues of K, where

$$\int_0^1 f(s)K(s,t)dt = \lambda f(s), \ 0 \leq t \leq 1$$

and the associated orthonormal eigenfunctions f_i form a complete set of the subspace S then the Kac and Siegert decomposition holds:

$$K(s,t) = \sum_{j=1}^{\infty} \lambda_j f_j(s) f_j(t), \ 0 < s,t < 1$$

We also have that

$$Z_j = \int_0^1 X(t) f_j(t) dt$$

are uncorrelated random variables with mean 0 and variance λ_j. The following theorem states some properties of this decomposition.

Theorem 6 (see Ch.5, [4]). *Suppose that X and K satisfies the properties above. Then*

- *i)* $\sum_{j=0}^{\infty} \lambda_j < \infty$
- *ii)* $\sum_{j=1}^{m} Z_j f_j \to_{\|\|_2} X$ *as* $m \to \infty$ *a.s.*
- *iii)* $Z_j =< X, f_j >$ *are with mean 0 and variance* λ_j
- *iv)* $\int_0^1 X^2(t)dt = \sum_{j=1}^{\infty} Z_j^2 = \sum_{j=1}^{\infty} \lambda_j Z_j^{*2}$ *where* $Z_j^* = \frac{Z_j}{\sqrt{\lambda_j}}$
- *v)* $E[X(t) - \sum_{j=1}^{m} Z_j f_j(t)]^2 \to 0$ *for each* t *as* $m \to \infty$
- *vi)* $X = \sum_{j=1}^{m} \sqrt{\lambda_j} f_j Z_j^*$ *with* $Z_j^* = \frac{Z_j}{\sqrt{\lambda_j}}$ *uncorrelated with mean 0 and variance 1.*

4 Simulation of Brownian Motion via IFSM

In the literature there are several methods of simulation of the trajectory of the Browian motion, i.e. the stochastic process $\{B(\omega, t), t \in [0, 1]\}$, such that $B(0) = 0$ a.s., $B(t) - B(s)$ is distributed with Gaussian law with zero mean and variance $t - s$, and with independent increments.

The Euler Method

In this case, the trajectory is obtained simulating the increments of B in the following way: $B(0) = 0$, $B(t_{i+1}) = B(t_i) + \sqrt{t_{i+1} - t_i} \cdot Z_i$, where the Z_i's are independent $\mathcal{N}(0, 1)$ random variables. In the other points the trajectory is built by linear interpolation of these simulated data.

The Kac-Siegert Method

Karhunen-Loève / Kac-Siegert decomposition of B is better for pathwise simulation

$$B(\omega, t) = \sum_{i=0}^{\infty} Z_i \phi_i(t), \quad 0 \leq t \leq 1$$

with

$$\phi_i(t) = \frac{2\sqrt{2}}{(2i+1)\pi} \sin\left(\frac{(2i+1)\pi t}{2}\right)$$

ϕ_i a basis of orthogonal functions and Z_i's are $\mathcal{N}(0, 1)$

The trajectory generated by Euler method is too simple and regular to mimic the roughness of the BM; moreover the simulated path is stochastically equivalent to the true trajectory only on the points of the grid used in the simulation. The Kac-Siegert decomposition of the BM is a pathwise approximation which can lead to a too smooth path (see figure 1); our idea is to use IFSM for generating fractal trajectories of the BM. There are applications in finance (for instance pricing of american options) in which the whole path matters; our IFSM approch produces a global approximation of the trajectory preserving the geometric fractal nature of the target.

This method can be also used to simulate paths of solutions of stochastic differential equations driven by Brownian motion (e.g. diffusion processes) replacing the linear behaviour of the Euler trajectory with a fractal object.

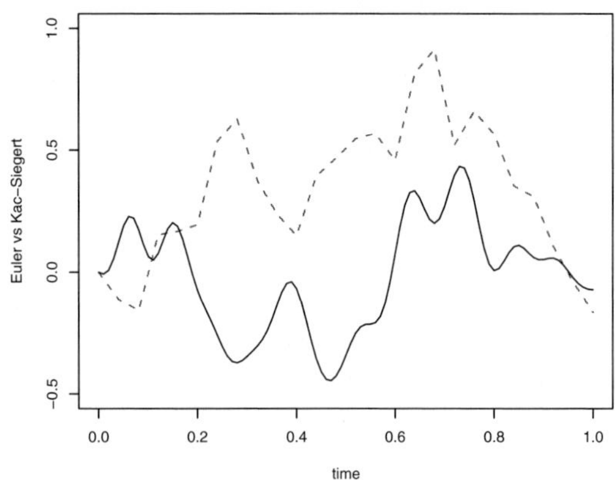

Fig. 1: Paths of Brownian motion simulated by the Euler scheme (dotted line) and using Kac-Siegert decomposition (continuous line). The same ($n = 25$) pseudo-random Gaussian numbers were used.

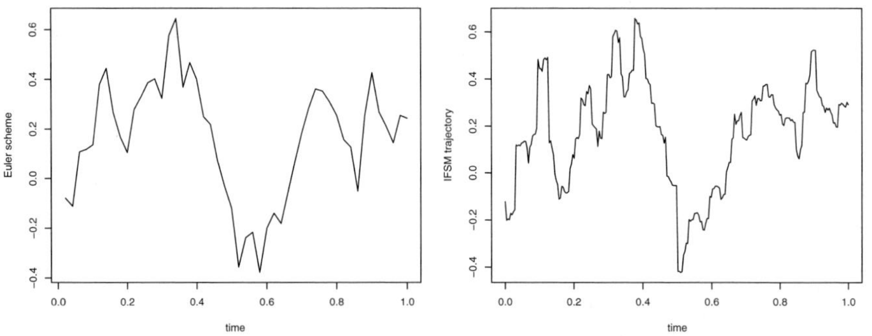

Fig. 2: Euler scheme versus IFSM trajectory of the Browninan motion. IFSM with wavelet type maps and $M = 8$. Both methods used the same 50 Gaussian random terms to generate the trajectory.

For the solution of the inverse problem for the BM, we choose the so-called wavelet type maps [2], that is:

$$w_{ij}^*(x) = \frac{x + j - 1}{2^i}$$

with $i = 1, 2, \ldots$ and $j = 1 \ldots 2^i$ For each fixed i, the family w_{ij}^* is a set of nonoverlapping maps. For these maps $c_i = 2^{-i} < 1$. We organize them as follows

$$w_1 = w_{11}^* \quad w_2 = w_{12}^* \quad w_3 = w_{21}^* \quad w_4 = w_{22}^* \ldots$$

To simulate a trajectory of B with non overlapping maps we then need to simulate the joint distribution of all this objects

1. $\displaystyle\int_0^1 B^2(t)dt$

2. $\displaystyle\int_0^1 B(t)dt$

3. $\displaystyle\int_0^1 B(t)B(w_i^{-1}(t))dt = \int_0^1 B(t)B\left(\frac{t - a_i}{s_i}\right)dt$

4. $\displaystyle\int_{w_i([0,1])} B(t)dt$

5. $\displaystyle\int_0^1 |B(t)|dt$

but it appears to be still a too difficult problem.

In practice, it is preferable to use all the above maps and not only the subset of non-overlapping maps. In this case, we need simulate the value of the trajectory of the Brownian motion on a fixed grid (using one of the known methods) and we use these points to approximate the integrals in the quadratic form. We then solve the constrained quadratic programming problem using standard algorithms (see e.g. [1]). Figure 2 bottom shows an example of trajectory generated using the IFSM approach using wavelet type maps for $i = 1, \ldots, M$, $M = 8$. Figure 2 top represents the Euler trajectory built on 50 Gaussian terms which has been used to build the IFSM. As one can notice the IFSM path shows more "fractal" complexity then the corresponding Euler path.

5 Conclusions

We have proposed a new method to generate paths of the Brownian motion. These IFSM paths seem to mimic more closely the fractal nature of the trajectory of the Brownian motion than existing schemes. At current stage we are not able to show formal property of the IFSM path in terms of strong and weak approximation (see [3]). Open source software for generating IFSM trajectories written in C and R language [5] is available via `ifs` package at `http://CRAN.R-project.org` for free download.

References

1. Byrd, R.H., Lu, P., Nocedal, J. and Zhu, C. (1995), "A limited memory algorithm for bound constrained optimization", *SIAM J. Scientific Computing*, 16, 1190-1208.
2. Forte, B., Vrscay, E.R. (1995), "Solving the inverse problem for function/image approximation using iterated function systems, I. Theoretical basis", *Fractal*, **2**, 3, 325-334.
3. Kloden, P., Platen, E., Shurtz, H. (2000), Numerical Solution of SDE through computer experiments, Springer, Berlin.
4. Shorack, G., Wellner, J.A. (1986), Empirical processes with applications to statistics, Wiley, New York.
5. R Development Core Team (2005), R: A language and environment for statistical computing. R Foundation for Statistical Computing, Vienna, Austria. ISBN 3-900051-07-0, URL http://www.R-project.org

Iterated Function Systems on Multifunctions

Davide La Torre[1], Franklin Mendivil[2] and Edward R. Vrscay[3]

[1] Department of Economics, Business and Statistics, University of Milan, Italy
   davide.latorre@unimi.it
[2] Department of Mathematics and Statistics, Acadia University, Wolfville, Nova
   Scotia, Canada
   franklin.mendivil@acadiau.ca
[3] Department of Applied Mathematics, University of Waterloo, Waterloo, Ontario,
   Canada
   ervrscay@uwaterloo.ca

Dedicated to the memory of Professor Bruno Forte

Summary. We introduce a method of iterated function systems (IFS) over the
space of set-valued mappings (multifunctions). This is done by first considering a
couple of useful metrics over the space of multifunctions $\mathcal{F}(X,Y)$. Some appropriate IFS-type fractal transform operators $T : \mathcal{F}(X,Y) \to \mathcal{F}(X,Y)$ are then defined
which combine spatially-contracted and range-modified copies of a multifunction u
to produce a new multifunction $v = Tu$. Under suitable conditions, the fractal transform T is contractive, implying the existence of a fixed-point set-valued mapping $\bar{u}$.
Some simple examples are then presented.

We then consider the inverse problem of approximation of set-valued mappings
by fixed points of fractal transform operators T and present some preliminary results.

1 Introduction

In this paper, we introduce a method of iterated function systems (IFS) over
spaces of set-valued mappings or *multifunctions*. The idea of studying the action of sets of contraction mappings in $\mathbb{R}^n$ can be traced back to a number of
very interesting historical papers. However, the landmark papers by Hutchinson [7] and Barnsley and Demko [2] showed how such systems of contractive
maps with associated probabilities – called "iterated function systems" by the
latter – acting in a parallel manner, either deterministically or probabilisti-
cally, could be used to construct fractal sets and measures.

This formulation of an IFS-type method over multifunction represents recent results of an ongoing research programme on the construction of appropriate IFS-type operators, or *generalized fractal transforms*, over various
spaces, i.e., function spaces and distributions [5, 6], vector-valued measures

[10], integral transforms [4] and wavelet transforms [9, 11]. Very briefly, and at the risk of sacrificing rigor, the action of a GFT T on an element u of the complete metric space (X, d) under consideration can be summarized as follows: (i) it produces a set of N spatially-contracted copies of u, (ii) it then modifies the values of these copies by means of a suitable range-mapping and finally (iii) it recombines these copies using an appropriate operator to produce the element $v \in X$, $v = Tu$. (In the case of fractal-wavelet transforms [9, 11], the copies of u in (i) are actually subtrees of a tree that are then copied onto lower positions of the tree.)

In each of the above-mentioned cases, the fractal transform T is guaranteed to be contractive when the parameters defining it satisfy appropriate conditions specific to the metric space of concern. In this situation, Banach's fixed point theorem guarantees the existence of a unique fixed point $\bar{u} = T\bar{u}$.

The *inverse problem* of fractal-based approximation is as follows: Given an element y, can we find a fractal transform T with fixed point $\bar{u}$ so that $d(y, \bar{u})$ is sufficiently small. However, the search for such transforms is enormously complicated. Thanks to a simple consequence of Banach's fixed point theorem known as the "Collage Theorem" (to be discussed below), most practical methods of solving the inverse problem seek to find an operator T for which the *collage distance* $d(u, Tu)$ is as small as possible.

In this paper, as stated above, we formulate some IFS-type fractal transform operators on the space of set-valued mappings over closed and bounded intervals of $\mathbb{R}^n$. We first consider a couple of metrics over these spaces and then establish the Lipschitz constants of the fractal transforms in these metrics. Some graphical examples are then presented.

Finally, we present an application of this method of "IFS over multifunctions" (IFSMF) to fractal image coding and present a simple example of an IFSMF-coded image multifunction.

2 Preliminary Results on Hausdorff Distance

In the following we will denote by $\mathcal{H}(Y)$ the space of all non-empty compact subsets of Y and by $d_h(A, B)$ the Hausdorff distance between A and B, that is

$$d_h(A, B) = \max\{\max_{x \in A} d(x, B), \max_{x \in B} d(x, A)\},$$

where $d(x, y)$ is the Euclidean norm and $d(x, A)$ is the usual distance between the point x and the set A, i.e.,

$$d(x, A) = \min_{y \in A} d(x, y).$$

It is well known that the space $(\mathcal{H}(Y), d_h)$ is a complete metric space if Y is complete [7]. We now prove some results concerning this metric.

Lemma 1. *Let* $A, B, I \subset \mathbb{R}^n$. *Then* $d_h(A + I, B + I) \leq d_h(A, B)$.

Proof. We see that

$$d(A+I, B+I) = \max_{a+i} \min_{b+j} \|(a+i)-(b+j)\|$$
$$\leq \max_{a+i} \min_{b} \|(a+i)-(b+i)\|$$
$$= \max_{a+i} \min_{b} \|a-b\| = d(A,B).$$

By symmetry we also have $d(B+I, A+I) \leq d(B,A)$, which gives the desired result. $\square$

Lemma 2. *Let $A_i, B_i \subset \mathbb{R}^n$ and $\lambda_i \geq 0$ for $i = 1, 2, \ldots, N$. Then*

$$d_h\left(\sum_i \lambda_i A_i, \sum_i \lambda_i B_i\right) \leq \sum_i \lambda_i \, d_h(A_i, B_i).$$

Proof. For simplicity we prove the case $i = 2$. Computing, we see that

$$d(\lambda_1 A_1 + \lambda_2 A_2, \lambda_1 B_1 + \lambda_2 B_2) = \max_{a_1,a_2} \min_{b_1,b_2} \|\lambda_1 a_1 + \lambda_2 a_2 - \lambda_1 b_1 - \lambda_2 b_2\|$$
$$\leq \max_{a_1,a_2} \min_{b_1,b_2} [\lambda_1 \|a_1 - b_1\| + \lambda_2 \|a_2 - b_2\|]$$
$$= \lambda_1 \max_{a_1} \min_{b_1} \|a_1 - b_1\| + \lambda_2 \max_{a_2} \min_{b_2} \|a_2 - b_2\|$$
$$= \lambda_1 d(A_1, B_1) + \lambda_2 d(A_2, B_2).$$

Similarly we have that $d(\lambda_1 B_1 + \lambda_2 B_2, \lambda_1 A_1 + \lambda_2 A_2) \leq \lambda_1 d(B_1, A_1) + \lambda_2 d(B_2, A_2)$. Since $d(A_1, B_1) \leq d_h(A_1, B_1)$ and $d(B_1, A_1) \leq d_h(A_1, B_1)$, we have the desired result. $\square$

It is easy to see that if A is convex and $\lambda_i \geq 0$ with $\sum_i \lambda_i = 1$ then $A = \sum_i \lambda_i A$. Using this observation and the previous result we easily get the following lemma.

Lemma 3. *Let $A, B, C \subset \mathbb{R}^n$, $\lambda_1, \lambda_2 \in [0,1]$ such that $\lambda_1 + \lambda_2 = 1$. Suppose that A, B, C are compact and A is convex. Then*

$$d_h(A, \lambda_1 B + \lambda_2 C) \leq \lambda_1 d_h(A, B) + \lambda_2 d_h(A, C).$$

Example 1. The previous lemma is not true without the convexity of the set A; for instance, take

$$A = \{(x,y) \in \mathbb{R}^2 : 0 \leq x \leq 1, y = 1\} \cup \{(x,y) \in \mathbb{R}^2 : x = 0, 1/2 \leq y \leq 1\}$$

$$\cup \{(x,y) \in \mathbb{R}^2 : x = 1, 1/2 \leq y \leq 1\}$$

and $B = (0,0)$, $C = (1,0)$, $\lambda_1 = \lambda_2 = 1/2$. Then

$$d_h(A, \lambda_1 B + \lambda_2 C) = 1 \geq \lambda_1 d_h(A, B) + \lambda_2 d_h(A, C) = 1/2.$$

3 Some IFS Operators on Multifunctions

The aim of this section is to introduce some IFS operators of the space of multifunctions. We recall that a setvalued mappings or multifunction $F : X \rightrightarrows Y$ is a function from X to the power set 2^Y. We recall that the graph of F is the following subset of $X \times Y$

$$\mathrm{graph}F = \{(x, y) \in X \times Y : y \in F(x)\}.$$

If $F(x)$ is a closed, compact or convex we say that F is closed, compact or convex valued, respectively. Let $(X, \mathbb{B}, \mu)$ be a finite measure space; a multifunction $F : X \to Y$ is said to be measurable if for each open $O \subset Y$ we have

$$F^{-1}(O) = \{x \in X : F(x) \cap O \neq \emptyset\} \in \mathbb{B}$$

A function $f : X \to Y$ is a selection of F if $f(x) \in F(x)$, $\forall x \in X$. In the following we will suppose that Y is compact and $F(x)$ is compact for each $x \in X$. Define

$$\mathcal{F}(X, Y) = \{F : X \to \mathcal{H}(Y)\}.$$

We place the following two metrics on $\mathcal{F}(X, Y)$; the first is

$$d_\infty(F, G) = \sup_{x \in X} d_h(F(x), G(x))$$

and the second (here μ is a finite measure on X and $p \geq 1$)

$$d_p(F, G) = \left(\int_X d_h(F(x), G(x))^p \, d\mu(x) \right)^{1/p}.$$

Proposition 1. *The space $(\mathcal{F}(X, Y), d_\infty)$ is a complete metric space.*

Proof. It is trivial to prove that $d_\infty(F, G) = 0$ if and only if $F = G$ and that $d_\infty(F, G) = d_\infty(G, F)$. Furthermore for all $F, G, L \in \mathcal{F}(X, Y)$ we have

$$\begin{aligned}
d_\infty(F, G) &= \sup_{x \in X} d_h(F(x), G(x)) \\
&\leq \sup_{x \in X} d_h(F(x), L(x)) + d_h(L(x), G(x)) \\
&\leq \sup_{x \in X} d_h(F(x), L(x)) + \sup_{x \in X} d_h(L(x), G(x)) \\
&= d_\infty(F, L) + d_\infty(L, G)
\end{aligned}$$

To prove that it is a complete, let F_n be a Cauchy sequence of elements of $\mathcal{F}(X, Y)$; so $\forall \epsilon > 0$ there exists $n_0(\epsilon) > 0$ such that for all $n, m \geq n_0(\epsilon)$ we have $d_\infty(F_n, F_m) \leq \epsilon$. So for all $x \in X$ and for all $n, m \geq n_0(\epsilon)$ we have $d_h(F_n(x), F_m(x)) \leq \epsilon$ and the sequence $F_n(x)$ is Cauchy in $\mathcal{H}(Y)$. Since it is complete there exists $A(x)$ such that $d_h(F_n(x), A(x)) \to 0$ when $n \to +\infty$. So for all $x \in X$ and for all $n, m \geq n_0(\epsilon)$ we have $d_h(F_n(x), F_m(x)) \leq \epsilon$ and sending $m \to +\infty$ we have $d_h(F_n(x), A(x)) \leq \epsilon$ that is $d_\infty(F_n, A) \leq \epsilon$. $\square$

Proposition 2. d_p *is a (pseudo) metric on* $\mathcal{F}(X, Y)$.

Proof. It is clear that $d_p(F, G) = 0$ iff $d_h(F(x), G(x)) = 0$ for μ almost all $x \in X$ which happens iff $F(x) = G(x)$ for μ almost all $x \in X$. It is also clear that d_p is symmetric. For the triangle inequality, notice that

$$
\begin{aligned}
d_p(F, G) &= \left(\int_X d_h(F(x), G(x))^p \, d\mu(x) \right)^{1/p} \\
&\leq \left(\int_X [d_h(F(x), H(x)) + d_h(H(x), G(x))]^p \, d\mu(x) \right)^{1/p} \\
&\leq \left(\int_X d_h(F(x), H(x))^p \, d\mu(x) \right)^{1/p} + \left(\int_X d_h(H(x), G(x))^p \, d\mu(x) \right)^{1/p} \\
&= d_p(F, H) + d_p(H, G). \qquad \square
\end{aligned}
$$

Notice that we only get a pseudo-metric since functions which differ only on a set of μ measure zero will clearly be zero distance apart. However, this is the usual situation with the L^p spaces.

Proposition 3. *Let* Y *be a compact interval of* $\mathbb{R}$ *and suppose that* $F(x)$ *is convex for each* $x \in X$ *and for all* $F \in \mathcal{F}(X, Y)$. *Suppose that all* $F \in \mathcal{F}(X, Y)$ *are measurable. Then* $\mathcal{F}(X, Y)$ *is complete under* d_p.

Proof. To prove that it is a complete, let F_n be a Cauchy sequence of elements of $\mathcal{F}(X, Y)$; so $\forall \epsilon > 0$ there exists $n_0(\epsilon) > 0$ such that for all $n, m \geq n_0(\epsilon)$ we have $d_p(F_n, F_m) \leq \epsilon$. Since $F_n(x)$ is compact and convex then $F_n(x) = [\min F_n(x), \max F_x(x)]$. The functions $\phi_n^*(x) = \min F_n(x)$ and $\phi_n^{**}(x) = \max F_n(x)$ are measurable and

$$
\|\phi_n^*(x) - \phi_m^*(x)\|_p \leq d_p(F_n, F_m)
$$

$$
\|\phi_n^{**}(x) - \phi_m^*(x)\|_p \leq d_p(F_n, F_m)
$$

and so ϕ_n^* and ϕ_n^{**} are Cauchy in $L^p(X)$. So there exists ϕ^* and ϕ^{**} such that $\phi_n^* \to \phi^*$ and $\phi_n^{**} \to \phi^{**}$ in the usual L^p metric. If we build the function $F(x) = [\phi^*(x), \phi^{**}(x)]$ then

$$
\begin{aligned}
d_p(F_n, F) &= \left(\int_X d_h(F_n(x), F(x))^p \, d\mu(x) \right)^{1/p} \\
&= \left(\int_X \max\{|\phi_n^*(x) - \phi^*(x)|^p, |\phi_n^{**}(x) - \phi^{**}(x)|^p\} \, d\mu(x) \right)^{1/p} \\
&\leq \left(\int_X |\phi_n^*(x) - \phi^*(x)|^p \, d\mu(x) \right)^{1/p} \\
&\quad + \left(\int_X |\phi_n^{**}(x) - \phi^{**}(x)|^p \, d\mu(x) \} \right)^{1/p} \qquad \square
\end{aligned}
$$

Having these preliminaries out of the way, in next sections we define a two IFS-type operators on $\mathcal{F}(X, Y)$.

3.1 The Union Operator

Let $w_i : X \to X$ be maps on X and $\phi_i : \mathcal{H}(Y) \to \mathcal{H}(Y)$ are Lipschitz continuous with respect to the Hausdorff metric and K_i are the corresponding Lipschitz constants. Define $T : \mathcal{F}(X,Y) \to \mathcal{F}(X,Y)$ by

$$T(F)(x) = \bigcup_i \phi_i(F(w_i^{-1}(x))).$$

Proposition 4. *If $K = \max_i K_i < 1$, then T is contractive in d_∞.*

Proof. We compute that

$$\begin{aligned}
d_\infty(T(F), T(G)) &= \sup_x \, d_h \left(\bigcup_i \phi_i(F(w_i^{-1}(x))), \bigcup_i \phi_i(G(w_i^{-1}(x))) \right) \\
&\leq \sup_x \max_i \, d_h \left(\phi_i(F(w_i^{-1}(x))), \phi_i(G(w_i^{-1}(x))) \right) \\
&\leq \sup_x \max_i K_i d_h \left(F(w_i^{-1}(x)), G(w_i^{-1}(x)) \right) \\
&\leq K \sup_z \, d_h(F(z), G(z)) = K d_\infty(F, G).
\end{aligned}$$

The result follows. $\square$

Proposition 5. *Assume that $d\mu(w_i(x)) \leq s_i d\mu(x)$ where $s_i \geq 0$. Then*

$$d_p(T(F), T(G)) \leq \left(\sum_i K_i^p s_i \right)^{1/p} d_p(F, G).$$

Proof. Computing, we get

$$\begin{aligned}
d_p(T(F), T(G)) &= \left\{ \int_X d_h \left[\bigcup_i \phi_i(F(w_i^{-1}(x))), \bigcup_i \phi_i(G(w_i^{-1}(x))) \right]^p d\mu(x) \right\}^{1/p} \\
&\leq \left\{ \int_X \max_i d_h \left[\phi_i(F(w_i^{-1}(x))), \phi_i(G(w_i^{-1}(x))) \right]^p d\mu(x) \right\}^{1/p} \\
&\leq \left\{ \int_X \max_i K_i \, d_h \left[F(w_i^{-1}(x)), G(w_i^{-1}(x)) \right]^p d\mu(x) \right\}^{1/p} \\
&= \left\{ \sum_i K_i^p \int_{M_i} d_h \left[F(w_i^{-1}(x)), G(w_i^{-1}(x)) \right]^p d\mu(x) \right\}^{1/p} \\
&\leq \left\{ \sum_i K_i^p \int_{w_i(X)} d_h \left[F(w_i^{-1}(x)), G(w_i^{-1}(x)) \right]^p d\mu(x) \right\}^{1/p} \\
&\leq \left\{ \sum_i K_i^p s_i \int_X d_h \left[F(z), G(z) \right]^p d\mu(z) \right\}^{1/p} \\
&= \left[\sum_i K_i^p s_i \right]^{1/p} d_p(F, G).
\end{aligned}$$

In the above, we have used the sets $M_i \subset w_i(X)$ defined by

$$M_i = \left\{ x \in X : d_h(F(w_i^{-1}(x)), G(w_i^{-1}(x))) \geq d_h(F(w_j^{-1}(x)), G(w_j^{-1}(x))) \text{ for all } j \right\}.$$

That is, the set M_i consists of all those points for which the ith preimage gives the largest Hausdorff distance. $\square$

Notice that if $X \subset \mathbb{R}$ and μ is Lebesgue measure and $w_i(x)$ satisfy $|w_i'(x)| \leq s_i$ then the condition $d\mu(w_i(x)) \leq s_i d\mu(x)$ is satisfied. This is the situation that is used in image processing applications.

3.2 The Sum Operator

With a similar setup as in the previous section, define the operator $T : \mathcal{F}(X,Y) \to \mathcal{F}(X,Y)$ by

$$T(F)(x) = \sum_i p_i(x)\phi_i(F(w_i^{-1}(x)))$$

where the sum depends on x and is over those i so that $x \in w_i(X)$. We require that the functions p_i satisfy that $\sum_i p_i(x) = 1$ (again, with the dependence of the sum on x).

The idea is to average the contributions of the various components in the areas where there is overlap.

Proposition 6. *We have*

$$d_\infty(T(F), T(G)) \leq \left[\sup_x \sum_i p_i(x) K_i \right] d_\infty(F, G).$$

Proof. We compute and see that

$$d_\infty(T(F), T(G))$$

$$= \sup_x d_h\left(\sum_i p_i(x)\phi_i(F(w_i^{-1}(x))), \sum_i p_i(x)\phi_i(G(w_i^{-1}(x))) \right)$$

$$\leq \sup_x \sum_i p_i(x) K_i d_h(F(w_i^{-1}(x)), G(w_i^{-1}(x)))$$

$$\leq \left[\sup_x \sum_i p_i(x) K_i \right] d_\infty(F, G). \qquad \square$$

Lemma 4. *Let $a_i \in \mathbb{R}$, $i = 1 \ldots n$. Then*

$$\left| \sum_i a_i \right|^p \leq C(n)^p \sum_i |a_i|^p,$$

with $C(n) = n^{(p-1)/p}$. Thus if $p = 1$, we can choose $C(n) = 1$.

Proposition 7. *Let $p_i = \sup_x p_i(w_i(x))$ and $s_i \geq 0$ be such that $d\mu(w_i(x)) \leq s_i d\mu(x)$. Then we have*

$$d_p(T(F), T(G)) \leq C(n) \left(\sum_i K_i^p s_i^p p_i^p \right)^{1/p} d_p(F, G).$$

Proof. We compute and see that

$$d_p(T(F), T(G))^p$$

$$= \int_X \left(d_h \left(\sum_i p_i(x)\phi_i(F(w_i^{-1}(x))), \sum_i p_i(x)\phi_i(G(w_i^{-1}(x))) \right) \right)^p d\mu(x)$$

$$\leq \int_X \left(\sum_i p_i(x) \; K_i \; d_h \left(F(w_i^{-1}(x)), G(w_i^{-1}(x)) \right) \right)^p d\mu(x)$$

$$\leq \int_{w_i(X)} C(n)^p \sum_i p_i(x)^p \; K_i^p \; \left(d_h \left(F(w_i^{-1}(x)), G(w_i^{-1}(x)) \right) \right)^p d\mu(x)$$

$$\leq C(n)^p \sum_i K_i^p s_i^p \int_X p_i(w_i(z))^p \; d_h \left(F(z), G(z) \right)^p \; d\mu(z)$$

$$\leq C(n)^p \left(\sum_i K_i^p s_i^p p_i^p \right) d_p(F, G)^p. \qquad \square$$

Notice that it is easy (but messy) to tighten the estimate in the Proposition.

4 Applications to Fractal Image Coding and the Inverse Problem

We now present some practical realizations and applications of IFSMF with particular focus on the coding of signals and images. The idea of this section is that to each pixel of an image is associated an interval which measures the "error" in the value for that pixel. In this situation, therefore, we restrict our set-valued functions so that they only take closed intervals as values. We also need to restrict the ϕ_i maps so that they map intervals to intervals.

Thus, we shall consider $X = [0, 1]^n$ for $n = 1$ or 2 and $Y = [a, b]$. For each x, let $\beta(x) \in \mathcal{H}$ be an interval in Y. Then we define $T : \mathcal{F}(X, Y) \to \mathcal{F}(X, Y)$ by

$$T(F)(x) = \beta(x) + \sum_i p_i(x) \; \alpha_i F(w_i^{-1}(x))$$

where $\alpha_i \in \mathbb{R}$.

Corollary 1. *We have the following inequalities*

$$d_\infty(T(F), T(G)) \leq \left[\sup_x \sum_i \alpha_i p_i(x) \right] d_\infty(F, G)$$

$$d_p(T(F), T(G)) \leq C(n) \left(\sum_i \alpha_i^p s_i^p p_i^p \right)^{1/p} d_p(F, G)$$

where $p_i = \sup_x p_i(w_i(x))$ and $s_i \geq 0$ be such that $d\mu(w_i(x)) \leq s_i d\mu(x)$.

Proof. We only need to see that

$$d_h \left(\beta(x) + \sum_i p_i(x)\alpha_i F(w_i^{-1}(x)), \beta(x) + \sum_i p_i(x)\alpha_i G(w_i^{-1}(x)) \right)$$
$$= d_h \left(\sum_i p_i(x)\alpha_i F(w_i^{-1}(x)), \sum_i p_i(x)\alpha_i G(w_i^{-1}(x)) \right)$$

from which point the proof is the same as the proof of Proposition 6. $\square$

In Figure 1 are presented the attractor multifunctions for two IFSMF with contractive affine IFS maps w_i. The top image corresponds to the attractor of the following IFSMF

$$w_1(x) = 0.6x, \qquad \phi_1(t) = 0.7t,$$
$$w_2(x) = 0.6x + 0.4, \quad \phi_2(t) = 0.5t,$$
$$0.5 \leq \beta(x) \leq 1.0.$$

The right image corresponds to the attractor of the IFSMF with the same w_i and ϕ_i maps but with

$$0 \leq \beta(x) \leq 1, \qquad 0 \leq x < 0.5,$$
$$0.5 \leq \beta(x) \leq 1.5, \qquad 0.5 \leq x \leq 1.$$

4.1 Fractal Block Coding and the Inverse Problem

The inverse problem can be formulated as follows: Given a multifunction $F \in \mathcal{F}(X, Y)$, find a contractive IFSMF operator $T : \mathcal{F}(X, Y) \to \mathcal{F}(X, Y)$ that admits a unique fixed point $\tilde{F} \in \mathcal{F}(X, Y)$ such that $d_\infty(F, \tilde{F})$ is small enough. As discussed in the introduction, it is in general a very difficult task to find such operators. A tremendous simplification is provided by the "Collage Theorem" [3, 1], which we now state with particular reference to IFSMF.

Theorem 1. *(Collage Theorem for IFMSF) Given $F \in \mathcal{F}(X, Y)$ suppose that there exists a contractive operator T such that $d_\infty(F, T(F)) < \epsilon$. If F^* is the fixed point of T and $c := \sup_x \sum_i \alpha_i p_i(x)$ then*

$$d_\infty(F, F^*) \leq \frac{\epsilon}{1 - c}$$

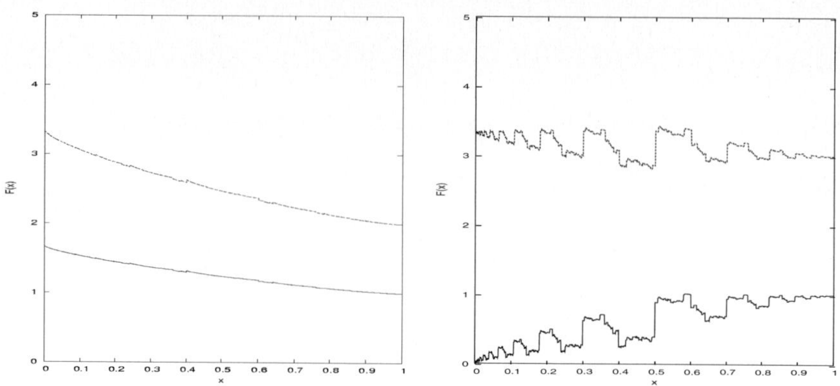

Fig. 1: Fixed-point attractor multifunctions $\bar{u}$ for the two IFSMF on $[0,1]$ given in the text. The upper and lower values of $\bar{u}(x)$ for $x \in [0,1]$ are sketched.

The inverse problem then becomes one of finding a contractive IFSMF operator that maps the "target" multifunction F as close to itself as possible.

Corollary 2. *Under the assumptions of the Collage Theorem we have the following inequality*

$$d_\infty(F, TF) \le \sum_i p_i \sup_{x \in X} \max\{\underline{A}_i(x), \bar{A}_i(x)\}$$

where $\underline{A}_i(x) = |\min F(x) - \min(\beta(x) + \alpha_i F(w_i^{-1})(x))|$, $\bar{A}_i(x) = |\max F(x) - \max(\beta(x) + \alpha_i F(w_i^{-1}(x)))|$ *and* $p_i = \sup_{x \in X} p_i(w_i(x))$.

Proof. In fact using a previous result on the Hausdorff distance and recalling that F is a closed interval multifunction,

$$d_\infty(F, TF) = d_\infty(F(x), \beta(x) + \sum_i p_i(x)\alpha_i F(w_i^{-1}(x)))$$

$$\le d_\infty(F(x), \sum_i p_i(x)(\beta(x) + \alpha_i F(w_i^{-1}(x))))$$

$$\le \sum_i p_i d_\infty(F(x), \beta(x) + \alpha_i F(w_i^{-1}(x)))$$

$$\le \sum_i p_i \sup_{x \in X} \max\{\underline{A}_i(x), \bar{A}_i(x)\}$$

where $\underline{A}_i(x) = |\min F(x) - \min(\beta(x) + \alpha_i F(w_i^{-1})(x))|$, $\bar{A}_i(x) = |\max F(x) - \max(\beta(x) + \alpha_i F(w_i^{-1}(x)))|$ and $p_i = \sup_{x \in X} p_i(w_i(x))$. $\square$

We now prove a similar result for the d_p metric.

Corollary 3. *Under the assumptions of the Collage Theorem we have the following inequality*

$$d_p(F, TF)^p \leq \|\min F - \min TF\|_p^p + \|\max F - \max TF\|_p^p$$

Proof. Computing, we have

$$d_p(F, TF)^p = \int_X \left(d_h(F(x), \beta(x) + \sum_i p_i(x)\alpha_i F(w_i^{-1}(x))) \right)^p d\mu(x)$$

$$\leq \int_X \left| \min F(x) - \min(\beta(x) + \sum_i p_i(x)\alpha_i F(w_i^{-1}(x))) \right|^p d\mu(x)$$

$$+ \int_X \left| \max F(x) - \max(\beta(x) + \sum_i p_i(x)\alpha_i F(w_i^{-1}(x))) \right|^p d\mu(x)$$

$$= \|\min F - \min TF\|_p^p + \|\max F - \max TF\|_p^p. \qquad \square$$

Most fractal block coding methods are based upon a method originally reported by Jacquin [8]. The pixel array defining the image is partitioned into a set of nonoverlapping *range subblocks* R_i. Associated with with each R_i is a larger *domain subblock* D_i, chosen so that the image function $u(R_i)$ supported on each R_i is well approximated by a greyscale-modified copy of the image function $u(D_i)$. In practice, affine greyscale maps are used:

$$u(R_i) \approx \phi_i(u(w_i(D_i))) = \alpha_i u(w_i(D_i)) + \beta_i, 1 \leq i \leq N$$

where $w_i(x)$ denotes the contraction that maps R_i to D_i (in discrete pixel space, the w_i maps will have to include a decimation that reduces the number of pixels in going from R_i to D_i). The greyscale map coefficients α_i and β_i are usually determined by least squares. The domain blocks D_i are usually chosen from a common *domain pool* $\mathcal{D}$. The domain block yielding the best approximation to $u(R_i)$, i.e., the lowest *collage error*,

$$\Delta_{ij} = \| u(R_i) - \phi_{ij}(u(w_{ij}(D_j))) \|, \quad 1 \leq j \leq M,$$

is chosen for the fractal coding (the L^2 norm is usually chosen).

In Figure 2 is presented the fixed point approximation $\bar{u}$ to the standard 512×512 *Lena* image (8 bits per pixel, or 256 greyscale values) using a partition of 8×8 nonoverlapping pixel blocks ($64^2 = 4096$ in total). The domain pool for each range block was the set of $32^2 = 1024$ 16×16 non-overlapping pixel blocks. (This is not an optimal domain pool – nevertheless it works quite well.) The image $\bar{u}$ was obtained by starting with the seed image $u_0 = 255$ (plain white image) and iterating $u_{n+1} = Tu_n$ to $n = 15$.

We now consider a simple IFSMF version of image coding, using the partition described above. Since the range blocks R_i are nonoverlapping, all coefficients $p_i(x)$ in our IFSMF operator will have value 1. From the *Lena* image function $u(x)$ used above, we shall construct a multifunction $U(x)$ so that

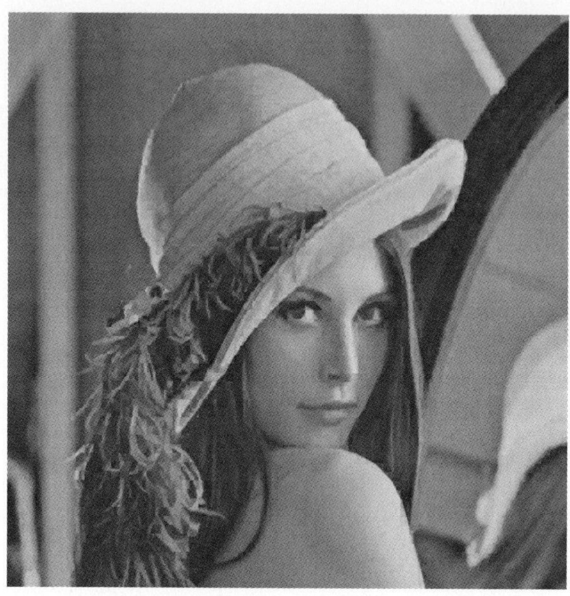

Fig. 2: The fixed point $\bar{u}$ of the fractal transform operator T described in the main text, designed to approximate the standard 512×512 (8bpp) *Lena* image.

$$U(x) = [u^-(x), u^+(x)].$$

The approximation of the multifunction range block $U(R_i)$ by $U(D_i)$ then takes the form of two coupled problems

$$u^-(R_i) \approx \alpha_i u^-(w_i(D_i)) + \beta_i^-(R_i),$$
$$u^+(R_i) \approx \alpha_i u^+(w_i(D_i)) + \beta_i^+(R_i), \quad 1 \le i \le N.$$

For simplicity, we assume that the $\beta^+(x)$ and $\beta^-(x)$ functions are piecewise constant over each block R_i. For a given domain-range block pair D_i/R_i, we then have a system of three equations in the unknowns α_i, β_i^- and β_i^+. The domain block yielding the best total L^2 collage distance,

$$\Delta_{ij} = \quad \| u^-(R_i) - \alpha_i u^-(w_{ij}(D_j)) - \beta_i^-(R_i) \|$$
$$+ \| u^+(R_i) - \alpha_i u^+(w_{ij}(D_j)) - \beta_i^+(R_i) \|, \quad 1 \le j \le M,$$

is selected for the fractal code. Corresponding to this fractal code will be the multifunction attractor $\bar{U}(x) = [\bar{u}^-(x), \bar{u}^+(x)]$.

To illustrate, we consider the multifunction constructed from the *Lena* image defined as follows,

$$U_{ij} = [u_{ij} - \delta_{ij}, u_{ij} + \delta_{ij}],$$

where

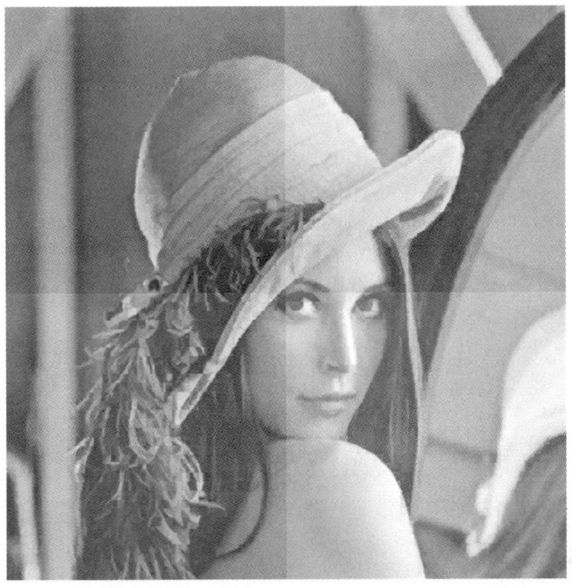

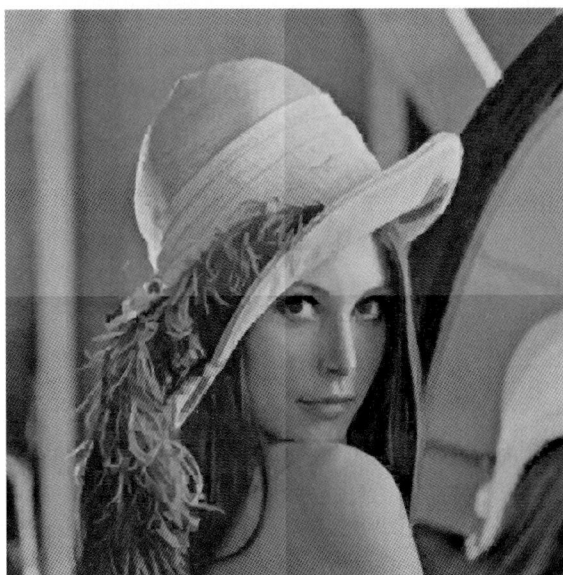

Fig. 3: The upper (top) and lower (bottom) functions, $\bar{u}^+$ and $\bar{u}^-$ respectively, of the attractor multifunction $\bar{U}$ produced by the IFSMF fractal coding procedure described in the main text.

$$\delta_{ij} = \begin{cases} 0, & 1 \leq i,j \leq 255, \\ 40, & 256 \leq i,j \leq 512, \\ 20, & \text{otherwise.} \end{cases}$$

In other words, the error or uncertainty in the pixel values is zero for the upper left quarter of the image, 20 for the upper right and lower left quarters and 40 for the lower right. In Figure 3 we show the lower and upper functions, $\bar{u}^-(x)$ and $\bar{u}^+(x)$, respectively, produced by a fractal coding of this multifunction.

Acknowledgements

This work has been written during a research visit by DLT to the Department of Applied Mathematics of the University of Waterloo, Canada. DLT thanks ERV for this opportunity. For DLT this work has been supported by COFIN Research Project 2004. This work has also been supported in part by research grants (FM and ERV) from the Natural Sciences and Engineering Research Council of Canada (NSERC), which are hereby gratefully acknowledged.

References

1. M.F. Barnsley, *Fractals Everywhere*, Academic Press, New York (1989).
2. M.F. Barnsley and S. Demko, Iterated function systems and the global construction of fractals, Proc. Roy. Soc. London Ser. A, **399**, 243–275 (1985).
3. M.F. Barnsley, V. Ervin, D. Hardin and J. Lancaster, Solution of an inverse problem for fractals and other sets, Proc. Nat. Acad. Sci. USA **83**, 1975–1977 (1985).
4. B. Forte, F. Mendivil and E.R. Vrscay, IFS operators on integral transforms, in *Fractals: Theory and Applications in Engineering*, ed. M. Dekking, J. Levy-Vehel, E. Lutton and C. Tricot, Springer Verlag, London (1999).
5. B. Forte and E.R. Vrscay, Theory of generalized fractal transforms, Fractal Image Encoding and Analysis, NATO ASI Series F, Vol 159, ed. Y.Fisher, Springer Verlag, New York (1998).
6. B. Forte and E.R. Vrscay, Inverse problem methods for generalized fractal transforms, in *Fractal Image Encoding and Analysis, ibid.*
7. J. Hutchinson: Fractals and self-similarity, Indiana Univ. J. Math., 30, 713–747 (1981).
8. A. Jacquin, Image coding based on a fractal theory of iterated contractive image transformations, IEEE Trans. Image Proc. **1**, 18–30 (1992).
9. F. Mendivil and E.R. Vrscay, Correspondence between fractal-wavelet transforms and iterated function systems with grey-level maps, in *Fractals in Engineering: From Theory to Industrial Applications*, ed. J. Levy-Vehel, E. Lutton and C. Tricot, Springer Verlag, London (1997).
10. F. Mendivil and E.R. Vrscay, Fractal vector measures and vector calculus on planar fractal domains, Chaos, Solitons and Fractals **14**, 1239–1254 (2002).
11. E.R. Vrscay, A generalized class of fractal-wavelet transforms for image representation and compression, Can. J. Elect. Comp. Eng. **23**, 69–84 (1998).

Part II

Mathematical Problems in Biology, Medicine and Ecology

Stochastic Modeling and Estimation
in a Neutron Lifetime Experiment

Grace L. Yang[1] and Kevin J. Coakley[2]

[1] Department of Mathematics, University of Maryland, College Park, Maryland,
USA 20742, gly@math.umd.edu
[2] National Institute of Standards and Technology, Boulder, Colorado, USA 80305,
kevin.coakley@nist.gov

Summary. A team of researchers demonstrated at the National Institute of Standards and Technology Cold Neutron Research Facility for the first time that ultra cold neutrons can be confined in a magnetic trap filled with liquid helium, see [6]. This technical breakthrough allows a more accurate measurement of the neutron lifetime and helps to answer questions fundamental to physics and astrophysics. Since the demonstration, an experimental protocol for data collection and statistical analysis has been under development.

The experiment is composed of two stages. In the first stage, ultra cold neutrons are generated and confined in the magnetic trap. In the second stage, decays of the trapped neutrons are recorded. During the first stage, nothing is observable. We do not know the number of neutrons available from the first stage for decay recording during the second stage. Furthermore, neutron lifetimes are only partially observable and are subject to contamination due to the presence of background events.

In this presentation, we give an overview of stochastic modeling of lifetime data from such experiment and statistical estimation of mean neutron lifetime. We model a neutron lifetime by a birth and death process. Models are used to account for missing or incomplete lifetimes and background contamination, and thereby correcting biases in the estimation of the mean neutron lifetime. Our statistical approach unifies many of the existing statistical methods used for studying radioactive decay processes. See , e.g. [3], [4].

The problem of lifetime estimation is extensively studied in the survival analysis of patients in biostatistics in which lifetime data are subject to censoring, truncation and length-biased (cross-sectional) sampling. In the context of renewal processes, Feller [2] called length-bias a renewal paradox. Neutron lifetime data are subject to similar sampling constraints. However, distinct characteristics of neutrons bring out some statistical problems that rarely encountered in the survival analysis about which we shall discuss.

1 Introduction

A highly accurate determination of the neutron lifetime is of fundamental importance in physics and astrophysics. Moreover, the neutron trapping technology has important applications in other fields such as material science. The neutron lifetime, in combination with other parameters of the neutron decay, can be used to test the Standard Model and to predict the light element abundances from Big-Bang Nucleosynthesis (BBN) theory. Currently, the experimental precision in the neutron lifetime is the primary source of uncertainty in these predictions. See [9].

Suppose X denotes the lifetime of a (free) neutron. It is assumed that X has a probability density

$$f(x) = \mu \exp(-\mu x), \quad \text{for } x > 0, \mu > 0,$$

where μ is the neutron (exponential) decay rate and $\tau = 1/\mu$ is the expected neutron lifetime. A neutron lifetime estimate is an estimate of τ. This estimation problem is conceptually simple. For instance, an estimate can be obtained by taking the average $\bar{X}$ of a number of measured neutron lifetimes. The difficulty lies in the measuring of lifetime X.

A free neutron is unstable. Experimental determination of the lifetime of a neutron is not straight forward. Neutron lifetimes are often not completely observable in an experiment and the estimate of τ varies with experimental protocol. Usually an estimate is determined by consensus. The currently accepted value of the mean lifetime of a free neutron is (885.7 ± 0.8) seconds. See [9].

To see the difficulties in measuring neutron lifetime, let us consider a standard type of a neutron lifetime experiment. In this experiment, a storage bottle is used to confine ultra cold neutrons (UCN). The bottle is filled with UCN from an external source and then after a fixed time, the number of UCN remaining in the bottle is counted with a UCN detector. Many factors affect measurements. They include: (a) the number of UCN in the bottle changes because of neutron (beta) decay and we do not know how many UCN in the bottle at any given time, (b) loss of neutrons due to collisions of neutrons with the container walls, (c) the efficiency of the UCN detectors is not 100%, and (d) contamination by the recordings of background events. In statistical terms, factor (a) means that we do not know the sample size, and (b) corresponds to right-censoring of a neutron lifetime measurement. That is, a lost neutron would have it's lifetime shortened by collision before decay occurs.

Under these circumstances, clearly we are unable to compute the simple average of lifetimes with fragmented lifetime observations and unknown sample size. Correction for missing and incomplete lifetime data and modeling of the sample size and background process are necessary for reducing bias in the estimate. Efforts toward correction include designing a better experimental protocol and constructing appropriate stochastic models.

Using magnetic fields to confine neutrons eliminates the wall loses inherent in material bottles, thereby significantly increases the number of trapped neutrons and decreases background events. The technique to produce and confine ultra cold neutrons is a magnetic trap (shown in Fig. 1) is regarded as a breakthrough experimental contribution. Currently, the uncertainty of the estimate of the neutron lifetime determined from analysis of all experimental values is dominated by a systematic error that cannot be reduced by prolonging the duration of the experiment. In contrast, systematic errors in the latest version of neutron lifetime experiment based on the Fig. 1 technique should be relatively negligible. Even so, there remain the issues of censoring, truncation, missing values and contamination which we shall address below.

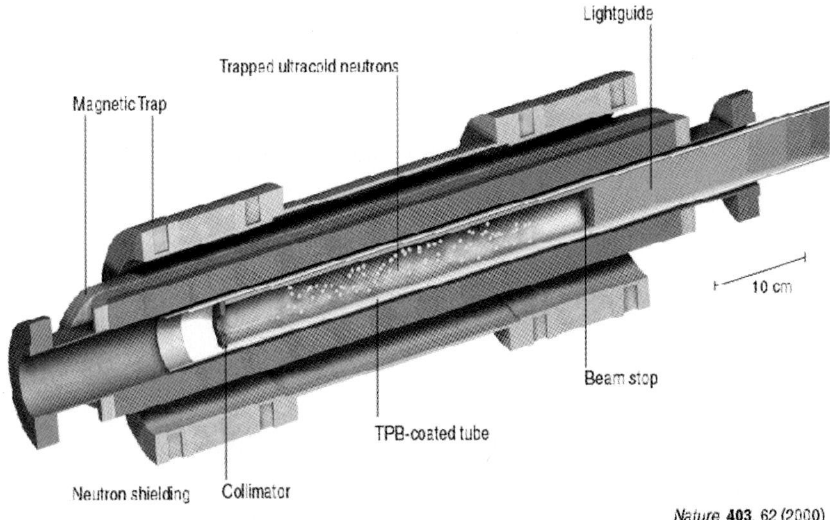

Fig. 1: At the NIST Center for Neutron Research, cold neutrons from a reactor are guided into a magnetic trap and can inelastically scatter in superfluid ^{4}He to produce ultracold neutrons. Above, we show a cross sectional perspective of the magnetic trap that confines these ultracold neutrons. See also Plate 8 on page 343

2 Stochastic Models for Two-stage Neutron Lifetime Experiment

We present stochastic models that were constructed in Yang and Coakley [7]. The neutron lifetime experiment is composed of two stages: the production stage and the recording stage. In the first stage, $[0, T_1]$, neutrons are produced and confined in a magnetic trap. The production terminates at time T_1. In the second stage, $[T_1, T_1 + T]$, neutron decay times as well as the background events are recorded. The estimation of the mean value of neutron lifetimes is based solely on the decay data obtained from the second stage, since nothing is observable in the first stage. We assume that neutrons are generated at a Poisson rate $\lambda > 0$. Once generated, they decay independently of one another at a rate μ with mean lifetime $\tau = 1/\mu$. This assumption entails that the number of neutrons, $N(t)$, not yet disintegrated at any time $t \geq 0$ is a Markovian birth and death process with "birth" rate λ and "death" rate μ. Then the number of neutrons at time T_1, $N(T_1)$, has a Poisson distribution with expected value

$$a = EN(T_1) = \frac{\lambda}{\mu}(1 - e^{-\mu T_1}). \tag{1}$$

Note that $N(t); t \geq 0$ is not observable. Fig.2 illustrates what can be recorded during the second stage. For clarity, we shall first assume that there are no background events.

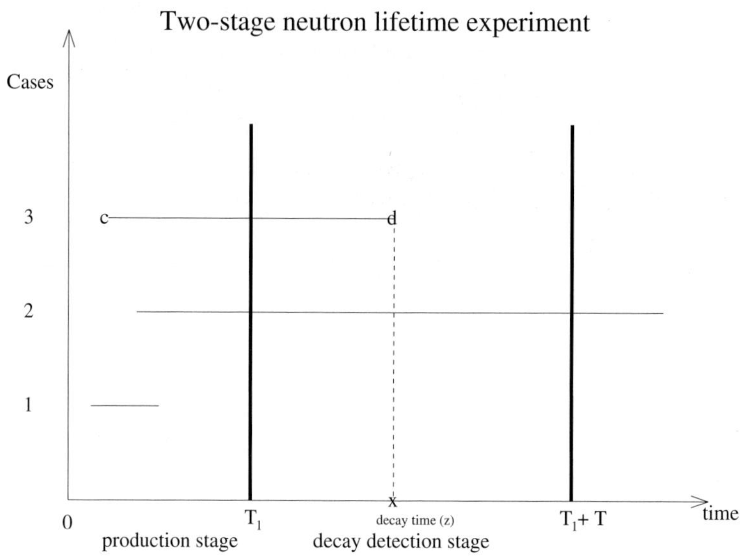

Fig. 2: Observed data (z) in a two-stage neutron lifetime experiment. We indicate the time line for the creation (c) and decay (d) for a particular neutron.

Horizontal lines represent 3 cases of lifetimes. Only when a neutron's decay time occurs in the second stage, it can be recorded as shown in case 3. In this case, we can compute its residual life (Y) as measured from T_1 to the decay time d but not the full lifetime X. If a neutron's decay time occurs in stage one (case 1) or beyond stage 2 (case 2), then it's lifetime cannot be recorded and we have a missing value in each of these cases. The recordings in the second stage are a set of residual lifetimes measured from time T_1, as

$$Y_1, \ldots, Y_{N(T_1)},$$

where $N(T_1)$ is the unobservable number of neutrons available at the beginning of the recording stage.

For notational simplicity, we shall suppress T_1 from here on by denoting $N(T_1)$ by N and the second stage $[T_1, T_1 + T]$ by $[0, T]$.

In actual experiments, background events are always present, the recorded values are not the $X's$, but contaminated values,

$$Z_{(1)} \le Z_{(2)} \le \ldots \le Z_{(M(T))}, \tag{2}$$

where a Z can be either the time of a true neutron decay or a background noise. The value $M(T)$ is the total number of recorded events during $[0, T]$ which is the sum

$$M(T) = S(T) + B(T), \tag{3}$$

where $S(T)$ is the number of true neutron decays among $N(T_1)$ neutrons and $B(T)$ is the number of background events recorded in $[0, T]$.

We shall assume that the number of background events in $(0, t]$, $B :=\{B(t), t > 0\}$, is a homogeneous Poisson process with rate $b > 0$ and independent of $S := \{S(t), t > 0\}$.

By assumption of Markovian birth and death process for $N(t)$, $\{S(t), t > 0\}$ is a non homogeneous Poisson process with mean

$$\xi(t) = a(1 - e^{-\mu t}).$$

It follows that the observable process $\{M(t) = B(t) + S(t); t \ge 0\}$ is a non homogeneous Poisson process with mean

$$EM(t) = \Psi(t) = bt + \xi(t) = a(1 - e^{-\mu t}) + bt, \quad \text{for } t \in [0, T]. \tag{4}$$

Neither S nor B can be observed separately. The estimation of mean neutron lifetime (τ) is based on the Z-data, or equivalently, realizations of $M(t) : t \in [0, T]$.

3 Likelihood Functions

We present two probability models. One for $Z_{(1)} \le Z_{(2)} \le \ldots \le Z_{(M(T))}$, and another for the binned Z-data. Both of them may serve as likelihood functions for parameter estimation.

3.1 Joint Probability Density of the $Z's$

From the intensity of $M(t)$,

$$\psi(t) = \Psi'(t) = b + a\mu e^{-\mu t}. \tag{5}$$

we obtain the joint density of $Z_{(1)} \leq Z_{(2)} \leq \ldots \leq Z_{(M(T))}$, with respect to Lebesgue measure,

$$L_1 = \prod_{i=1}^{M(T)} \psi(z_{(i)}) e^{-\Psi(T)}, \tag{6}$$

where $\Psi(T)$ is defined by (5).

The model L_1 differs from that used in survival analysis in several unobservable quantities and in $M(T), z_{(i)}$. Both $M(T)$ and $z_{(i)}$ are contaminated observations.

In survival analysis, statistical analysis is carried out with a known sample size N, say it is equal to n, while in our neutron experiment, the sample size N is not known. To compare them, let us suppose that N is observable and $N = n$ in the neutron experiment. Then conditioning on the event $[N = n]$, the intensity of the process $M(t)$ at time $t \geq Z_{(i)}$ is $b + [n - S(Z_{(i)}-) + 1]\mu$, in which $S(Z_{(i)}-)$ is not observable. Furthermore, under the same conditioning, $\{M(t)\}$ is no longer Markovian which greatly complicates the model and statistical analysis. However, the situation becomes a lot simpler if the background process $B(t)$ is absent. Then $X = Z$, and conditioning on the event $N = n$, the model in (6) reduces to

$$\frac{n!}{(n - S(T))!} \mu^{-S(T)} \exp[- \sum_{j=1}^{S(T)} x_{(j)}\mu - (n - S(T))\mu T].$$

This is the classical Type I censoring model initially studied by Epstein and Sobel [1].

3.2 Poisson Regression Model for Count Data

In practice, it is considerably easier and less expensive to collect binned data than to record exact values of the $Z's$. Partition the time interval of the second stage into subintervals, $(t_k - t_{k-1}]$, for $k = 1, \ldots, K + 1$, where $t_0 = 0, t_K = T, t_{K+1} = \infty$. Note that the last interval (t_K, t_{K+1}) has infinite length. The total number of recorded events in the $k - th$ time interval is the sum

$$\nu_k = N_k + B_k,$$

of N_k number of neutron decays and B_k number of background events in the kth interval. As in $M(T)$, it is the sum but not the individual component N_k or B_k that is observable.

$N(t)$ being a Poisson process implies that N_k for $k = 1, \ldots, K + 1$, are independent Poisson random variables. It follows that the $\nu_k's$ are independent Poisson random variables with expected value

$$r_k(\theta) = E[\nu_k] = ap_k + b(t_k - t_{k-1}), \quad \text{for } k = 1, \dots, K+1,$$

where

$$p_k = e^{-\mu t_{k-1}} - e^{-\mu t_k}.$$

Note that ν_{K+1} is not observable. The observed binned data are $\nu_1, \dots, \nu_K$. The joint probability of $\nu_k, k = 0, \dots, K$ is

$$L_2 = \prod_{k=1}^{K} \frac{e^{-r_k(\theta)}(r_k(\theta))^{\nu_k}}{\nu_k!}, \tag{7}$$

where $\theta = (a, b, \tau)$.

This defines a Poisson regression model.

Either model L_1 (in (6)) or model L_2 (in (7)) can be used for estimation of the parameter θ. The intensity function $\psi(t)$ and the expected values $r_k(\theta)$ are well-behaved smooth functions. The parameter θ is identifiable in both models. The choice between the two depends on what kind of data is available. Usually, only binned data are available. Having both models allows us to study the information loss by going from exact decay times to binned observations.

Standard estimation methods such as maximum likelihood and minimum chi-squares are applicable which, in our case, yield asymptomatically efficient estimates $\hat{\theta}$ for θ. Consider first model L_1. The data for estimation comes from repeated experiments. Suppose that there are m repeated experiments. We introduce subscript c to denote the $c-th$ experiment, for $c = 1, \dots, m$. Then L_{1c}, $Z_{c(i)}$ and $M_c(T)$ denote the respective values of $L_1, Z_{(i)}, M(T)$ for the $c-th$ experiment.

The joint probability density of the data $Z_{c(i)}$ for $i = 0, 1, \dots, M_c(T), c = 1, \dots, m$ from all m experiments is the product,

$$L_1(\theta) = \prod_{c=1}^{m} L_{1c} = \prod_{c=1}^{m} \left(\left[\prod_{i=1}^{M_c(T)} \psi(z_{c(i)}) \right] e^{-\Psi(T)} \right),$$

where ψ and Ψ are defined by (4) and (5).

Similarly, the joint probability of the binned data is given by

$$L_2(\theta) = \prod_{c=1}^{m} \prod_{k=1}^{K} \frac{e^{-r_k(\theta)}(r_k(\theta))^{\nu_{ck}}}{\nu_{ck}!}, \tag{8}$$

where ν_{ck} is the value of ν_k in the $c-th$ experiment.

The maximum likelihood estimate $\hat{\theta}$ of θ computed from $L_1(\theta)$ has an asymptotically normal distribution;

$$\sqrt{m}(\hat{\theta} - \theta) \quad \text{converges in distribution to } \mathcal{N}(\mathbf{0}, (\mathbf{B'B})^{-1}),$$

as $m \to \infty$, with information matrix

$$\mathbf{B'B} = \left(-E_\theta \frac{\partial^2 log L_1}{\partial\theta_i\partial\theta_j}\right), \tag{9}$$

where L_1 is given by (6).

The information matrix was computed analytically in Yang and Coakley [7].

Similarly, the maximum likelihood estimate $\hat{\theta}$ of θ based on the likelihood $L_2(\theta)$ in eq.(8) has an asymptotically normal distribution as in eq.(9), but with the information matrix computed for L_2 as given in eq.(7). Both of these models have no closed forms for these estimates. Their information matrices are also too complicated for analytical comparison. We resort to numerical computations with simulated data to study the biases and variances of these estimates. These two models have been extensively used in the design and statistical analysis of the neutron lifetime experiment at The National Institute of Standards and Technology. In our numerical studies, T is treated as an experimental parameter. We studied the reduction in bias and variance in the estimator of τ as T increases. The information loss from using binned data is examined by looking at the ratio of the variances of the estimates computed from both models. Numerical studies suggest that by appropriately chosen bin widths, the loss of information in using binned data is not very significant. The reader is referred to [7] for the study of bias and variance reduction and information loss from using binned data. A method of selecting appropriate time lengths, T_1 and T for the two stages of the experiment was developed in a form of contour plot by Coakley [5].

4 Concluding Remarks

We presented two models for analyzing neutron lifetime data collected from a two-stage experiment. In these models we have, for simplicity, modeled the background process by a homogeneous Poisson process. As is well known that in some situations the rate of background event is non stationary in time [8]. It would be interesting and important to generalize our models to include a non stationary background process.

Acknowledgments

The research of Grace L. Yang is partially supported by a grant from the National Science Foundation. Contributions to this work by staff of the National Institute of Standards and Technology, an agency of the US Government, are not subject to copyright laws.

References

1. Epstein, B., Sobel, M.: Life testing. Journal of the American Statistical Association, **48**, 486–502, (1953)
2. Feller, W.: *An Introduction to Probability Theory and Its Applications,* **Vol.II**, Wiley, New York (1966)
3. Cleveland, B.: Nuclear. Instr. and Methods Phys. Res. A **214**, 451, (1983)
4. Baker, S., Cousins, R.D.: Nuclear. Instr. and Methods Phys. Res A **221**, 437, (1984)
5. Coakley, K.J.: Statistical planning for a neutron lifetime experiment using magnetically trapped neutrons. Nuclear. Instr. and Methods A, 406, p. 451-463 (1998)
6. Huffman, P.R., Brome, C.R., Butterworth, J.S., Coakley, K.J., Dewey, M.S., Dzhosyuk, S.N., Golub, R., Green, G.L., Habicht, K., Lamoreaux, S.K., Mattoni,C.E.H., McKinsey, D.N., Wietfeldt, F.E., and Doyle, J.M.: Magnetic trapping of neutrons. Nature, **403**, 62–64 (2000)
7. Yang, G.L., Coakley, K.J.: Likelihood models for two-stage neutron lifetime experiments. Physical Review C, **63**, 014602/1–16 (2001).
8. Coakley, K.J., Yang, G.L.: Estimation of the neutron lifetime: Comparison of methods which account for background. Physical Review C, **65**, 064612/1–7 (2002)
9. Dzhosyuk, S.N.: Magnetic Trapping of Neutrons for Measurement of the neutron lifetime. Ph.D thesis, Department of Physics, Harvard University, Cambridge, Massachusetts, (2004)

The Transport of Specific Monoclonal Antibodies in Tumour Cords

Alessandro Bertuzzi[1], Antonio Fasano[2], Alberto Gandolfi[1], and Carmela Sinisgalli[1]

[1] Istituto di Analisi dei Sistemi ed Informatica "A. Ruberti" – CNR, Viale Manzoni 30, 00185 Roma, Italy
`{bertuzzi,gandolfi,sinisgalli}@iasi.cnr.it`
[2] Dipartimento di Matematica "U. Dini", Università di Firenze, Viale Morgagni 67/A, 50134 Firenze, Italy
`fasano@math.unifi.it`

1 Introduction

Blood flow in tumour vasculature carries oxygen and nutrients necessary for cell life and proliferation, and allows delivery of therapeutic agents within the tumour. To reach their target cells, these agents must extravasate and be transported by diffusion and by the convection associated to the movement of extracellular fluid. Convective transport may become important for therapeutic agents with large molecular weight or size, such as the monoclonal antibodies or the viruses used as vectors in gene therapy [11]. The high interstitial fluid pressure, exhibited by most solid tumors, is thought to be a barrier for fluid extravasation and efficient convective transport.

Monoclonal antibodies, able to bind specifically to antigens located on tumour cell membrane, have been proposed for cancer therapy, either because of their possible direct cytotoxicity or because antibodies can be conjugated to radionuclides or toxins [2]. A mathematical model that describes the transport of monoclonal antibodies by diffusion and convection in spherical tumors, under the assumption of a continuous distribution of fluid and solute sources in the tumor mass, was proposed in [1]. Fujimori et al. [9] studied the transport of antibodies in a cylinder of tumour tissue around a central blood vessel. In that paper, convection was modelled in a very simplified way, but the binding of antibodies to cell membrane antigen was taken into account.

In the present work, we analyse the transport of antibodies within a cylindrical arrangement of tumour cells around a blood vessel and surrounded by necrosis (tumour cord, see [14, 10, 12]). We describe in more detail the diffusive and convective transport and the binding of bivalent (IgG) antibodies to cell membrane molecules. For the fluid motion and the interstitial pressure, we use the model previously proposed [5, 6], with some refinements in the description of the necrotic region.

2 The Mathematical Model of Tumour Cords

In this section we summarize the tumor cord model proposed in [5, 6], and give an refined description of the necrotic region. We consider an ideal regular array of parallel and identical tumor cords inside the tumor mass (a geometry similar to the Krogh model of microcirculation), each cord being separated from others by a region of necrosis. We assume cylindrical symmetry around the axis of the central blood vessel, the radial coordinate r varying between the radius r_0 of the vessel and the outer boundary B of the necrotic region that surrounds each cord. The radius of the interface between cord and necrosis is denoted by ρ_N. Because of the radial symmetry of the system of cords, no exchange of matter occurs through the boundary $r = B$. This boundary is mobile since blood vessels are assumed to be displaced as the tumor mass is growing or regressing. The axial coordinate z will range in the interval $[-H, H]$. All the quantities involved depend at most on r, z, and the time t. Only one species of nutrient is considered, and we identify this critical nutrient with oxygen, denoting by σ its local concentration.

2.1 The Cord

In the general case of treated tumours, three components are present in the cord : 1) viable cells, which are subdivided into proliferating (P) and quiescent cells (Q); 2) dead cells produced by treatment; 3) extracellular fluids that fill the interstitial space. We will denote the fractions of volume occupied locally by these components by ν_P, ν_Q, ν_A, and ν_E, respectively. Supposing no voids, we have

$$\nu_P + \nu_Q + \nu_A + \nu_E = 1 \,.$$

As in [3, 4], it is assumed that (i) the volume fraction of extracellular fluid in the cord is constant; (ii) dead cells move at the same velocity as living cells; (iii) cell velocity is radial; (iv) σ, ν_P, ν_Q, ν_A, and the velocity $\mathbf{u}$ of the cellular component do not depend on z; (v) all cells die if σ reaches a death threshold σ_N. In view of assumptions (iii) and (iv), we have $\mathbf{u} = (u(r, t), 0)$. The velocity of the fluid component is denoted by $\mathbf{v} = (v_r(r, z, t), v_z(r, z, t))$.

Under the assumption that all the components have the same constant mass density, the mass balance equations, for $r_0 < r < \rho_N(t)$, can be written as follows:

$$\frac{\partial \nu_P}{\partial t} + \nabla \cdot (\nu_P \, \mathbf{u}) = \chi \nu_P + \gamma(\sigma)\nu_Q - \lambda(\sigma)\nu_P - \mu_P(r,t)\nu_P \,, \tag{1}$$

$$\frac{\partial \nu_Q}{\partial t} + \nabla \cdot (\nu_Q \, \mathbf{u}) = -\gamma(\sigma)\nu_Q + \lambda(\sigma)\nu_P - \mu_Q(r,t)\nu_Q \,, \tag{2}$$

$$\frac{\partial \nu_A}{\partial t} + \nabla \cdot (\nu_A \, \mathbf{u}) = \mu_P(r,t)\nu_P + \mu_Q(r,t)\nu_Q - \mu_A\nu_A \,, \tag{3}$$

$$\nu_E \nabla \cdot \mathbf{v} = \mu_A\nu_A - \chi\nu_P \,. \tag{4}$$

In (1)–(4), χ is the rate of volume increment due to cell proliferation; $\gamma(\sigma)$ and $\lambda(\sigma)$ are the rates of the transitions $Q \to P$ and $P \to Q$, respectively, assumed as in [8] to be regulated by the oxygen concentration; μ_P and μ_Q are death rates representing the killing effects of treatment by drugs or radiation; μ_A is the rate of volume loss due to degradation of dead cells to a liquid waste. According to the experimental evidence, the function $\lambda(\sigma)$ will be nonincreasing and $\gamma(\sigma)$ nondecreasing. In particular, we assign two threshold values for σ, $\sigma_Q < \sigma_P$, and we assume $\lambda = \lambda_{max}$ and $\gamma = \gamma_{min}$ for $\sigma \leq \sigma_Q$, $\lambda = \lambda_{min}$ and $\gamma = \gamma_{max}$ for $\sigma \geq \sigma_P$, with $\lambda_{max} > \lambda_{min} \geq 0$ and $\gamma_{max} > \gamma_{min} \geq 0$. In the interval (σ_Q, σ_P), $\lambda(\sigma)$ decreases linearly and $\gamma(\sigma)$ increases linearly.

We set $\nu^{\star} = \nu_P + \nu_Q + \nu_A = 1 - \nu_E$, where $\nu^{\star}$ is constant in view of assumption (i), and we derive the equation for the composite velocity by summing (1)–(4),

$$\nabla \cdot (\nu^{\star}\mathbf{u} + (1 - \nu^{\star})\mathbf{v}) = 0 \,. \tag{5}$$

By summing (1)–(3), we obtain the equation for $u(r,t)$,

$$\nu^{\star} \frac{1}{r} \frac{\partial}{\partial r}(ru) = \chi\nu_P - \mu_A(\nu^{\star} - \nu_P - \nu_Q) \,. \tag{6}$$

Equation (6) is complemented by the boundary condition

$$u(r_0, t) = 0 \,.$$

This equality implies that no boundary condition is required for (1)–(3).

We assume that diffusion in a quasi-stationary regime is the dominant transport mechanism for oxygen, because of the high oxygen diffusivity [14]. Thus we have the following equation for σ:

$$\Delta\sigma = f_P(\sigma)\nu_P + f_Q(\sigma)\nu_Q \,,$$

with the boundary conditions

$$\sigma(r_0, t) = \sigma_b \,,$$

$$\left. \frac{\partial\sigma}{\partial r} \right|_{r=\rho_N(t)} = 0 \,,$$

where $f_P(\sigma)$, $f_Q(\sigma)$ denote the ratio between the consumption rate per unit volume of P and Q cells, respectively, and the diffusion coefficient. We set

$f_P(\sigma) \geq f_Q(\sigma)$ and require $f_Q(\sigma_N) > 0$. At the inner boundary $r = r_0$, we prescribe the (constant) oxygen blood concentration $\sigma_b > \sigma_P$, although a more realistic flux condition might be imposed.

To determine the interface $r = \rho_N(t)$, we recall that necrotic material cannot be converted back to live cells and that assumption (v) precludes to have live cells when σ is smaller than σ_N. Thus the following inequalities must be satisfied:

$$u(\rho_N,t) - \dot{\rho}_N \geq 0\,,$$
$$\sigma(\rho_N,t) \geq \sigma_N\,.$$

As pointed out in [5], two regimes are possible, one with $u(\rho_N,t)-\dot{\rho}_N>0$ and the other with $u(\rho_N,t)-\dot{\rho}_N=0$, that must satisfy the constraint

$$\left(u(\rho_N,t)-\dot{\rho}_N\right)\left(\sigma(\rho_N,t)-\sigma_N\right) = 0\,.$$

Switching between the two regimes is possible during the evolution of the cord that follows the treatment.

The extracellular fluid motion was described in [5, 6] by deriving an approximate equation for the longitudinal average of $v_r(r,z,t)$:

$$v(r,t) = \frac{1}{2H} \int_{-H}^{H} v_r(r,z,t)\, dz\,.$$

This was achieved by approximating the volumetric efflux of liquid from the cord ends according to

$$(1 - \nu^\star)[v_z(r,H,t) - v_z(r,-H,t)] = 2\zeta_{\text{out}}\,(p(r,t) - p_\infty)\,, \tag{7}$$

where ζ_{out} represents the conductivity of the tissues traversed by the outgoing flux, p_∞ is a "far field" pressure (identifiable with the pressure in the lymphatic vessels), and $p(r,t)$ is the longitudinal average of fluid pressure. Thus, starting from (5), the following equation for the average radial velocity $v(r,t)$ is obtained:

$$\frac{1}{r}\frac{\partial}{\partial r}(rv) = -\frac{1}{1-\nu^\star}\left[\chi\nu_P - \mu_A(\nu^\star-\nu_P-\nu_Q) + \frac{\zeta_{\text{out}}}{H}(p - p_\infty)\right]. \tag{8}$$

Assuming that extracellular fluid flow is governed by Darcy law, the longitudinal average of the radial component of Darcy equation,

$$(1 - \nu^\star)(v - u) = -\kappa\frac{\partial p}{\partial r}\,,$$

yields the following equation for p:

$$p(r,t) = p_0(t) - \frac{1-\nu^\star}{\kappa}\int_{r_0}^{r}[v(r',t) - u(r',t)]\, dr'\,, \tag{9}$$

with $p_0(t) = p(r_0^+, t)$. The pressure $p_0(t)$ is actually unknown, and (9) requires a condition at $r = \rho_N(t)$, which we will see below. Equation (8) is complemented by the boundary condition at the vessel wall,

$$(1 - \nu^\star) v(r_0, t) = \zeta_{\text{in}} (p_b - p_0(t)),$$

where ζ_{in} is the hydraulic conductivity of the wall and $p_b > p_\infty$ represents the longitudinal mean of hydraulic pressure in the blood, corrected with the jump of osmotic pressure.

2.2 The Necrotic Region

The necrotic region (N) is composed of dead cells and liquid, with volume fractions denoted by ν_N and ν_E ($\nu_N + \nu_E = 1$). Dead cells degrade to liquid with rate constant μ_N. Thus, for $\rho_N(t) < r < B(t)$, mass balance yields:

$$\frac{\partial \nu_N}{\partial t} + \nabla \cdot (\nu_N \mathbf{u}) = -\mu_N \nu_N, \tag{10}$$

$$\frac{\partial \nu_E}{\partial t} + \nabla \cdot (\nu_E \mathbf{v}) = \mu_N \nu_N, \tag{11}$$

where $\mathbf{u}$ and $\mathbf{v}$ still represent the velocities of the cellular and, respectively, of the liquid component. As above, $\mathbf{u} = (u(r,t), 0)$. Assumption (i) is relaxed, by allowing ν_E (and then ν_N) to change with time. We assume that the pressure of the liquid, p_N, is spatially uniform. From (10), we obtain

$$\frac{1}{r} \frac{\partial}{\partial r} (ru) = -\mu_N - \frac{\dot{\nu}_N}{\nu_N}, \tag{12}$$

and, since $\nabla \cdot (\nu_N \mathbf{u} + \nu_E \mathbf{v}) = 0$, we have

$$\nabla \cdot \mathbf{v} = \frac{\nu_N}{1 - \nu_N} \left(\mu_N + \frac{\dot{\nu}_N}{\nu_N} \right). \tag{13}$$

We consider the longitudinal average, $v(r,t)$, of the radial component of $\mathbf{v}$ and make the following assumption (that parallels (7))

$$(1 - \nu_N)[v_z(r, H, t) - v_z(r, -H, t)] = 2\zeta_{\text{out}}^N (p_N(t) - p_\infty),$$

where $\zeta_{\text{out}}^N \geq \zeta_{\text{out}}$ is the conductivity of the tissues traversed by the flux outgoing from necrotic region. Proceeding as above, from (13) we obtain

$$\frac{1}{r} \frac{\partial}{\partial r} (rv) = \frac{1}{1 - \nu_N} \left[\mu_N \nu_N + \dot{\nu}_N - \frac{\zeta_{\text{out}}^N}{H} (p_N - p_\infty) \right]. \tag{14}$$

Equations (12) and (14) are complemented by the following boundary conditions at $r = \rho_N$:

$$\nu_N(t)(u(\rho_N^+,t) - \dot\rho_N) = \nu^\star(u(\rho_N^-,t) - \dot\rho_N)\,,$$
$$(1 - \nu_N(t))(v(\rho_N^+,t) - \dot\rho_N) = (1 - \nu^\star)(v(\rho_N^-,t) - \dot\rho_N)\,.$$

The dynamics of ν_N, p_N, and B was derived in [6] on the basis of the following assumptions: 1) the cellular fraction cannot not exceed a maximal value smaller than one, since necrotic cells retain some structural integrity before degradation; 2) the fluid pressure cannot exceed a given increasing function of B, denoted by $\Psi(B)$, because of the elastic reaction to displacement of the tissues that surround the whole tumour; 3) when ν_N is strictly smaller than the maximal value (taken equal to $\nu^\star$), the reaction of surrounding tissues is supported by the liquid component and the pressure is equal to $\Psi(B)$. In summary:

$$\nu_N(t) \leq \nu^\star\,,$$
$$p_N(t) \leq \Psi(B(t))\,,$$
$$\left(\nu_N(t) - \nu^\star\right)\left(p_N(t) - \Psi(B(t))\right) = 0\,.$$

As discussed in [6], two regimes are possible. In the first one we have $\nu_N(t) < \nu^\star$, $p_N(t) = \Psi(B(t))$ and

$$\frac{dB^2}{dt} = 2\rho_N[(1 - \nu^\star)v(\rho_N,t) + \nu^\star u(\rho_N,t)] - \frac{\zeta_{\text{out}}^N}{H}(B^2 - \rho_N^2)(p_N - p_\infty)\,, \quad (15)$$

$$\frac{d\nu_N}{dt} = \frac{1}{B^2 - \rho_N^2}\left[2\rho_N\nu^\star(u(\rho_N,t) - \dot\rho_N) - 2\nu_N(B\dot B - \rho_N\dot\rho_N)\right] - \mu_N\nu_N\,. \quad (16)$$

Taking into account that matter cannot cross the boundary $r = B(t)$, (15) can be derived from the mass balance of dead cells plus liquid in N, and (16) from the mass balance of dead cells, whose total volume is $2H\pi(B^2 - \rho_N^2)\nu_N$. In the second regime we have instead $\nu_N(t) = \nu^\star$, $p_N(t) \leq \Psi(B(t))$ and

$$p_N(t) = p_\infty + \frac{H}{\zeta_{\text{out}}^N}\left[\frac{2\rho_N(1 - \nu_N)[v(\rho_N,t) - u(\rho_N,t)]}{B^2 - \rho_N^2} + \mu_N\right]\,, \quad (17)$$

$$\frac{dB^2}{dt} = 2\rho_N u(\rho_N,t) - \mu_N(B^2 - \rho_N^2)\,. \quad (18)$$

Equation (18) is derived from the mass balance of dead cells, by taking into account that $\nu_N = \nu^\star$ in this case, whereas $p_N(t)$, according to (17), is such that the outgoing flux keeps the volume fraction of liquid at the value $1 - \nu^\star$. During the evolution, switching between the above regimes may occur when one of the two constraints (on ν_N or on p_N) can no longer be satisfied.

2.3 The Steady State

In the absence of treatment ($\mu_P = \mu_Q = 0$), the only cell populations present in the cord are the viable proliferating and quiescent subpopulations, and

$\nu_P + \nu_Q = 1$. In this condition, the model admits a stationary state defined by the constants ρ_N, B, ν_N, p_0, p_N, and by the time-independent functions $\nu_P(r)$, $\sigma(r)$, $p(r)$, defined in the interval (r_0, ρ_N), and $u(r)$, $v(r)$ in (r_0, B). Existence and uniqueness of the stationary solution were proved in [5] for a simplified version of the model in which the whole necrotic region was treated as a liquid. The behaviour of the steady-state solutions was explored numerically in [6].

3 Transport of Antibodies in the Cord at Steady State

Although the monoclonal antibodies (Ab) used for cancer therapy are usually conjugated to radionuclides or toxins, here we restrict to considering the transport and binding of antibodies (assumed to have negligible mass) deprived of cytotoxic action. The cord steady state will then be not perturbed. The transport of free Ab molecules occurs by diffusion and convection in the interstitial space only. We will consider IgG antibodies possessing two equivalent binding sites, and the antigen is assumed to be monovalent and able to diffuse on the cell membrane, so that antibodies can form single or double bonds.

Let us denote the extracellular free Ab concentration by c, and the surface concentrations of antibodies bound monovalently or bivalently by $\hat{b}_1$ and $\hat{b}_2$, respectively. Let $\hat{S}$ be the (constant) surface concentration of total antigen. Free and bound antigens in the extracellular fluid are disregarded (negligible antigen shedding or loss of the binding ability when the antigen molecules are in solution [13]). By writing the mass balance in the toroidal volume element $(r, r + dr) \times (z, z + dz)$ of the cord, we obtain

$$\frac{\partial}{\partial t}(c\nu_E) - \nu_E D\nabla c + \nabla \cdot (c\nu_E f\mathbf{v}) = -2k_a c\hat{s}\alpha^\star + k_d\hat{b}_1\alpha^\star, \tag{19}$$

$$\frac{\partial}{\partial t}(\hat{b}_1\alpha^\star) + \nabla \cdot (\hat{b}_1\alpha^\star\mathbf{u}) = 2k_a c\hat{s}\alpha^\star - k_d\hat{b}_1\alpha^\star - \hat{k}'_a\hat{s}\hat{b}_1\alpha^\star + 2k_d\hat{b}_2\alpha^\star, \tag{20}$$

$$\frac{\partial}{\partial t}(\hat{b}_2\alpha^\star) + \nabla \cdot (\hat{b}_2\alpha^\star\mathbf{u}) = \hat{k}'_a\hat{s}\hat{b}_1\alpha^\star - 2k_d\hat{b}_2\alpha^\star, \tag{21}$$

with

$$\hat{s} = \hat{S} - \hat{b}_1 - 2\hat{b}_2. \tag{22}$$

In the above equations, D is the effective interstitial diffusivity, f is the retardation factor (i.e., the ratio of solute velocity to fluid velocity), $\alpha^\star$ is the area of cellular surface per unit volume, $2k_a$ is the rate constant for forming the first bond between the antibody molecule and the antigen, k_d is the dissociation rate constant of a bond (any bond is assumed to be independent), and $\hat{k}'_a$ is the rate constant for forming the second bond (see [7]). In the case of delivery of the antibody Fab fragment, which is monovalent, the equations have to be changed accordingly. We disregard the possible internalization of bound Ab, that however could be easily accounted for.

158   A. Bertuzzi, A. Fasano, A. Gandolfi, C. Sinisgalli

Consistently with assumption (iv), we assume that Ab concentration in the central vessel, c_b, is independent of z, and that also c, $\hat{b}_1$, $\hat{b}_2$ are independent of z. After defining the quantities

$$b_1 = \hat{b}_1 \frac{\alpha^\star}{\nu_E}\,, \quad b_2 = \hat{b}_2 \frac{\alpha^\star}{\nu_E}\,, \quad S = \hat{S}\frac{\alpha^\star}{\nu_E}\,, \quad k'_a = \hat{k}'_a \frac{\nu_E}{\alpha^\star}\,,$$

by taking (5) and (6) into account and performing the longitudinal mean over $(-H, H)$, (19)–(22) become

$$\frac{\partial c}{\partial t} - \frac{D}{r}\frac{\partial}{\partial r}\left(r\frac{\partial c}{\partial r}\right) + fv(r)\frac{\partial c}{\partial r} = f\chi\frac{\nu_P(r)}{1-\nu^\star}c - 2k_a cs + k_d b_1\,, \tag{23}$$

$$\frac{\partial b_1}{\partial t} + u(r)\frac{\partial b_1}{\partial r} = -\chi\frac{\nu_P(r)}{\nu^\star}b_1 + 2k_a cs - k_d b_1 - k'_a sb_1 + 2k_d b_2\,, \tag{24}$$

$$\frac{\partial b_2}{\partial t} + u(r)\frac{\partial b_2}{\partial r} = -\chi\frac{\nu_P(r)}{\nu^\star}b_2 + k'_a sb_1 - 2k_d b_2\,, \tag{25}$$

with

$$s = S - b_1 - 2b_2\,.$$

We recall that the functions $u(r)$, $v(r)$, and $\nu_P(r)$ are solutions of the model at the steady state.

At $r=r_0$, we impose for c the following boundary condition that accounts for both diffusive and convective extravasation:

$$-D\frac{\partial c}{\partial r}\bigg|_{r=r_0} + fv(r_0)c(r_0,t) = \frac{P}{\nu_E}(c_b(t) - c(r_0,t))\frac{\mathrm{Pe}}{e^{\mathrm{Pe}}-1} + v(r_0)(1 - \sigma_f)c_b(t)\,,$$

where Pe (Peclet number) is given by

$$\mathrm{Pe} = \nu_E v(r_0)(1 - \sigma_f)/P\,,$$

P is the permeability of the vessel wall, and σ_f is the filtration reflection coefficient. The second boundary condition for c requires the description of the antibody transport in the necrotic region.

Because few information is available on the antibody binding to dead cells, in the simulations that follow we assume for simplicity that antibodies in the region N can bind to the surface of dead cells with the same binding constants as in the living cord (however, different values can also be used). Moreover, a full representation of antigen and antibody fate upon cell degradation would be very complex. Therefore, two extreme simplifications, both consistent with the assumption of neglecting free and bound antigen in the extracellular fluid, have been adopted: antigen and bound antibodies are destroyed upon the degradation of the cell (Model 1), or antigen is destroyed and bound antibody becomes free immediately after degradation (Model 2). Proceeding as above, and using (12), the following equations are obtained for $r \in (\rho_N, B)$ in the case of Model 1:

$$\frac{\partial c}{\partial t} - \frac{D}{r}\frac{\partial}{\partial r}\left(r\frac{\partial c}{\partial r}\right) + fv(r)\frac{\partial c}{\partial r} = -f\mu_N\frac{\nu_N}{1-\nu_N}c - 2k_a c\tilde{s} + k_d\tilde{b}_1\,, \qquad (26)$$

$$\frac{\partial \tilde{b}_1}{\partial t} + u(r)\frac{\partial \tilde{b}_1}{\partial r} = 2k_a c\tilde{s} - k_d\tilde{b}_1 - \tilde{k}_a'\tilde{s}\tilde{b}_1 + 2k_d\tilde{b}_2\,, \qquad (27)$$

$$\frac{\partial \tilde{b}_2}{\partial t} + u(r)\frac{\partial \tilde{b}_2}{\partial r} = \tilde{k}_a'\tilde{s}\tilde{b}_1 - 2k_d\tilde{b}_2\,, \qquad (28)$$

with $\tilde{s} = \tilde{S} - \tilde{b}_1 - 2\tilde{b}_2$ and having defined:

$$\tilde{b}_1 = \hat{b}_1\frac{\alpha_N}{1-\nu_N}\,, \quad \tilde{b}_2 = \hat{b}_2\frac{\alpha_N}{1-\nu_N}\,, \quad \tilde{S} = \hat{S}\frac{\alpha_N}{1-\nu_N}\,, \quad \tilde{k}_a' = \hat{k}_a'\frac{1-\nu_N}{\alpha_N}\,.$$

In the above definitions, α_N denotes the area of cellular surface per unit volume in the N region. Taking $\alpha_N/\alpha^\star = \nu_N/\nu^\star$, we have

$$\tilde{S} = \frac{\nu_N}{\nu^\star}\frac{1-\nu^\star}{1-\nu_N}S\,, \quad \tilde{k}_a' = \frac{\nu^\star}{\nu_N}\frac{1-\nu_N}{1-\nu^\star}k_a'\,.$$

In the case of Model 2, equation (26) is substituted by:

$$\frac{\partial c}{\partial t} - \frac{D}{r}\frac{\partial}{\partial r}\left(r\frac{\partial c}{\partial r}\right) + fv(r)\frac{\partial c}{\partial r} = -f\mu_N\frac{\nu_N}{1-\nu_N}c - 2k_a c\tilde{s} + k_d\tilde{b}_1$$
$$+ \mu_N(\tilde{b}_1 + \tilde{b}_2)\,.$$

At $r = \rho_N$, we impose

$$c(\rho_N^+) = c(\rho_N^-)\,,$$

that, from the continuity of the flux of free antibodies and the assumption that retardation factor is equal in the cord and in the region N, implies

$$(1-\nu_N)\frac{\partial c}{\partial r}\bigg|_{r=\rho_N^+} = (1-\nu^\star)\frac{\partial c}{\partial r}\bigg|_{r=\rho_N^-}\,.$$

Furthermore, we have

$$\tilde{b}_i(\rho_N^+,t) = \frac{\nu_N}{\nu^\star}\frac{1-\nu^\star}{1-\nu_N}b_i(\rho_N^-,t)\,, \quad i=1,2\,.$$

Finally, at $r = B$, we impose

$$\frac{\partial c}{\partial r}\bigg|_{r=B} = 0\,.$$

4 Nondimensional Variables and Parameters

In the numerical solution, we use the following nondimensional variables:

$$t' = t\chi, \qquad r' = \frac{r}{r_0}, \qquad z' = \frac{z}{H},$$

$$u' = \frac{u}{\chi r_0}, \qquad v' = \frac{v}{\chi r_0}, \qquad p' = \frac{p - p_\infty}{p_b - p_\infty}, \qquad \sigma' = \frac{\sigma}{\sigma_b}.$$

All the Ab concentrations (c_b, c, b_1, b_2, $\tilde{b}_1$ $\tilde{b}_2$) are rescaled by S. All the rate costants, χ, γ, λ, μ_N, k_d are rescaled by χ. The association rate constants are rescaled by χ/S. For the other parameters we have

$$\kappa' = \kappa \frac{p_b - p_\infty}{\chi r_0^2}, \qquad \zeta'_{\mathrm{in}} = \zeta_{\mathrm{in}} \frac{p_b - p_\infty}{\chi r_0}, \qquad \zeta'_{\mathrm{out}} = \zeta_{\mathrm{out}} \frac{p_b - p_\infty}{\chi H},$$

$$D' = \frac{D}{\chi r_0^2}, \qquad P' = \frac{P}{\chi r_0}.$$

For the sake of simplicity, the primes will be omitted and we will use the same symbols for the nondimensional and the dimensional quantities.

5 Numerical Results

In this section we give examples of the distribution of bound antibody computed according to the proposed model. For the numerical solution of the steady state of the tumour cord, we refer to [6]. To approximate the nonlinear elasticity of biological tissues, the function $\Psi(B)$ was chosen as $\Psi(B) = e(B - 1)^2$ in the nondimensional form, with e a given elasticity coefficient. As in [6], the nondimensional values of the cord parameters were chosen, whenever possible, according to dimensional values available in the literature. Concerning the parameters of Ab transport, the values of diffusivity and vessel permeability were chosen according to the following dimensional values: $D = 1.3 \times 10^{-8}\,\mathrm{cm}^2/\mathrm{s}$ and $P/\nu_E = 5.7 \times 10^{-7}\,\mathrm{cm/s}$ [9]. Moreover, $f = 0.75$ and $\sigma_f = 0.8$ [1]. For the time course of Ab concentration in plasma, we have set

$$c_b(t) = c_{b0}\left(m e^{-t/\tau_1} + (1 - m)e^{-t/\tau_2}\right),$$

with values of m, τ_1 and τ_2 as in [9]. Equations (23)–(25) and (26)–(28) were solved by means of a finite difference method that combines a modified Crank-Nicholson scheme for c with the solution of the equations for the bound concentration over the characteristic lines. Zero initial conditions were assumed.

Figure 1, upper left panel, shows for Model 1 the distributions of bound ($b_1 + b_2$) and free Ab in a high-affinity case with $K = k_a/k_d = 50$ (the corresponding dimensional value is $5 \times 10^7\,\mathrm{M}^{-1}$ if $S = 10^{-6}\,\mathrm{M}$). In this case, antibodies in the cord are mainly in the bound state and their concentration declines with r. The lower left panel shows the time course of b_1 and b_2 at $r = r_0$ and $r = \rho_N$. The doubly bound Ab largely prevails, expecially at the cord periphery where the free Ab concentration is very small. Note the marked time delay of the maximal bound concentration at the periphery with respect to the inner region of the cord. The panels on the right of Fig. 1 depict the case of a reduced affinity, with $K = 2$. The bound Ab is much smaller, but more uniform with r. Since the free Ab concentration is higher, b_1 is close to b_2 (lower panel). The delay of the maximum of bound Ab at the periphery is decreased, highlighting the role of binding in reducing the velocity of Ab penetration.

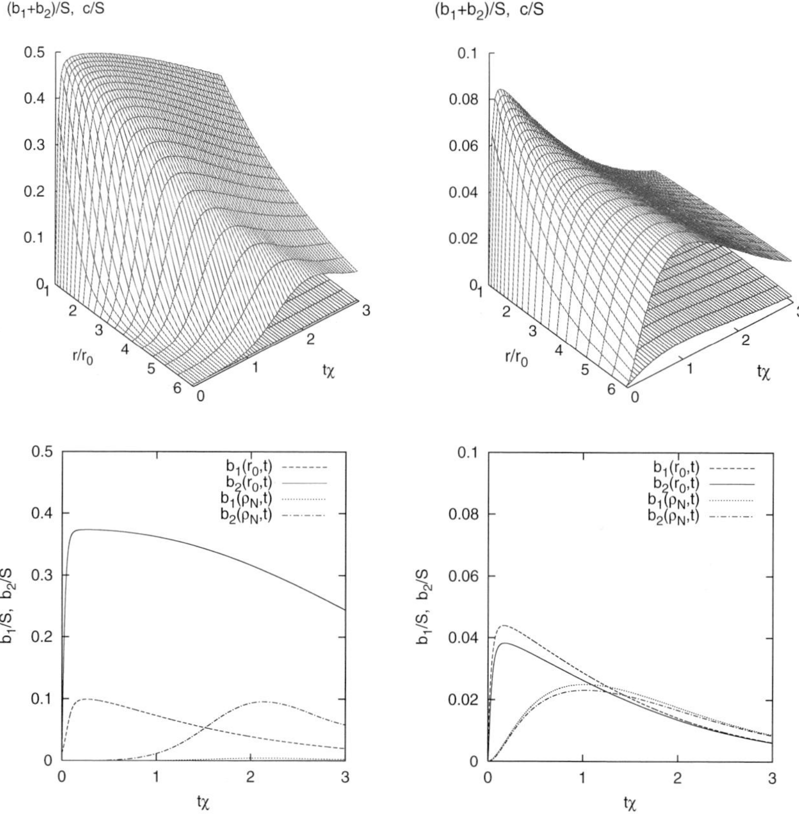

Fig. 1: Distribution of bound and free Ab (upper panels, in both panels the lower surface represents free Ab); time course of b_1 and b_2 at $r = r_0$ and $r = \rho_N$ (lower panels). Left panels: $k_a = k'_a = 1000$, $k_d = 20$. Right panels: $k_a = k'_a = 100$, $k_d = 50$. Other parameters: $\zeta_{in} = 400$, $\zeta_{out} = \zeta_{out}^N = 0.5$, $\kappa = 10000$, $e = 12 \times 10^{-3}$, $\mu_N = 1$, $D = 400$, $P = 5$, $c_{b0} = 0.1$.

In Fig. 2 the time course of the bound Ab at $r = \rho_N$, computed by Model 1, is compared with that computed by Model 2. In addition to the cord of Fig. 1 ($\rho_N = 6.23$, $B = 9.42$, $\nu_N = 0.315$), we have considered the Ab transport in a cord with a reduced necrotic region ($\rho_N = 6.23$, $B = 7.37$, $\nu_N = 0.509$), obtained by changing the values of $\zeta_{\text{out}} = \zeta_{\text{out}}^N$, e, and μ_N. It can be seen that the predictions obtained according to the two models for Ab transport in the N region present only moderate differences, except in the case of high affinity and reduced necrotic region. At $r = r_0$, these differences are very small (not shown). These results suggest that the fate of antibodies after cell degradation is not particularly relevant, apart from cases in which both the degradation rate and the amount of bound Ab are large. Note that a larger necrotic region introduces a smoothing in the time course of bound Ab concentration at $r = \rho_N$, at least in the low affinity case, since the necrotic region acts as a storage chamber for antibodies.

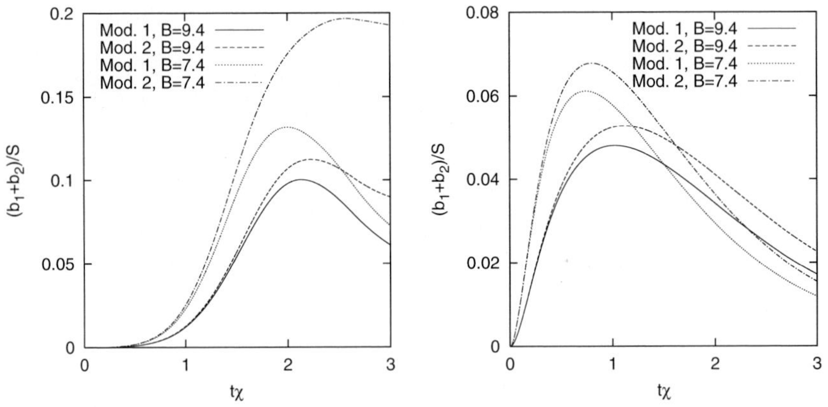

Fig. 2: Time course of bound Ab at $r = \rho_N$ computed by Model 1 and Model 2. Left panel: $k_a = k_a' = 1000$, $k_d = 20$; right panel: $k_a = k_a' = 100$, $k_d = 50$. In the case with $B = 7.37$, parameters as in Fig. 1, except $\zeta_{\text{out}} = \zeta_{\text{out}}^N = 2$, $e = 20 \times 10^{-3}$, $\mu_N = 2$.

In the simulations of Fig. 1, taken as the reference cases, the cord steady state was characterized by $p_0 = 0.86$ and a mean interstitial fluid velocity of 90.93. Because of the high value of Darcy's constant κ, it is $p_0 \simeq p_N$, so the fluid pressure is fairly uniform throughout the system. The computation of the diffusive and convective terms revealed a rather significant contribution of convection to the transport. To test the influence of a reduced convection, we decreased $\zeta_{\text{out}} = \zeta_{\text{out}}^N$ from 0.5 to 0.065 and increased e from 12×10^{-3} to 14×10^{-3}. In this way we had $p_0 = 0.98$ and a quite small interstitial fluid velocity (mean value equal to 7.02), while the radius B was almost unchanged ($B = 9.36$). In the high-affinity case, the maximum of bound Ab at $r = r_0$ is only slightly reduced (88% of the reference value, simulation by Model 1), whereas the reduction is greater at the cord periphery (26%). In the low-affinity case, the reduction of the maximum is more uniform with r, in particular it is 70% at $r=r_0$ and 65% at $r=\rho_N$. By contrast, an increased convection was obtained lowering p_0 to 0.52, by setting $\zeta_{\text{out}}=\zeta_{\text{out}}^N=3$ and $e=7\times10^{-3}$ (mean value of v equal to 324.8 and $B=9.36$). In the high-affinity case, the maximum of bound Ab at $r=r_0$ is slightly increased (110% of the reference value), whereas the increment is very marked at the cord periphery (344%). We note that in the inner cord the increment is not so large because the binding sites are almost saturated. In the low-affinity case, the increment of the maximum is still more uniform, in particular 131% at $r=r_0$ and 158% at $r=\rho_N$.

As a concluding remark, we observe that the high binding to cell surface antigens results in a "barrier" to Ab penetration, generating a more heterogeneous Ab distribution, since the binding in the inner region of the cord produces a marked decrease of free Ab concentration as r increases (see also [9]). In our simulations, convective transport appears to be significant especially at the periphery of the cord, although, even at very high interstitial pressures, the overall transport is not suppressed. However, further investigations that explore other parameter combinations are necessary to elucidate the importance of this phenomenon on Ab transport.

References

1. Baxter, L.T., Jain, R.K.: Transport of fluid and macromolecules in tumors. I. Role of interstitial pressure and convection. Microvasc. Res., **37**, 77–104 (1989)
2. Berinstein, N.L.: Biological therapy of cancer. In: Tannock, I.F., Hill, R.P. (eds) The Basic Science of Oncology. McGraw-Hill, New York, 420–442 (1998)
3. Bertuzzi, A., d'Onofrio, A., Fasano, A., Gandolfi, A.: Regression and regrowth of tumour cords following single-dose anticancer treatment. Bull. Math. Biol., **65**, 903–931 (2003)
4. Bertuzzi, A., Fasano, A., Gandolfi, A.: A free boundary problem with unilateral constraints describing the evolution of a tumour cord under the influence of cell killing agents. SIAM J. Math. Anal., **36**, 882–915 (2004)
5. Bertuzzi, A., Fasano, A., Gandolfi, A.: A mathematical model for tumour cords incorporating the flow of interstitial fluid. Math. Mod. Meth. Appl. Sci., **15**, 1735–1777 (2005)
6. Bertuzzi, A., Fasano, A., Gandolfi, A., Sinisgalli, C.: Interstitial pressure and extracellular fluid motion in tumour cords. Math. Biosci. Engng., **2**, 445–460 (2005)
7. DeLisi, C.: Antigen Antibody Interactions. Lecture Notes in Biomathematics, Vol. 8. Springer-Verlag, Berlin (1976)
8. Friedman, A.: A hierarchy of cancer models and their mathematical challenges. Discrete Contin. Dyn. Syst. Ser. B, **4**, 147–159 (2004)
9. Fujimori, K., Covell, D.G., Fletcher, J.E., Weinstein, J.N.: Modeling analysis of the global and microscopic distribution of immunoglobulin G, F(ab')$_2$, and Fab in tumors. Cancer Res., **49**, 5656–5663 (1989)

10. Hirst, D.G., Denekamp, J.: Tumour cell proliferation in relation to the vasculature, Cell Tissue Kinet., **12**, 31–42 (1979)
11. Jain, R.K.: Delivery of molecular medicine to solid tumors: lessons from in vivo imaging of gene expression and function. J. Controlled Release, **74**, 7–25 (2001)
12. Moore, J.V., Hasleton, P.S., Buckley, C.H.: Tumour cords in 52 human bronchial and cervical squamous cell carcinomas: Inferences for their cellular kinetics and radiobiology. Br. J. Cancer, **51**, 407–413 (1985)
13. Nagata, S., Ise, T., Onda, M., Nakamura, K., Ho, M., Raubitschek, A., Pastan, I.H.: Cell membrane-specific epitopes on CD30: Potentially superior targets for immunotherapy. Proc. Natl. Acad. Sci. USA, **102**, 7946–7951 (2005)
14. Tannock, I.F.: The relation between cell proliferation and the vascular system in a transplanted mouse mammary tumour. Br. J. Cancer, **22**, 258–273 (1968)

Structural Adaptation in Normal and Cancerous Vasculature

Philip K. Maini[1], Tomás Alarcón[2], Helen M. Byrne[3], Markus R. Owen[3], and James Murphy[3]

[1] Centre for Mathematical Biology, Mathematical Institute, University of Oxford, Oxford OX1 3LB, UK maini@maths.ox.ac.uk
[2] Bioinformatics Unit, Department of Computer Science, University College London, Gower Street, London WC1E 6BT, UK t.alarcon@cs.ucl.ac.uk
[3] Centre for Mathematical Medicine, School of Mathematical Sciences, University of Nottingham, Nottingham NG7 2RD, UK helen.byrne@nottingham.ac.uk, markus.owen@nottingham.ac.uk

Dedicated to Professor Vincenzo Capasso on the occasion of his 60th birthday

Summary. The dynamics of cancerous tissue growth involves the complex interaction of a number of phenomena interacting over a range of temporal and spatial scales. While several processes involved have been studied, the adaptation of the vasculature within a growing tumour has thus far received little attention. We consider a hybrid cellular automaton model which analyses the interaction between the tumour vascular network and tissue growth. We compute the temporal behaviour of the cancerous cell population under different hypotheses of structural adaptation in the vasculature. This may provide a possible method of determining experimentally which adaptation mechanisms are at work.

1 Introduction

The main function of vasculature is to ensure adequate and efficient nutrient delivery to tissue. To achieve this, blood vessels must be able to structurally adapt in response to signals from the tissue they perfuse. Experimental and theoretical studies have significantly advanced our understanding of the possible design principles and adaptation mechanisms at work in normal vessels [7], but there are still many open questions, and how these aspects of vasculature design change under diseased or abnormal conditions largely remains a mystery.

In normal vasculature, design principles based on an optimality assumption were first proposed by Murray [8], whereby the structure of the vascular system is postulated to arise from the balance between blood metabolic energy consumption and energy dissipated by blood flow. Murray's design principle has been shown to imply that the wall shear stress (WSS) must be constant over the vascular network and experimental data appear to validate these predictions for arteries [15]. However, more recent experimental studies by Pries et al. [10] have shown that the WSS is not constant in smaller arterioles and capillaries, thus contradicting these predictions. Based on these results, they proposed a design principle whereby the vascular system must adapt to a sigmoidal WSS-pressure curve. A design principle based on Murray's optimality principle and recent blood-rheological data [3] has been shown to reproduce the non-constant WSS-pressure relationship found by Pries et al. [10].

Adaptation of the normal vascular system to a number of stimuli has been extensively analysed by Pries et al. [11, 12]. They have considered a model which accounts for adaptation in response to haemodynamic signals (WSS and pressure [13]) and metabolic stimulus, and have also considered both upstream and downstream signalling between vessels. The actual mechanistic bases for these stimuli are largely unknown, although there is some evidence that the downstream signal is carried by ATP molecules, whereas the upstream signal consists of changes in the membrane potential of endothelial cells that are propagated along the vessel walls.

In contrast to normal vasculature, which appears well organised according to the principles mentioned above, tumour vasculature appears to be very disorganised in all respects. Vessels lack the well-defined anatomical structure of their normal counterparts and are leaky. Blood flow in tumour vascular beds is also quite disorganised compared to normal circulation. In addition, there is evidence of signalling between tumour cells and normal vessels that induces a dematuration process within normal vessels as tumour malignancy progresses and co-opts normal vessels [14]. The significance of understanding how these changes affect circulation is obvious when one considers that the vasculature delivers drugs to the tumour.

In a first attempt towards a model of tumour vasculature, we aim to assess which of the normal adaptation mechanisms are more likely to be absent in tumour vasculature. To this end, we use the multi-scale model framework proposed in [2] to assess the effects of different adaptation cues. In effect, we "turn off" individual elements of the normal adaptation mechanism proposed by Pries et al. [12] and determine predicted outcomes. We hope that by experimental observation of tumour dynamics, one might then be able to deduce what structural adaptation mechanisms are at work.

2 Summary of the Multi-scale Model

The model we use integrates phenomena occurring on very different time and length scales TLSs (see Fig. 1). These features include blood flow and structural adaptation of the vascular network, transport into the tissue of

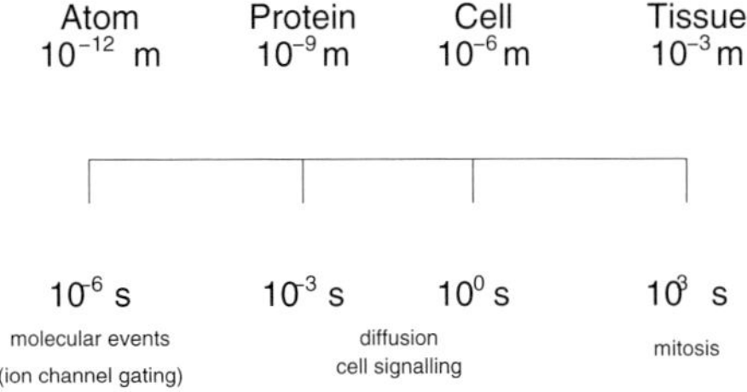

Fig. 1: Time and length scales involved in our model [6].

blood-borne oxygen, competition between cancer and normal cells, cell division, apoptosis, VEGF (growth factor) release, and the coupling between them. In this section we present an overview of the main features of the integrated model without entering into a detailed description of the sub-models which form its component parts.

The modelling framework we use is based on the hybrid cellular automaton concept which has been used to model several aspects of tumour development (see [1, 5, 9]). We extend this approach to account not only for the presence of a diffusive substance (such as oxygen or glucose) as in previous papers, but also to include intracellular and tissue-scale phenomena, and the coupling between them. To this end, we have organised our model into three layers: vascular, cellular, and intracellular, which correspond, respectively, to the tissue, cellular and intracellular TLSs, (see Fig. 2). For a full account of the details we refer the reader to [2].

In the top layer, we deal with the structure of the vascular network and blood flow (see [1] for more details). We consider a hexagonal vascular network (similar to the one observed in liver). Each individual vessel is assumed to undergo structural adaptation (i.e. changes in radius) in response to different stimuli until the network reaches a quasi-equilibrium state. Through this structural adaptation process we compute the blood flow rate, the pressure drop and the haematocrit (i.e. relative volume of red blood cells) distribution in each vessel. Between the vascular layer and the cellular layer, i.e. coupling the dynamics at the cellular level to blood flow and vascular adaptation, we have the transport of blood-borne oxygen into the tissue. This process is modelled by a reaction-diffusion equation. The distribution of haematocrit is the source of oxygen, whereas the distribution of cells (provided by the cellular layer) gives us the (spatially distributed) sink of oxygen.

In the intermediate layer, we focus on cell-cell interactions (competition) and spatial distribution of cells. We consider two types of cells: normal and cancerous, which are modelled as individual elements. These two populations compete for space and resources. Cancerous phenotypes are usually better competitors, which results in the cancer population taking over. Competition between the two types of cells is introduced by a very simple rule, which, in turn, couples this middle layer to the intracellular layer. Apoptosis (programmed cell death) is controlled by the expression of p 53 (whose dynamics is dealt with in the intracellular layer): when the level of p 53 in a cell exceeds some threshold the cell undergoes apoptosis. However, this threshold is fixed according to the local spatial distribution of cells, which links the spatial distribution (cellular layer) with the apoptotic process (intracellular layer).

In the bottom layer, we consider intracellular processes, in particular cell division, apoptosis, and VEGF secretion. In this layer, we use ordinary differential equations (ODEs) to model the relevant biochemistry. One issue we focus on is how the external conditions modulate the dynamics of these intracellular phenomena and, in particular, how the level of extracellular oxygen affects the division rate, the expression of p 53 (which regulates apoptosis) and the production of VEGF. Since the spatial distribution of oxygen depends on both the spatial distribution of cells (cellular layer) and on the distribution of haematocrit (vascular layer), these processes at the intracellular level are linked to the behaviour of the other two layers: cell proliferation and apoptosis alter the spatial distribution of the cells (see Fig. 2); the cellular and the intracellular layers modulate the process of vascular structural adaptation through another transport process: diffusion of VEGF into the tissue and its absorption by the endothelial cells (ECs) lining the vessels.

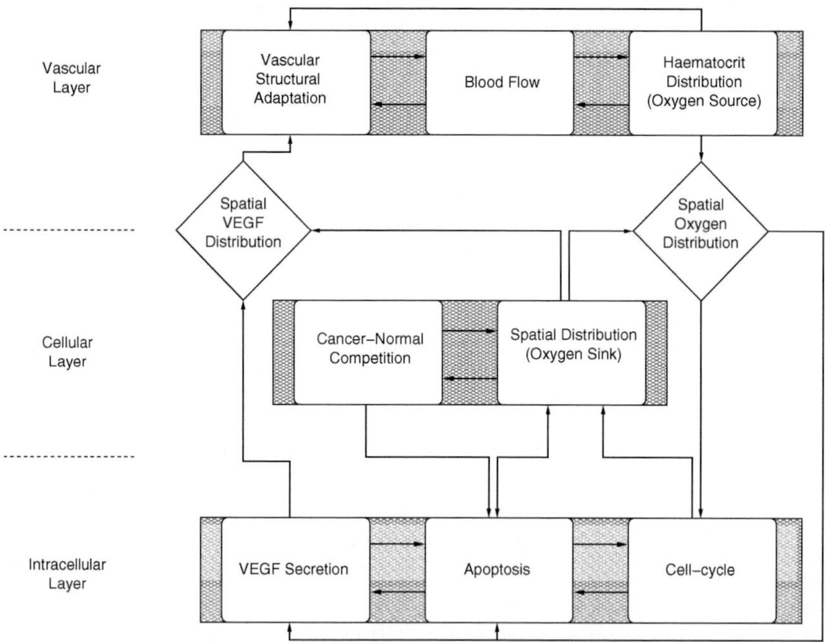

Fig. 2: Diagrammatic representation of the layer structure of our model.

3 Structural Adaptation in Normal Vasculature

In a series of papers, Pries, Secomb and co-workers have put together a model for vascular structural adaptation [11, 12]. According to this model, structural adaptation in normal vasculature occurs by adapting vessel radii to different stimuli:

$$\Delta R = S_{\mathrm{tot}} R \Delta t$$

where R is vessel radius, Δt the time step, and S_{tot} is the total stimulus, given by the sum of the different stimuli. According to [11], there are three types of stimuli, and we briefly describe each one in turn. They assume a *haemodynamic* stimulus, which forces the vessels to adapt to blood flow conditions. The main signals involved in haemodynamic adaptation appear to be wall shear stress, τ_w, and pressure, P [13], although each of these magnitudes seems to play a different role: whereas increased WSS generally induces radius increase, increased pressure leads to decrease in vessel radius [12]. Accordingly, Pries et al. [12] postulate the following form for the haemodynamic stimulus, S_{h}:

$$S_{\mathrm{h}} = \log(\tau_w + \tau_r) - k_p \log(\tau_e(P))$$

where τ_r is a constant introduced to avoid singular behaviour for low WSS, k_p is a constant and $\tau_e(P)$ is the level of WSS expected from the actual value of the intravascular pressure [12].

The second stimulus is the so-called *metabolic* stimulus. It is well known that, as part of their normal functionality, vessels respond and adapt to the metabolic needs of the surrounding tissue. Pries et al. [11] considered the following functional form for the metabolic stimulus, S_{m}:

$$S_{\mathrm{m}} = k_m \log\left(1 + \frac{\dot{Q}_r}{\dot{Q}H}\right) \tag{1}$$

where k_m is a constant, $\dot{Q}_r$ is a reference blood flow and H is the haematocrit. In [2], a modification of Eq. (1) was proposed in order to explicitly take into account the effect on the vasculature of VEGF, V (produced by nutrient-deprived cells) whereby the constant k_m was replaced by a function of V:

$$k_m(V) = k_m^0 \left(1 + \frac{V}{V_0 + V}\right) \tag{2}$$

where k_m^0 and V_0 are constants.

The third stimulus is actually a pair of stimuli, the so-called *conducted* stimuli, which consist of signals generated by the vessels and propagate either downstream or upstream. They are assumed to be necessary to maintain a fully functional vascular system. These signals are usually emitted under stress conditions, and therefore are closely related to the metabolic stimulus described above. Although most of the underlying biological details of these signalling mechanisms are unknown, the downstream stimulus is hypothesised to be transmitted by a chemical which is released into the blood (a good candidate seems to be ATP released by red blood cells under hypoxic conditions [4]) and thereby carried downstream by the flow. The upstream transmission of information seems to be along the vessel walls, perhaps by spread of changes in membrane potential through gap junctions [12].

4 Deconstructing Normal Vasculature

We now examine, in turn, the effect on tumour cell population dynamics of these stimuli. Specifically, we focus on those stimuli which are most likely to be absent in tumour vascular networks.

4.1 Adaptation Decoupled from VEGF Production

For completeness and later comparison, we first carry out simulations with $k_m = k_m^0$ independent of VEGF in Eq. (1). No conducted stimuli are introduced, so S_tot is given by:

$$S_\text{tot} = S_\text{h} + S_\text{m} - k_s$$

where k_s is the so-called *shrinking tendency* which accounts for vessel shrinkage in the absence of stimuli [11].

The results obtained are shown in Fig. 3. As we can see, the growth of the tumour does not have any impact on the vascular network, as tumour growth and vascular adaptation are effectively decoupled. It is worth noting the formation of a necrotic core in the centre of the growing tumour. We see that the flow is evenly distributed along the pathways running parallel to the diagonal as a consequence of the boundary conditions which are flow inward at the bottom left-hand corner, flow outward at the top right-hand corner, and zero flux elsewhere.

4.2 Adaptation Coupled to VEGF Production

We now account for the coupling between vasculature and VEGF, by taking in Eq. (1) $k_m = k_m(V)$ as given by Eq. (2). No conducted stimuli are introduced, so S_tot is given by:

$$S_\text{tot} = S_\text{h} + S_\text{m} - k_s.$$

In this case (see Fig. 4) the behaviour of the system resembles more closely what we would expect in a tumour: there are extensive hypoxic regions within the tumour, but no noticeable necrotic regions. We also see that this model, as

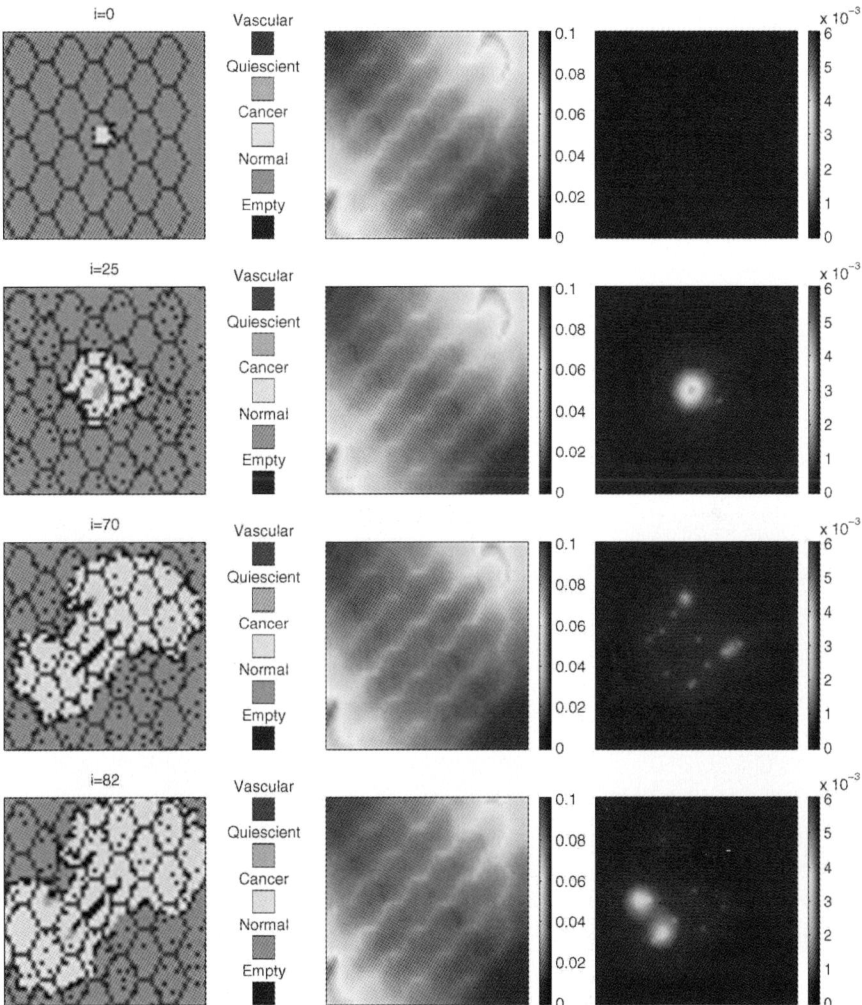

Fig. 3: Four snapshots showing simulations with no VEGF coupling and no conducted stimuli. Time increases from top to bottom. The left column corresponds to the evolution of the colonies of normal and cancerous cells, the central column to the distribution of oxygen and the right column to VEGF distribution. See also Plate 4 on page 339

in the previous case, leads to parallel circulatory pathways running along the diagonal. However, in this case, due to the coupling between VEGF production and vascular adaptation, there is only one pathway that takes most of the flow. This continues until eventually an instability occurs whereby there is basically only one pathway that carries all the flow. This may well contribute to the dynamic and rather unstable spatial patterns formed by real tumours.

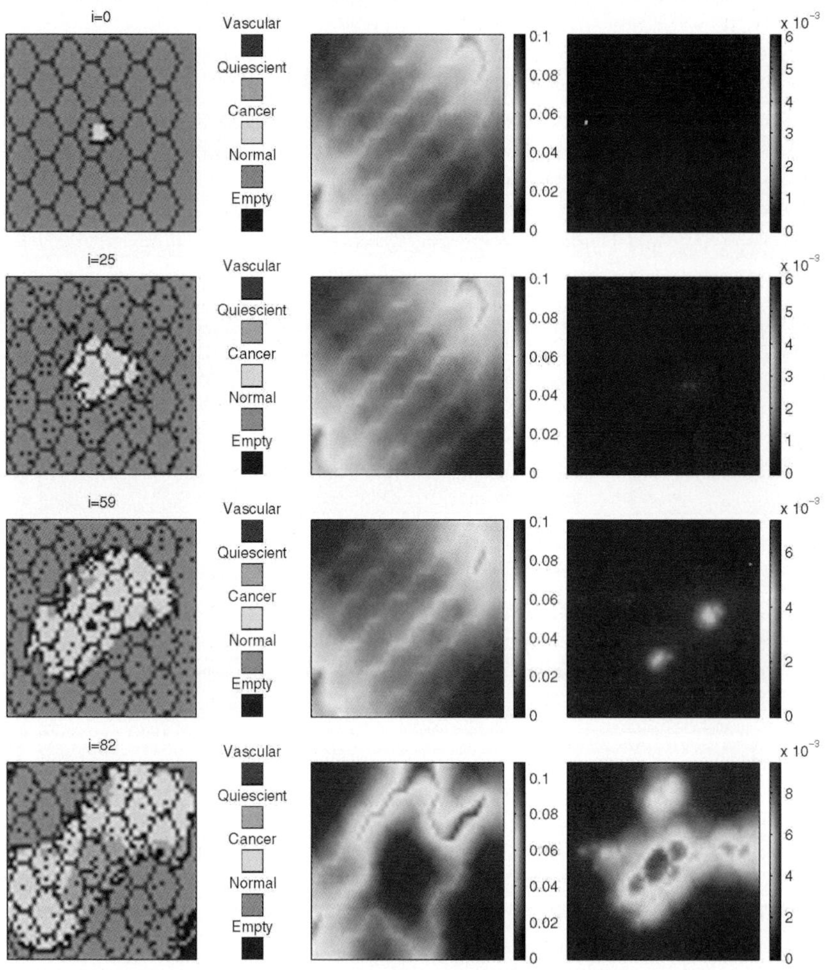

Fig. 4: Four snapshots showing simulations with vascular adaptation coupled to VEGF released by hypoxic cells. Time increases from top to bottom. The left column corresponds to the evolution of the colonies of normal and cancerous cells, the central column to the distribution of oxygen and the right column to VEGF distribution. See also Plate 5 on page 340

4.3 Inclusion of Downstream Signalling

The mechanism we propose for downstream transmission of signals differs somewhat from that proposed by Pries et al. [12]. Whereas they consider that the downstream stimulus is long-range and propagates from any vessel of the network to any other vessel downstream of it, we will assume that the downstream stimulus is only transmitted to the nearest neighbour, i.e. to the vessels immediately downstream of the one releasing the signal. The mechanism proposed by Pries et al. [12] relies on the fact that the chemical carrying the signal has a long half-life time in blood, which allows it to stay in the circulation for a significant length of time. Our mechanism, on the contrary, is based on the assumption that the chemical has a short half-life time. Because the identity and properties of the actual chemical are unknown, both mechanisms are feasible *a priori*.

The intensity of the downstream stimulus, S_d, is assumed to depend on the current of the signalling chemical along a particular vessel (vessel "1", say). If the vessels upstream (vessels "2" and "3") of vessel 1 are irrigating hypoxic regions, they will be receiving signals from the tissue in the form of secreted VEGF. If this is the case, i.e. if the concentration of VEGF in any of the vessels 2 or 3 is larger than zero, then these vessels will produce a (constant) amount of signalling chemical, ρ_0. The chemical produced in vessels 2 and 3 will enter vessel 1 and its current along vessel 1 will be (due to mass conservation):

$$J_1 = \rho_1(V)\dot{Q}_2 + \rho_2(V)\dot{Q}_2$$

where $\rho_i(V) = \rho_0$ if $V \neq 0$ in vessel $i = 1, 2$ and $\rho_i(V) = 0$ if $V = 0$ in vessel $i = 1, 2$. Using now the formula given in [12], S_d is given by:

$$S_\mathrm{d} = \log\left(1 + \frac{J_1}{\dot{Q} + \dot{Q}_{ref}}\right)$$

where $\dot{Q}_{ref}$ is a constant introduced to avoid singular behaviour. The total stimulus is then given by

$$S_\mathrm{tot} = S_\mathrm{h} + S_\mathrm{m} + S_\mathrm{d} - k_s$$

with $k_m = k_m(V)$ as in Eq. (2), i.e. the coupling between vascular adaptation and VEGF production is taken into account.

The corresponding results are shown in Fig. 5. Comparing the results to those obtained in Section 4.2, we see that this vasculature yields tumours with smaller hypoxic regions which release lower concentrations of VEGF. Related to this behaviour, we also observe differences in the vasculature and blood flow with respect to the two previous cases (Sections 4.1 and 4.2). In this case, the flow is initially distributed within disconnected pathways along the diagonal, but eventually blood flow is established along paths connecting the diagonal pathways (which are still the main flow paths). This generates a more homogeneous pattern of blood flow and oxygen concentration which leads to smaller hypoxic regions and therefore to a much more stable spatial pattern.

Therefore the inclusion of "first-neighbour" downstream signalling yields a more "normal-looking" vasculature and more static spatial pattern within the tumour. This leads to the conclusion that this mechanism of vascular adaptation is quite likely to be absent in tumour circulation.

4.4 Inclusion of Upstream Signalling

Following Pries et al. [12], the intensity of the upstream stimulus, S_{u}, is assumed to depend on a signal produced by vessels in hypoxic regions ($V > 0$). The "amount" of signal produced is assumed to be proportional to the length of the vessel, L_s. As in [12], we further assume the existence of a dissipative mechanism in the upstream signal propagation, which will be modelled by an exponential decay. At a given node of the network, the current of upstream stimulus produced by each "outgoing" vessel (defined as one such that the corresponding current has a negative value) is given by:

$$J_c^o = L_s e^{-L_s/L}$$

where L is a constant.

The total current, J_c, is the sum over all the outgoing vessels at a given node of the corresponding values of J_c^o. The upstream stimulus at each of the incoming vessels at the corresponding node is given by [12]:

$$S_{\mathrm{u}} = k_m k_c \frac{J_c}{J_c + J_0}$$

where J_0 is a constant. The total stimulus is then given by

$$S_{\mathrm{tot}} = S_{\mathrm{h}} + S_{\mathrm{m}} + S_{\mathrm{u}} - k_s.$$

Typical results are shown in Fig. 6. Comparing the results to those obtained in Section 4.3, we see that this mechanism yields a vasculature in which the circulation is heavily concentrated around the regions under hypoxic stress, in contrast to the situation observed in Fig. 5, in which the action of the downstream stimulus tends to homogenise the pattern of flow. The way in which this flow concentration around hypoxic regions is achieved is different from the one shown in Fig. 4, corresponding to an adaptation mechanism without long-range stimuli. In Fig. 4 we see that when several hypoxic regions appear within the tumour mass the adaptation mechanism reacts by creating large parallel vessels running through the hypoxic regions from inlet to outlet. In the present case (see Fig. 5), the pattern of flow when a number of hypoxic regions appear is much more homogeneous and "normal looking". Therefore we suggest that this mechanism is quite likely to be absent in tumour vasculature.

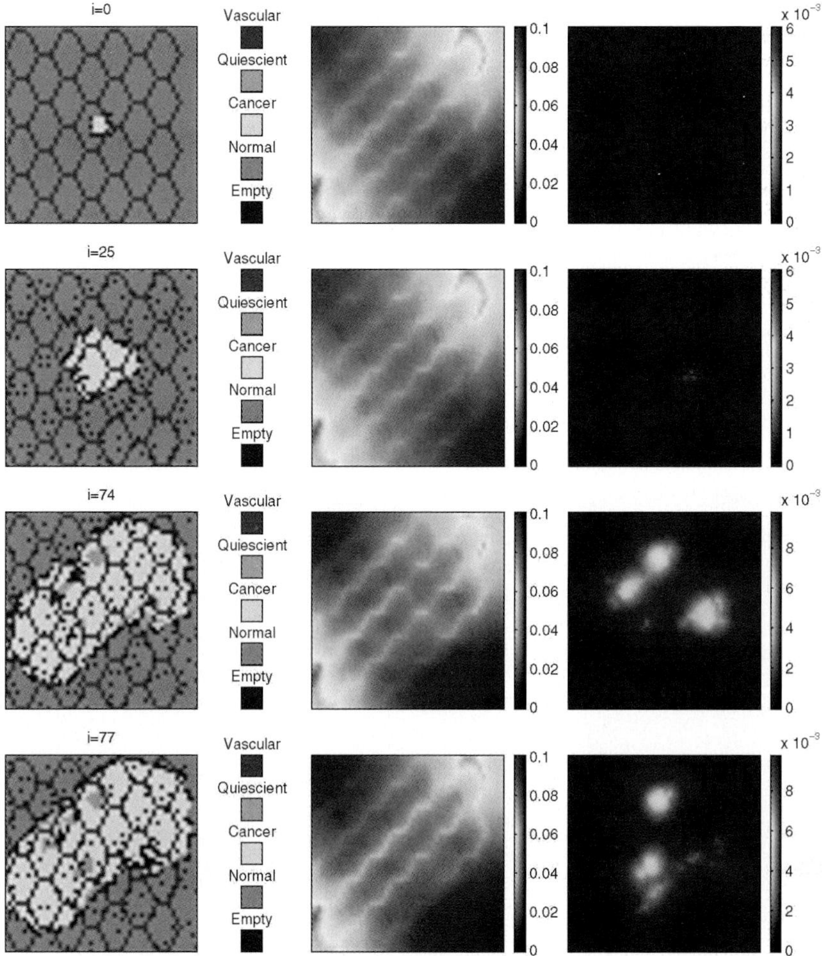

Fig. 5: Four snapshots showing simulations with a structural adaptation mechanism coupled to VEGF released by hypoxic cells plus "nearest-neighbour" downstream stimulus. The left column corresponds to the evolution of the colonies of normal and cancerous cells, the central column to the distribution of oxygen and the right column to VEGF distribution. See also Plate 6 on page 341

5 Conclusions and Discussion

We have used a previously developed hybrid cellular automaton model to explore the effects on tumour cell dynamics of different vasculature structural adaptation mechanisms. We summarise our new results as follows:

- Only vasculature in which adaptation is decoupled from VEGF can support a necrotic core, with a size which appears to correlate with total

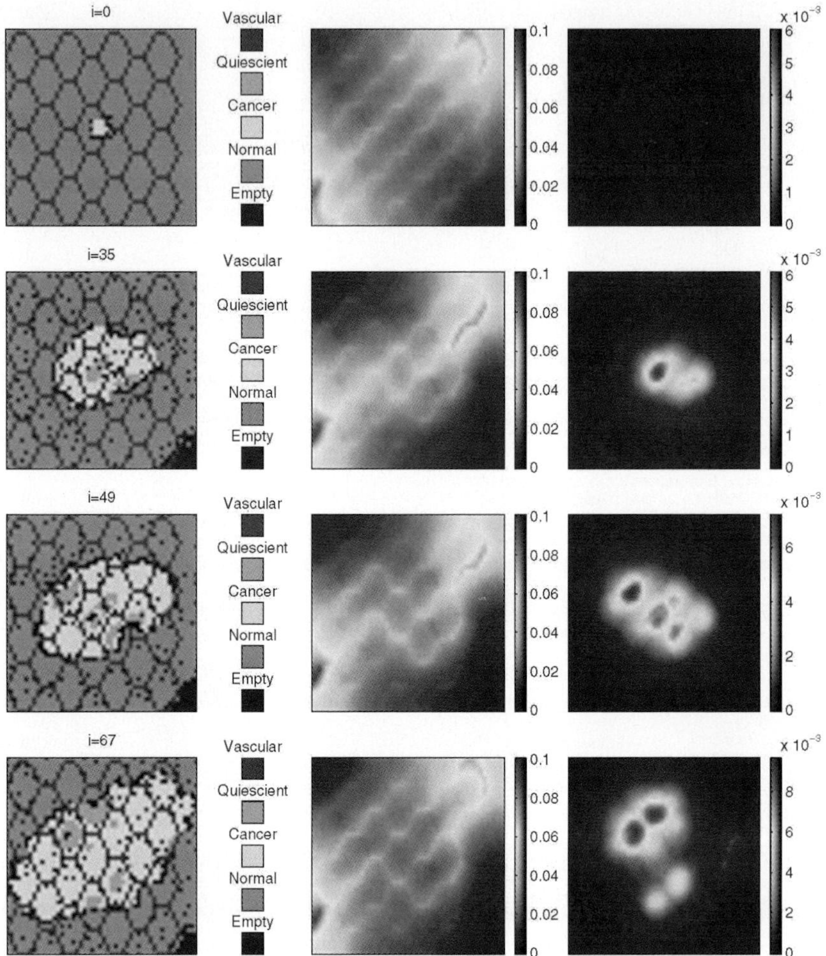

Fig. 6: Four snapshots showing simulations with a structural adaptation mechanism coupled to VEGF released by hypoxic cells plus "nearest-neighbour" upstream stimulus. The left column corresponds to the evolution of the colonies of normal and cancerous cells, the central column to the distribution of oxygen and the right column to VEGF distribution. See also Plate 7 on page 342

tumour size (see Fig. 3). This is due to the inability of the tumour to induce sufficient vasculature to supply extra oxygen to that particular region.

- The vasculature generated by assuming coupling between vascular adaptation and VEGF production appears to produce the most spatially heterogeneous pattern of flow and oxygen. Eventually the system evolves to one pathway carrying almost all of the flow.

- When introducing nearest-neighbour downstream signalling, the distribution of flow and oxygen becomes more homogeneous, yielding a much more stable spatial pattern within the tumour.
- Upstream signalling yields concentration of flow and oxygen around the hypoxic regions, although the patterns of flow look much more homogeneous than in the case without downstream and upstream stimuli.
- The size of hypoxic regions appears to correlate with the homogeneity of flow and oxygen distributions. Heterogeneous distributions (Fig. 4) yield larger hypoxic regions.

While in the above we have compared spatial distributions of key components in response to different stimuli, we can also easily compute how the total number of cells changes over time. In Fig. 7 we observe how the total number of cells and their temporal dynamics depend quite critically on the adaptation mechanism assumed. Intriguingly, the model predicts oscillatory behaviour in cancerous cell population.

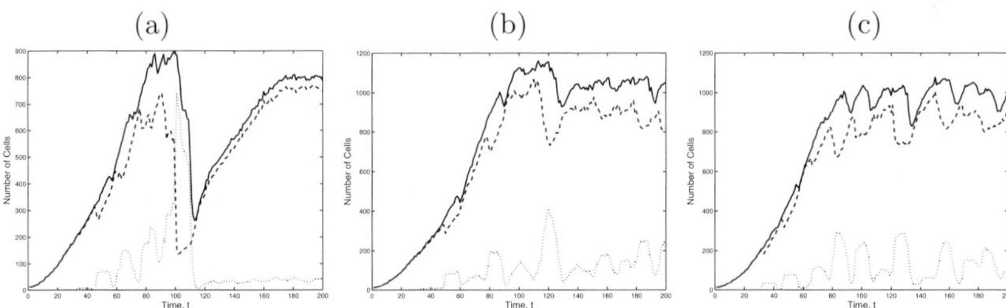

Fig. 7: Number of cells as a function of time for the different vascular adaptation mechanisms considered. Panel (a) shows the results for a VEGF-sensitive vasculature with no conducted stimuli. Panels (b) and (c) incorporate, in addition to VEGF coupling, downstream stimulus and upstream stimulus, respectively. Key: solid line corresponds to the total number of cancerous cells (quiescent plus proliferating), dashed line to the number of proliferating cancerous cells and dotted line to the number of quiescent cancerous cells.

There are many future directions in which this preliminary work must be extended to capture more realistically the biology of vasculature adaptation and cancerous cell dynamics. For example, the approach that we have used is based on empirical evidence of structural adaptation in large vessels. It is unclear if this holds in general for blood vessels. We will need to develop an adaptation principle which is more mechanistically based, allowing it to be verified more easily experimentally. However, the present study has yielded a number of experimentally testable predictions which may help elucidate some of the key underlying processes of adaptation which are absent or work abnormally in tumour vasculature.

Acknowlededgments

TA would like to thank the EPSRC for financial support (grant GR/509067).

References

1. T. Alarcón, H.M. Byrne, P.K. Maini. *A cellular automaton model for tumour growth in a heterogeneous environment.* J. theor. Biol. **225**, 257–274 (2003).
2. T. Alarcón, H.M. Byrne, P.K. Maini. *A multiple scale model for tumour growth.* SIAM Multiscale Model. Simul. **3**, 440–475 (2005).
3. T. Alarcón, H.M. Byrne, P.K. Maini. *A design principle for vascular beds: The effects of complex blood rheology.* Microvasc. Res. **69**, 156–172 (2005).
4. D.M. Collins, W.T. McCullough, M.L. Ellsworth. *Conducted vascular responses: Communication across the capillary bed.* Microvasc. Res. **56**, 43–53 (1998).
5. A. Deutsch, S. Dormann. *Modeling of avascular tumor growth with a hybrid cellular automaton.* In Silico Biol. **2**, 1–14 (2002).
6. P.J. Hunter, P. Robbins, D. Noble. *The IUPS human physiome project.* Pflügers Archiv- Eur. J. Physiol. **445**, 1–9 (2002).
7. M. LaBarbera. *Principles of design of fluid transport systems in zoology.* Science. **249**, 992–1000 (1990).
8. C.D. Murray. *The physiological principle of minimom work I The vascular system and the cost of blood volume.* Proc. Nat. Acad. Sci. USA. **12**, 207 (1977).
9. A.A. Patel, E.T. Gawlinski, S.K. Lemieux, R.A. Gatenby. *A cellular automaton model of early tumor growth and invasion: The effects of native tissue vascularity and increased anaerobic tumor metabolism.* J. theor. Biol. **213**, 315–331 (2001).
10. A.R. Pries, T.W. Secomb, P. Gaehtgens. *Design principles of vascular beds.* Circ. Res. **77**, 1017–1023 (1995).
11. A.R. Pries, T.W. Secomb, P. Gaehtgens. *Structural adaptation and stability of microvascular networks: theory and simulations.* Am. J. Physiol. **275**, H349–H360 (1998).
12. A.R. Pries, B. Reglin, T.W. Secomb. *Structural adaptation of microvascular networks: functional response to adaptive responses.* Am. J. Physiol. **281**, H1015–H1025 (2001).
13. N. Resnick, H. Yahav, A. Shay-Salit, M. Shushy, S. Schubert, L.C.M. Zilberman, E. Wofovitz. *Fluid shear stress and the vascular endothelium: for better and for worse.* Progress Biophys. Mol. Biol. **81**, 177–199 (2003).
14. G.D. Yancopoulos, S. Davis, N.W. Gale, J.S. Rudge, S.J. Wiegand, J. Holash. *Vascular-specific growth factors and blood vessel formation.* Nature. **407**, 242–248 (2000).
15. M. Zamir. *Shear forces and blood vessel radii in vardiovascular-system.* J. Gen. Physiol. **69**, 449–461 (1977).

Approximation of 2D and 3D Models of Chemotactic Cell Movement in Vasculogenesis

Fausto Cavalli[1], Andrea Gamba[2], Giovanni Naldi[1], and Matteo Semplice[1]

[1] Dipartimento di Matematica, Università di Milano, via Saldini 50, 20133 Milano, Italy {cavalli,naldi,semplice}@mat.unimi.it
[2] Dipartimento di Matematica, Politecnico di Torino, Corso Duca degli Abruzzi 24, 10129 Torino, Italy
andrea.gamba@polito.it

Cell migration plays a central role in a wide variety of biological phenomena. In the case of chemotaxis, cells (or an organism) move in response to a chemical gradient. Chemotaxis underlies many events during embryo development and in the adult body. An understanding of chemotaxis is not only gained through laboratory experiments but also through the analysis of model systems, which often are more amenable to manipulation. This work is concerned with the relaxation schemes for the numerical approximation of a 2D and 3D model for cell movement driven by chemotaxis. More precisely, we consider models arising in the description of blood vessels formation and network formation starting from a random cell distribution.

1 A Model for Vasculogenesis

1.1 Brief Biological Background

It is well known that the embryonic heart and vasculature are the first organs which start functioning with largely the same main purpose as in the adult: blood transport. The origin and assembly of embryonic blood vessels not only involve multiple sources of precusor cells, but are also influenced by various combinations of proliferation, migration, differentiation, competition between cell-cell and cell-matrix interactions [7, 15, 27, 28].

The process of formation of this initial vascular network is called vasculogenesis. As the organism develops, subsequent growth and remodelling of the vascular network occur mainly via angiogenesis, whereby vessels sprout from existing vessels into surrounding tissues [20, 22].

In this work we consider a numerical simulation of a model of the vasculogenesis phenomenon in order to describe the de novo blood vessel formation from the mesoderm. The vasculogenetic process is driven by the recruitment of undifferentiated mesodermal cells in the embryonic body to the endothelial lineage and the de novo assembly of such cells into blood vessels. Results from a number of technical advances and studies (for a review see, for example, [7, 21]) have defined the following as essential steps in the process:

1. the birth of angioblasts (the endothelial cell precursors);
2. the aggregation of angioblasts;
3. the elongation of angioblasts into chord-like structures;
4. the organization of isolated vascular segments into a capillary-like network and, concomitant with this step, their endothelialization and lumenization.

It is also important to note that blood vessels formed by vasculogenesis are initially free of smooth muscle cells, pericytes, and other associated cells; they may remain as nascent endothelial tubes for a considerable period of time.

In order to study and identify the factors influencing blood vessel formation, several mathematical models have been presented, see for example [4, 8, 14, 26, 16]. In this work we consider a mathematical model that describes biochemical interactions during blood vessel formation. The model consists of a system of non-linear partial differential equations and is based on the theory presented by Gamba et al. in [9] and by Serini et al. in [23].

1.2 Mathematical Model

As recent experiments (see [3]) show, the process of formation of a vascular network starting from a distribution of seeded cells can be tracked. The motion of each cell appears to be directed towards the areas of high concentration of cells. This fact suggests that chemotactic factors play a role in guiding cell motion. In chemotaxis phenomena, motile cells sense and respond directionally to chemical gradients due to some biochemical factor.

Here the cell population is described by a continuous density $n(\mathbf{x}, t)$, where $\mathbf{x} \in \mathbb{R}^d$ $(d = 2, 3)$ is the space variable, while $t \geq 0$ is the time variable. The population density moves with velocities $\mathbf{v}(\mathbf{x}, t)$, that are triggered either by chemical gradients of a soluble factor or by random motion. The chemoattractant is described by a scalar chemical concentration field $c(\mathbf{x}, t)$. Moreover, the chemical factor is supposed to be released by the cells themselves, diffuse, and degrade in finite time, in agreement with experimental observations. These assumptions give rise to the following system (see [9]):

$$\frac{\partial n}{\partial t} + \nabla \cdot (n\mathbf{v}) = 0 \tag{1a}$$

$$\frac{\partial \mathbf{v}}{\partial t} + \mathbf{v} \cdot \nabla \mathbf{v} = \mu(c)\nabla c - \nabla p(n) - \beta \mathbf{v} \tag{1b}$$

$$\frac{\partial c}{\partial t} = D\Delta c + g(n, c) - \frac{c}{\tau} \tag{1c}$$

Here $\mu(c)$ measures the cell response to the chemotactic factor, while D and τ are respectively the diffusion coefficient and the characteristic degradation time of the soluble chemoattractant. Finally the function $g(n, c)$ determines the rate of release of the chemical factor.

A simple model may be obtained by assuming a constant cell sensitivity $\mu(c) = \mu_0$ and that the release of the chemoattractant is linearly proportional to the cell density: $g(n, c) = \alpha n$, with constant rate $\alpha > 0$. A more realistic description may be obtained including saturation effects via non-linearities in the function $g(n, c)$ or by considering non-constant functions $\mu(c)$. (For the details, please refer to Section 3.)

The term $\nabla p(n)$ is a density dependent pressure where $p(n)$ is zero for low densities, and increases for densities above a suitable threshold. This pressure is a phenomenological term which tries to model short range interaction between cells and the fact that cells do not compenetrate and have some degree of rigidity. Finally, the friction term mimics the adhesion of the cells to the substrate.

Initial conditions are given as a set of uniform randomly distributed bumps in the density field, with zero velocities and zero concentration of the chemoattractant. Starting from these conditions, equations (1) are integrated numerically.

The two-dimensional model has a clear biological counterpart: it may be directly compared with "in vitro" experiments of self-organization of endothelial cells seeded on a matrigel plate that are observed to evolve forming a network-like structure (see [23] and references therein). Quantitative comparisons may be achieved by studying the percolation properties of the network observable in the final state of $n(\mathbf{x})$ when the initial cell density is varied and by measuring the average vessel length in the final state (see [9]).

Since 1997, the biologists' community has become aware of the importance of the extracellular structures for the behaviour of the cells. M. Weawer at al., in their seminal paper [29], showed that a line of cancer cells has two completely different behaviours in a 2D and inside a 3D culture. Since then much work has been done in this direction, proving the need of three-dimensional cell cultures to reproduce more faithfully the biochemical activity of living beings (see the review papers [1, 6]).

It is known that in the early stages of development almost all intraembryonic mesodermal tissues contain migrating endothelial precursors, which appear to be randomly scattered (see e.g. [5]). Therefore in the three dimensional version of our model (1) we use initial conditions that represent a randomly scattered distribution of cells. Thus, model (1) is a candidate to describe experiments of vasculogenetic processes, both "in vivo" and in three dimensional cell cultures.

2 Relaxation Approximation

In order to solve numerically system (1), we consider schemes which are based on a suitable relaxation approximation. Such a scheme permits to reduce non-linear second order equations or quasilinear conservation laws to first order semi-linear hyperbolic systems with stiff terms. In the case of approximation of a scalar conservation law

$$\frac{\partial u}{\partial t} + \frac{\partial}{\partial x} f(u) = 0, \tag{2}$$

Jin and Xin [12] have proposed the following system

$$\frac{\partial u}{\partial t} + \frac{\partial j}{\partial x} = 0 \tag{3a}$$

$$\frac{\partial j}{\partial t} + a\frac{\partial u}{\partial x} = -\frac{1}{\epsilon}(j - f(u)), \tag{3b}$$

where j plays the role of a physical flux, ϵ is a small positive parameter, called relaxation time, and a is a suitable positive constant. The first order approximation of the conservation law (3) is

$$\frac{\partial u}{\partial t} + \frac{\partial}{\partial x} f(u) = \epsilon\frac{\partial}{\partial x}\left((a - f'(u)^2)\frac{\partial u}{\partial x} \right), \tag{4}$$

which can be derived using the Chapman-Enskog expansion. It is also clear that (4) is dissipative, provided that the subcharacteristic condition $a > f'(u)^2$ is satisfied. We would expect that appropriate numerical discretization of the relaxation system (3) yields accurate approximation to the original equation (2) when the relaxation parameter ϵ is sufficiently small.

In view of its numerical approximation, the main advantage of the relaxation system (3) over the original equation (2) lies in the linear structure of the characteristic fields and in the localized low order term. In particular this linear structure avoids the use of time consuming Riemann solvers. Moreover, proper implicit time discretizations can be exploited to overcome the stability constraints due to the stiffness and to avoid the use of non-linear solvers.

In recent years several relaxation approximations to partial differential equations of various type have been proposed, from kinetic schemes for gas dynamics to general relaxation schemes for conservation laws and diffusive relaxation schemes for convection-diffusion and reaction-diffusion problems [2, 13, 19]. For example, let's consider the following one-dimensional equation

$$\frac{\partial u}{\partial t} + \frac{\partial}{\partial x} f(u) = \frac{\partial^2}{\partial x^2} p(u),$$

where p and f are given smooth functions such that $p(0) \geq 0$ and $p'(u) > 0$. By introducing a new variable j, one can couple j and u in the following semi-linear hyperbolic system:

$$\frac{\partial u}{\partial t} + \frac{\partial j}{\partial x} = 0 \tag{5a}$$

$$\frac{\partial j}{\partial t} + \frac{1}{\epsilon}\frac{\partial u}{\partial x} = -\frac{1}{\epsilon}k(u)(j - f(u)). \tag{5b}$$

Here ϵ is the relaxation parameter and $k(u) = p'(u)^{-1}$. As usual, when $\epsilon \ll 1$, system (5) is said to be stiff. In order to consider also degenerate diffusion problems, a different relaxation system can be introduced with a third variable w,

$$\frac{\partial u}{\partial t} + \frac{\partial j}{\partial x} = 0 \tag{6a}$$

$$\frac{\partial j}{\partial t} + \frac{1}{\epsilon}\frac{\partial w}{\partial x} = -\frac{1}{\epsilon}(j - f(u)) \tag{6b}$$

$$\frac{\partial w}{\partial t} + a\frac{\partial j}{\partial x} = -\frac{1}{\epsilon}(w - p(u)), \tag{6c}$$

with a suitable positive constant a to control the stability condition.

The numerical passage from the relaxation system to the non-linear diffusion equation is realized by using semi-implicit or fully implicit time discretization combined with upwind and central differences in space. If we consider, as a prototype for the numerical scheme, the linear diffusion equation $\frac{\partial u}{\partial t} - \frac{\partial^2 u}{\partial x^2} = 0$, it suffices to consider the following relaxation system (also called Maxwell-Cattaneo system)

$$\frac{\partial u}{\partial t} + \frac{\partial j}{\partial x} = 0 \tag{7a}$$

$$\frac{\partial j}{\partial t} + \frac{1}{\epsilon}\frac{\partial u}{\partial x} = -\frac{1}{\epsilon}j. \tag{7b}$$

In this simple case, an analysis of the drawbacks of the different numerical approaches is described in [17]. Let Δt and Δx be respectively the time step and the uniform grid spacing. The standard semi-implicit discretization in conservative form, for small values of ϵ, leads to a modified equation with a numerical dissipation rate of order $\Delta x/2\epsilon$. Then, if $\Delta x \geq \epsilon$ the numerical dissipation will be comparable with, or dominate, the physical dissipation. We also have to solve in time the stiffness of this numerical dissipation term and hence the CFL condition is of the type $\Delta t \simeq \epsilon\Delta x$. Clearly, this is too restrictive near the parabolic regime $\epsilon \ll \Delta x$ where a condition of the type $\Delta t \simeq \Delta x^2$ is expected. A different upwind selection for the numerical flux which avoids unacceptable CFL condition and permits high order extension, is proposed in [17]. However the modified scheme was difficult to generalize to nonlinear diffusion. A more general and reliable numerical recipe is considered in [13, 18]. The main idea consists in splitting the scales by rewriting the relaxation system as

$$\frac{\partial u}{\partial t} + \frac{\partial j}{\partial x} = 0 \tag{8a}$$

$$\frac{\partial j}{\partial t} + \lambda(\epsilon)\frac{\partial u}{\partial x} = -\frac{1}{\epsilon}\left(j + (1 - \epsilon\lambda(\epsilon))\frac{\partial u}{\partial x}\right), \tag{8b}$$

where $\lambda(\epsilon)$ is such that $0 \le \lambda(\epsilon) \le 1/\epsilon$. This restriction on λ guarantees the positivity of both λ and $(1 - \epsilon\lambda)$. Now, as it is usually done for kinetic equations or hyperbolic systems with relaxation, (8) can be split into two subproblems:

$$\frac{\partial u}{\partial t} + \frac{\partial j}{\partial x} = 0 \tag{9a}$$

$$\frac{\partial j}{\partial t} + \lambda(\epsilon)\frac{\partial u}{\partial x} = 0 \tag{9b}$$

and

$$\frac{\partial u}{\partial t} = 0 \tag{9c}$$

$$\frac{\partial j}{\partial t} = -\frac{1}{\epsilon}\left(j + (1 - \epsilon\lambda(\epsilon))\frac{\partial u}{\partial x}\right). \tag{9d}$$

We remark that the standard splitting does not work for (7) because, when $\epsilon \to 0$, we obtain the equilibrium equations

$$j = 0 \quad \text{and} \quad \frac{\partial u}{\partial x} = 0,$$

that are inconsistent with the diffusive limit.

Summarizing, we can consider relaxation approximation both for conservation laws and for diffusion equations. Hence we can adopt the same approach for the whole model of vasculogenesis. In the case of multidimensions, a similar discretization can be applied to each space dimension [12, 13, 18]. Then, since the structure of the multidimensional diffusive relaxation system is similar to the 1D system, the numerical implementation for higher dimensional problems, based on dimensional splitting, is not much harder than for 1D problems.

Very fine grids have to be used, in order to resolve the details of the field $n(\mathbf{x}, t)$, which might have hundreds of small bumps, each representing a single cell. The computational cost may be reduced by using parallel computing: the semilinearity of relaxation systems, together with appropriate discretizations, gives rise to parallel algorithms with almost optimal scaling properties.

3 Numerical Results

As in [9, 23] we perform two-dimensional numerical simulations of model (1) on a square box with side of lentgh $L = 1$mm, with periodic boundary conditions. The relaxation system is numerically solved by considering the splitting scheme (9) for the pure convective step and the relaxation step. These steps are combined in a second order Runge Kutta scheme (see [11, 12]). For the numerical discretization of the transport step, in order to achieve an accuracy of $O(\Delta x^2)$, we use a second order TVD scheme with suitable slope limiter (see [10, 24]).

Biochemical experiments suggests the values of $D = 10^{-3} \text{mm}^2/\text{sec}$ and $\tau = 4000\text{sec}$ for the diffusion constant and the decay rate of the chemoattractant. We fix the other constant parameters by dimensional analysis and the consideration of the characteristic scales of the system. In particular, for the two-dimensional model, we choose: $\mu_0 = 10^{-11} \text{mm}^4/\text{sec}^3$, $\alpha = 1\,\text{sec}^{-1}$, $\beta = 10^{-3}\,\text{sec}^{-1}$.

The pressure function is taken to be

$$p(n) = \begin{cases} C_p(n - n_0)^3 & n > n_0 \\ 0 & n \leq n_0 \end{cases}$$

where $n_0 = 6.0$ and the areas where $n(\mathbf{x}) < 6$ (lighter gray in Figures 1, 2, 4 and 5) represent locations where network chords are thinner (one may see this effect on the plates of the "in vitro" experiments, as in Figure 3).

With this naive setting, we observe that the initial random distribution of cells evolve into a network that, however, represents only a transient state: eventually large blobs of matter arise. Figure 1 represents this situation: the cell density is shown at time $t = 0, 60$ and 150 minutes.

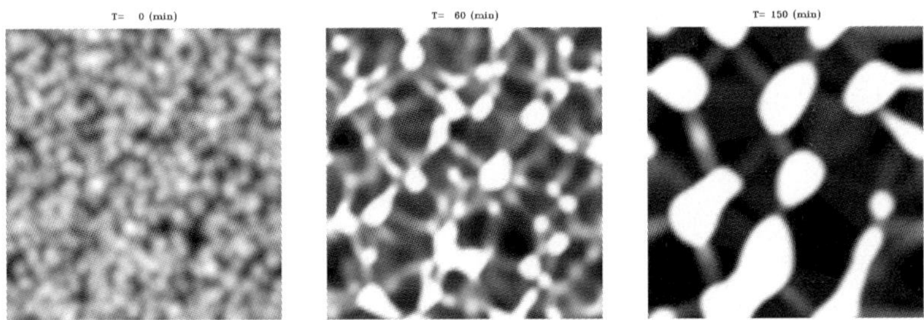

Fig. 1: Transient network state. With a linear emisison rate $g(n, c) = \alpha n$ and constant $\mu(c) = \mu_0$, the network state is only transient. These images plot the cell density distribution at time $t = 0, 60, 150$ minutes. The initial distribution is random with a mean density of $200\text{cell}/\text{mm}^2$.

It is natural, from a biological point of view, to suppose that saturation effects play a role. One may think that, when the background concentration of chemoattractant is high, the cells react more weakly to its gradient or that they emit less chemoattractant when its concentration in the surrounding space is already significant. These effects may be incorporated in our model using a non-constant sensitivity $\mu(c)$, a non-linear emission rate $g(n,c)$, or both. We choose a threshold c_0 and then functions like

$$\mu(c) = \mu_0(1 - \tanh(c - c_0)) \tag{10a}$$
$$g(n,c) = \alpha n(1 - \tanh(c - c_0)) \tag{10b}$$

The net effect is that the sensitivity of the cells and respectively their production of chemoattractant is strongly damped when the concentration c reaches the threshold c_0. We did not observe a significant dependence on the exact form of the damping function, provided that it approximates a step function that is nonzero only when $c < c_0$. With the above choices we obtain a network state that is not transient any more: the system settles onto it (see Figures 2, 4, 5).

In Figures 2,4 and 5 we present the results obtained with $c_0 = 1000$. For comparison purposes, the initial random distrubution of cells is the same as in Figure 1 and it is not shown. Using (10a), we observe that the state reached at time $t = 60$min is not significantly modified any more in the evolution (Figure 2). The density $n(\mathbf{x}, t)$ reaches a state that consists of blobs of matter linked by thinner chords, which is remarkably similar to the final state obtained in "in vitro" experiments (Figure 3). The numerical tests indicate that this network-like state is stable, unlike the case of Figure 1.

On the other hand, (10b) and a constant $\mu(c)$, is less effective in bringing the system to a network-like state, but the final state presents thinner chords, as is shown in Figure 4. This is to be expected since (10b) acts on equation (1c), where it competes with the decay term.

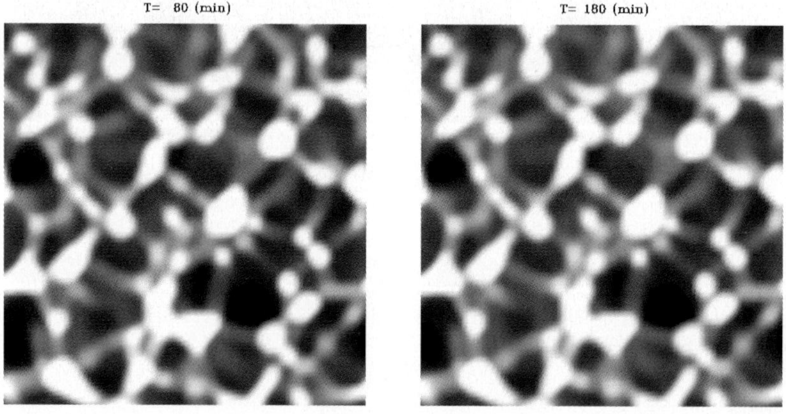

Fig. 2: Results of the numerical evolution of system (1), together with (10a) and linear $g(n,c) = \alpha n$. The images plot the cell density distribution at time $t = 60, 180$ minutes. The initial distribution is the same as in Figure 1.

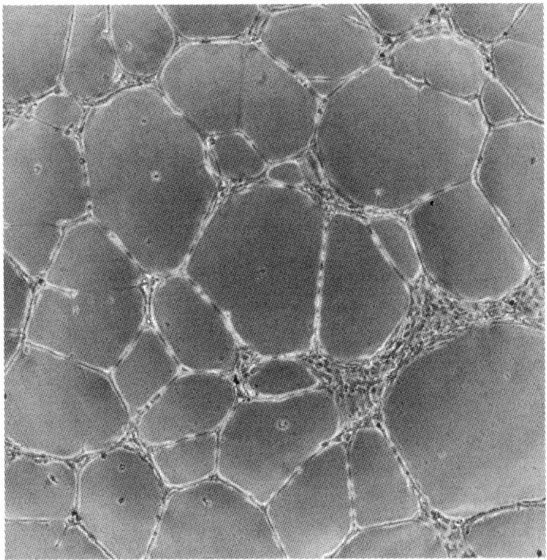

Fig. 3: In vitro experiment of self-organization of endothelial cells seeded on a matrigel plate of $2 \times 2\text{mm}^2$. (Thanks to G. Serini, IRCC, Candiolo - Torino)

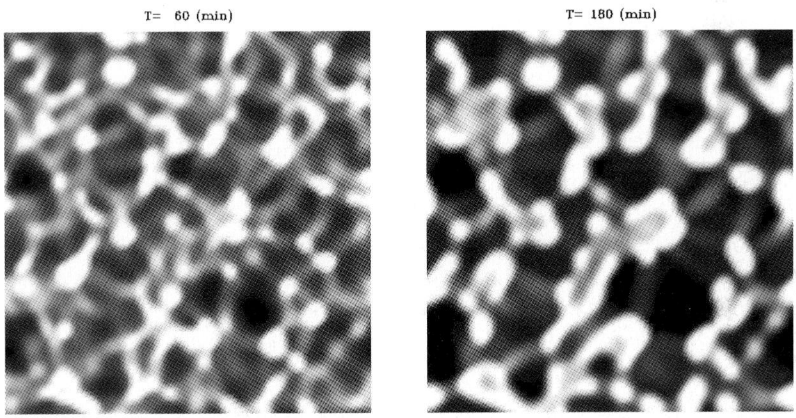

Fig. 4: Results of the numerical evolution of system (1), together with (10b) and constant $\mu(c) = \mu_0$. The images plot the cell density distribution at time $t = 60, 180$ minutes. The initial distribution is the same as in Figure 1.

Finally, Figure 5 shows that using both equations (10), with the same threshold c_0, the behaviour of Figure 2 prevails.

We observe here that in Nature several effects are reasonably expected to concur to the stabilization of network structures. Along with saturation effects, mechanical interactions also produce network stabilization ([25]).

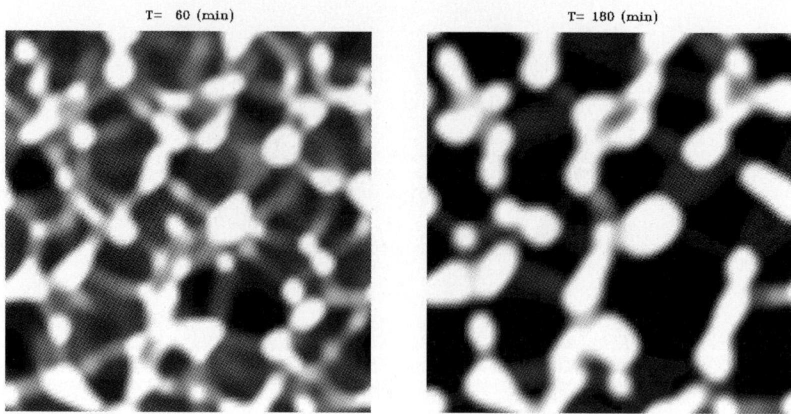

Fig. 5: Results of the numerical evolution of system (1), together with both (10a) and (10b). The images plot the cell density distribution at time $t = 60, 180$ minutes. The initial distribution is the same as in Figure 1.

In three dimensions we used the same parameter setting as in the two-dimensional case. Due to the computational costs, the algorithm has been implemented on a high performance cluster for parallel computation installed at the Department of Mathematics of the University of Milano (see http://cluster.mat.unimi.it/).

We observed that, starting with an initial random distribution of cells, the cell density evolves towards a network-like state. Figure 6 shows this state: it is transient since, in this simulation, we used a linear function $g(n, c)$ and constant $\mu(c)$, but we expect that incorporating (10), the good results of the two-dimensional case should be reproduced here as well.

Our choice of a numerical algorithm that performs only linear operations and local function evaluations allows us to obtain very good scaling properties in the parallel implementation, as shown in Figure 7.

4 Conclusions

In oder to gain understanding of the role of chemotaxis in the self-organization of cells, we performed numerical simulations aimed at reproducing the case of chemotaxis-driven vasculogenesis in two and three space dimensions. Our model does not simulate the individual cells but rather a continuous spatial distribution of matter, whose bumps do represent the cells. This allows us to use the tools of partial differential equations to describe the mathematical model (1).

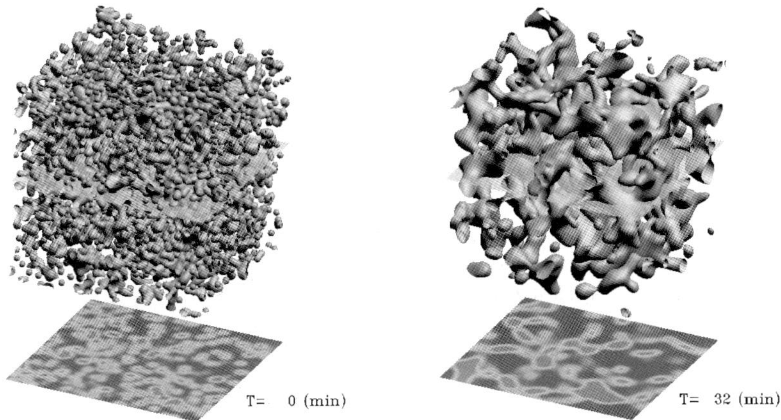

Fig. 6: Transient network state in 3D. These are the cell density distributions at time $t = 0, 32$ minutes. This was obtained with linear $g(c)$ and constant μ. The images represent an isosurface plot together with a gray-level cross section at the indicated location.

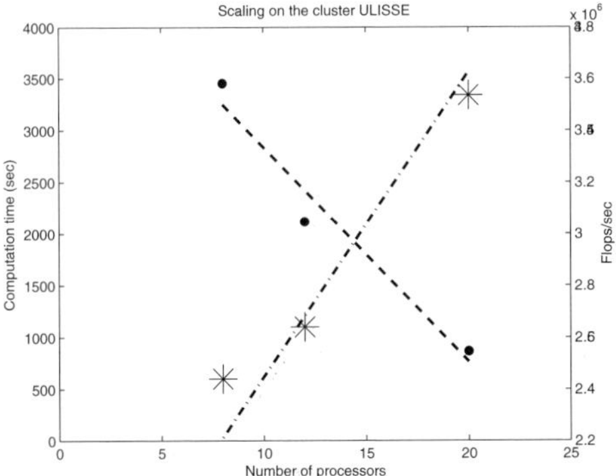

Fig. 7: Scaling of the 3D algorithm on the cluster ULISSE. The dots represent the execution time (in seconds) and the asterisks the Mflops/sec for our numerical algorithm. The dashed and dash-dot line are their respective linear interpolations.

Proper spatial and temporal approximations (Section 2) allow us to perform numerical simulations with an algorithm that performs only linear operations and local function evaluations without severe restrictions on the time step, despite the non-linearity of the original equations. This is also important for the implementation on parallel computers: the memory usage and the execution time of the algorithm decrease linearly with the number of processors and this allows us to reduce the computation time down to reasonable values.

The two-dimensional model has already proven to give results in good agreement with "in vitro" experiments of vasculogenesis. Our numerical tests indicate that the version that we present here possesses a stationary state; hence the model allows to investigate on the mechanisms that may play a role in bringing the biological system to stop its evolution when a proper pre-vascular network is formed. We proposed and compared mechanisms based on varying the sensitivity of the cells to the chemotactical signals and on varying the emission of the soluble chemoattractant.

Regarding the three dimensional model, we are currently working on the comparison of the numerical simulations with experimental data. Moreover we are working on the analysis of the numerical algorithms (stability and CFL condition for the non-linear relaxation).

References

1. A. Abbott: Biology's new dimension. Nature **424**, 870–872, (2003).
2. D. Aregba-Driollet, R. Natalini, S.Q. Tang: Diffusive kinetic explicit schemes for nonlinear degenerate parabolic systems. Math. Comp. **73**, 63–94, (2004).
3. P. Carmeliet: Mechanisms of angiogenesis and arteriogenesis. Nature Medicine **6**, 389–395, (2000).
4. M.A. Chaplain: Mathematical modelling of angiogenesis. J. Neuro. **50**, 37, (2000).
5. O. Cleaver and P. Krieg: Molecular mechanisms of vascular development. In R.P. Harvey and N. Rosenthal (eds): Heart development. Academic Press (1999), 221–252.
6. E. Cukierman, R. Pankov, D.R. Stevens, K.M. Yamada: Taking Cell-Matrix Adhesions to the Third Dimension. Science **294**, 1708–1712 (2001)
7. C.J. Drake, J.E. Hungerford and C.D. Little: Morphogenesis of the First Blood Vessels. Ann. New York Acad. Sci. **857**, 155–179, (1998).
8. E.A. Gaffney, K. Pugh, P.K. Maini and F. Arnold: Investigating a simple model of cutaneous wound healing angiogenesis. J. Math. Biol. **45**, 337–374, (2002).
9. A. Gamba, D. Ambrosi, A. Coniglio, A. De Candia, S. Di Talia, E. Giraudo, G. Serini, L. Preziosi and F. Bussolino: Percolation, Morphogenesis, and Burgers Dynamics in Blood Vessels Formation Phys. Rev. Lett. **90**, 118101 (2003).
10. A. Harten: High Resolution Schemes for Hyperbolic Conservation Laws. J. Comp. Phys. **49**, 357–393, (1983).
11. S. Jin and Z. Xin: Runge-Kutta Methods for Hyperbolic Conservation Laws with Stiff Relaxation Terms. J. Comp. Phys. **122**, 51–67, (1995).
12. S. Jin and Z. Xin: The Relaxation Schemes for Systems of Conservation Laws in Arbitrary Space Dimensions. Comm. Pure and Appl. Math. **48**, 235–276, (1995).
13. S. Jin, L. Pareschi and G. Toscani: Diffusive Relaxation Schemes for Discrete-Velocity Kinetic Equations. SIAM J. Numer. Anal. **35**, 2405–2439, (1998).
14. H.A. Levine, B.D. Sleeman and M. Nilsen-Hamilton: Mathematical modeling of the onset of capillary formation initiating angiogenesis. J. Math. Biol. **42**, 195–238, (2001).
15. C.D. Little: Vascular morphogenesis: in vivo, in vitro, in mente. Birkhäuser, Boston (1998).

16. R. MH Merks, A. Newman and J.A. Glazier: Cell-Oriented Modeling of in Vitro Capillary of Blood Vessel Growth. Lecture Notes in Computer Science **3305**, 425–434, (2004).
17. G. Naldi and L. Pareschi: Numerical Schemes for Kinetic Equations in Diffusive Regimes. Appl. Math. Lett. **11**, 29, (1998).
18. G. Naldi and L. Pareschi: Numerical Schemes for Hyperbolic Systems of Conservation Law with Stiff Diffusive Relaxation. SIAM J. Numer. Anal. **37**, 1246–1270, (2000).
19. G. Naldi, L. Pareschi and G. Toscani: Relaxation schemes for PDEs and applications to fourth order diffusion equations. Surveys in Mathematics Applied to Industry **10**, 315, (2002).
20. L. Pardanaud, F. Yassine,and F. Dieterlen-Lievre: Relationship between vasculogenesis, angiogenesis and haemopoiesis during avian ontogeny. Development **105**, 473–485, (1989).
21. T.J. Poole, E.B. Finkelstein and C.M. Cox: The role of FGF and VEGF in angioblast induction and migration during vascular development. Dev. Dynam. **220**, 1–17, (2001).
22. W. Risau, H. Sariola, H.G. Zerwes, J. Sasse, P. Ekblom, R. Kemler and T. Doetschmann: Vasculogenesis and angiogenesis in embryonic-stem-cell-derived embryoid bodies. Development **102**, 471–478, (1988).
23. G. Serini, D. Ambrosi, E. Giraudo, L. Preziosi and F. Bussolino: Modeling the early stages of vascular network assembly. The EMBO Journal **22**, 1771–1779, (2003).
24. P.R. Sweby: High Resolution Schemes Using Flux Limiters for Hyperbolic Conservation Laws. SIAM J. Num. Anal. **21**, 995–1011, (1984).
25. A. Tosin, D. Ambrosi and L. Preziosi: Mechanics and chemotaxis in the morphogenesis of vascular networks. To appear in Bull. Mat. Biol. (2006)
26. S. Tong and F. Yuan: Numerical simulations of angiogenesis in the cornea. Microvasc. Res. **61**, 14–27, (2001).
27. B.M. Weinstein: What guides early embryonic blood vessel formation? Dev. Dynam. **215**, 2–17, (1999).
28. J. Wilting, S. Brand,H. Kurz and B. Christ: Development of the embryonic vascular system. Cell. Mol. Biol. Res. **41**, 219–232, (1995).
29. V.M. Weaver, O.W. Petersen, F. Wang, C.A. Larabell, P. Briand, C. Damsky, M.J. Bissell: Reversion of the malignant phenotype of human breast cells in three-dimensional culture and in vivo by integrin blocking antibodies. J. Cell. Biol. **137**, 231–245 (1997).

Homogenization Closure For A Two-Dimensional Effective Model Describing Fluid-Structure Interaction in Blood Flow

Andro Mikelić[1] and Sunčica Čanić[2]

[1] Institut Camille Jordan, UFR Mathématiques, Université Claude Bernard Lyon 1, Site de Gerland, Bt. A, 50, avenue Tony Garnier, 69367 Lyon Cedex 07, France
`Andro.Mikelic@univ-lyon1.fr`
[2] Department of Mathematics, University of Houston, 4800 Calhoun Rd., Houston TX 77204-3476,USA
`canic@math.uh.edu`

This paper is dedicated to Professor Vincenzo Capasso for his 60th birthday

1 Introduction

We study the flow of a viscous incompressible fluid through a long and narrow elastic tube whose walls are modeled by the Navier equations for a curved, linearly elastic membrane.

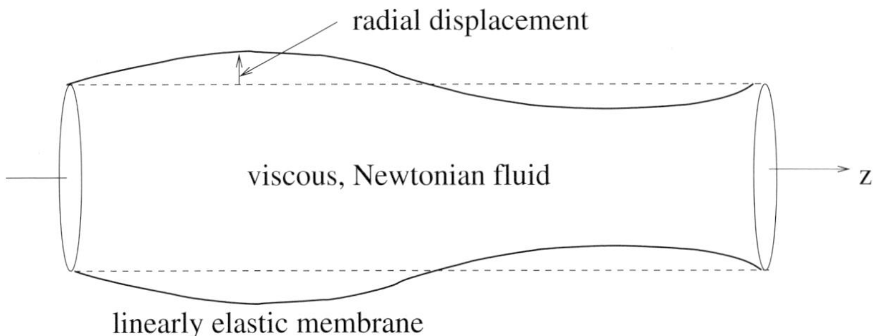

Fig. 1: Domain Sketch.

The flow takes place in $\Omega_\varepsilon = \{ x \in \mathbb{R}^3; x = (r\cos\vartheta, r\sin\vartheta, z), r < R + \eta^\varepsilon(z,t), 0 < z < L \}$ and is governed by a given time dependent pressure drop between the inlet and the outlet boundary, giving rise to a non-stationary incompressible flow modeled by the Navier-Stokes equations. The aspect ratio $\varepsilon = \frac{R}{L}$ is "small" ($\approx 3 \cdot 10^{-2}$).

We suppose that the lateral boundary of the cylinder $\Sigma_\varepsilon = \{r = R + \eta^\varepsilon\} \times (0, L)$ behaves as a linearly elastic membrane of thickness h, that the longitudinal displacement is zero, and that the radial displacement satisfies Navier's equation

$$-F_r = \frac{h(\varepsilon)E(\varepsilon)}{1 - \sigma^2} \frac{\eta^\varepsilon}{\varepsilon^2 R^2} + p_{ref}\frac{\eta^\varepsilon}{R} - h(\varepsilon)G(\varepsilon)k(\varepsilon)\frac{\partial^2 \eta^\varepsilon}{\partial z^2} + \rho_w h(\varepsilon)\frac{\partial^2 \eta^\varepsilon}{\partial t^2}, \qquad (1)$$

In (1), η^ε is the radial displacement from the reference state in Lagrangian coordinates (see Figure 1), $h = h(\varepsilon)$ is the membrane thickness, ρ_w the wall volumetric mass, $E = E(\varepsilon)$ is the Young modulus, $0 < \sigma < 1$ is the Poisson ratio, $G = G(\varepsilon)$ is the shear modulus and $k = k(\varepsilon)$ is Timoshenko shear correction factor (see [QTV:00]). F_r is the radial component of the external forces, coming from the stresses induced by the fluid, given by

$$-F_r = ((p^\varepsilon - p_{ref})I - 2\mu D(v^\varepsilon))\mathbf{n}e_r \left(1 + \frac{\eta^\varepsilon}{R}\right)\sqrt{1 + \left(\frac{\partial \eta^\varepsilon}{\partial z}\right)^2}. \qquad (2)$$

where $D(v^\varepsilon)$ is the rate of strain tensor. Equation (2) is valid on Σ_ε. At the wall Σ_ε we require continuity of velocity: the fluid velocity v^ε is linked with the velocity of the lateral wall Σ_ε by

$$v_r^\varepsilon(R + \eta^\varepsilon, z, t) = \frac{\partial \eta^\varepsilon}{\partial t}; \quad \text{and} \quad v_z^\varepsilon(R + \eta^\varepsilon, z, t) = 0 \,\forall t \in \mathbb{R}_+.$$

A time-dependent pressure head data at the inlet and at the outlet boundary drive the problem and we assume the following initial and boundary conditions

$$p^\varepsilon + \rho(v_z^\varepsilon)^2/2 = P_j(t) + p_{ref}, \text{ with } j = 1 \text{ for } z = 0, \, j = 2 \text{ for } z = L, \, \forall t$$

$$v_r^\varepsilon|_{z=0,L} = 0, \, \eta^\varepsilon = 0 \text{ for } z = 0, \, \eta^\varepsilon = 0 \text{ for } z = L, \, \forall t.$$

We will assume that the pressure drop $A(t) = P_1(t) - P_2(t) \in C_0^\infty(0, +\infty)$.

The Eulerian formulation of an incompressible viscous flow is given by the axially symmetric Navier-Stokes equations for $\mathbf{v}^\varepsilon = (v_r^\varepsilon, v_z^\varepsilon)$ and p^ε:

$$\rho\left\{\frac{\partial \mathbf{v}^\varepsilon}{\partial t} + (\mathbf{v}^\varepsilon\nabla)\mathbf{v}^\varepsilon\right\} - \mu\Delta\mathbf{v}^\varepsilon + \nabla p^\varepsilon = 0 \quad \text{in} \quad \Omega_\varepsilon \times \mathbb{R}_+,$$

Initially, the cylinder is filled with fluid and the entire structure is in an equilibrium. The equilibrium state has an initial reference pressure $P_0 = p_{ref}$ and the initial velocity zero. Furthermore, the initial data are given by

$$\eta^\varepsilon = \frac{\partial \eta^\varepsilon}{\partial t} = 0 \quad \text{on} \quad \Sigma_\varepsilon(0) \times \{0\}. \qquad (3)$$

We study the behavior of this coupled fluid-structure system (1)-(3) in the limit when $\varepsilon \to 0$. We derive the asymptotic equations that describe: (a) the flow occurring at the leading order time scale and (b) the oscillations of the membrane caused by a response of the elastic material. Since they occur at different time scales we introduce the scaling $\tilde{t} = \omega^\varepsilon t$. Classical 1D models lead to the variants of the shallow water model and require an **ad hoc** closure assumption. In this paper we will present effective equations which are obtained using homogenization, from the system (1)-(3), in the limit $\varepsilon \to 0$, without making any **ad hoc** assumptions.

2 Uniform a Priori Estimates

First we note that existence of solutions to the system (1)-(3) is an open problem. Recent references, containing existence results for the short time/small data can be found in [7] and [1].

We suppose existence of a smooth solution and study the energy estimate. The energy estimate, containing precise dependence on ε, is obtained in [6]. In order to capture the waves of the coupled fluid-structure response to the outside forcing, the authors introduced the new time $\tilde{t} = \omega^\varepsilon t$. The characteristic frequency ω^ε is calculated in [5] by requiring that the effects of both the pressure head data, $P_1(t)$ and $P_2(t)$, as well as the pressure drop data, $A(t)$, are seen in the solution. It was found that

$$\tilde{t} = \omega^\varepsilon t; \quad \omega^\varepsilon = \frac{1}{L}\sqrt{\frac{RC}{2\rho}} \tag{4}$$

Notice that $c = L\omega^\varepsilon$ is the characteristic wave speed (the local pulse wave velocity or sound speed). Expression (4) leads to the same characteristic wave speed as in [8].

We start by introducing the norms that will be used to measure the size of the inlet and the outlet boundary data. Define

$$\mathcal{C} = \frac{h(\varepsilon)E(\varepsilon)}{R^2(1-\sigma^2)}\left(1 + \frac{p_{ref}}{R(\varepsilon)}\frac{R}{h(\varepsilon)}(1-\sigma^2)\right); \quad \hat{P} = \frac{A(t)}{L}z + P_1(t)$$

$$\mathcal{P}^2 \equiv \sup_{z,t}|\tilde{P}|^2 + (\sup_z \int_0^t |\frac{\partial}{\partial t}\hat{P}|\, d\tau)^2 + T \int_0^t |A(\tau)|^2$$

We test the system (1)-(3) by a solution $(v_r^\varepsilon, v_z^\varepsilon, \eta^\varepsilon)$. After lengthy calculations the precise energy inequality is obtained. For details we refer to [6]. The precise energy inequality implies the following *a priori* estimate:

Proposition 1. *Solution $(v_r^\varepsilon, v_z^\varepsilon, \eta^\varepsilon)$ of problem (1)-(3) satisfies the following a priori estimates*

$$\frac{1}{L}\|\eta^{\varepsilon}(\tilde{t})\|^{2}_{L^{2}(0,L)} \leq \frac{32}{C^{2}}\mathcal{P}^{2} \tag{5}$$

$$\frac{1}{LR^{2}\pi}\|v^{\varepsilon}\|^{2}_{L^{2}(\Omega_{\varepsilon}(\tilde{t}))} \leq \frac{32}{\rho RC}\mathcal{P}^{2} \tag{6}$$

$$\int_{0}^{\tilde{t}}\left\{\|\frac{\partial v^{\varepsilon}_{r}}{\partial r}\|^{2}_{L^{2}(\Omega_{\varepsilon}(\tilde{t}))} + \|\frac{\partial v^{\varepsilon}_{z}}{\partial z}\|^{2}_{L^{2}(\Omega_{\varepsilon}(\tilde{t}))}\right\}d\tau \leq \frac{4\pi R^{2}}{\mu}\sqrt{\frac{2}{\rho RC}}\mathcal{P}^{2} \tag{7}$$

$$\int_{0}^{\tilde{t}}\left\{\|\frac{\partial v^{\varepsilon}_{z}}{\partial r}\|^{2}_{L^{2}(\Omega_{\varepsilon})} + \|\frac{v^{\varepsilon}_{r}}{r}\|^{2}_{L^{2}(\Omega_{\varepsilon}(\tilde{t}))} + \|\frac{\partial v^{\varepsilon}_{r}}{\partial z}\|^{2}_{L^{2}(\Omega_{\varepsilon})}\right\}d\tau \leq \frac{4R^{2}}{\mu}\sqrt{\frac{2}{\rho RC}}\mathcal{P}^{2} \tag{8}$$

The a priori estimates (5)-(8) provide a basis for asymptotic analysis in terms of the parameters of the problem.

Table 1: Table with parameter values.

PARAMETERS	AORTA/ILIACS	LATEX TUBE
Char. radius $R(m)$	0.006-0.012	0.011
Dyn. viscosity $\mu(\frac{kg}{ms})$	3.5×10^{-3}	3.5×10^{-3}
Young's modulus E(Pa)	$10^{5} - 10^{6}$	1.0587×10^{6}
Wall thickness h(m)	$1 - 2 \times 10^{-3}$	0.0009
Wall density $\rho_S(kg/m^{2})$	1.1,	1.1
Fluid density $\rho(kg/m^{3})$	1050	1000

3 From Asymptotic Expansions to Reduced Equations

3.1 Asymptotic Expansion

Introduce the non-dimensional independent variables $\tilde{r}$ and $\tilde{z}$

$$r = R\tilde{r}, \qquad z = L\tilde{z},$$

and recall that the time scale for the problem is determined by $t = \frac{1}{\omega^{\varepsilon}}\tilde{t}$. Based on the a priori estimates, we introduce the following asymptotic expansions

$$v^{\varepsilon} = V\left\{\tilde{v}^{0} + \varepsilon\tilde{v}^{1} + ...\right\}, \quad V = \sqrt{\frac{1}{R\rho C}}\mathcal{P}$$

$$\eta = \Xi\left\{\tilde{\eta}^{0} + \varepsilon\tilde{\eta}^{1} + ...\right\}, \quad \Xi = \frac{1}{C}\mathcal{P}$$

$$p = \rho V^{2}\left\{\tilde{p}^{0} + \varepsilon\tilde{p}^{1} + ...\right\}.$$

The approximate values of the scaling parameters, based on our parameters with $E = 6 \times 10^{5}$ Pa are $V = 0.5$ m/s, $\omega = 113$ and $\Xi = 0.00025$ m.

After ignoring the terms of order ε^2 and smaller, the leading-order asymptotic equations describing the conservation of axial and radial momentum, and the incompressibility condition in non-dimensional variables read

$$Sh\frac{\partial \tilde{v}_z}{\partial \tilde{t}} + \tilde{v}_z\frac{\partial \tilde{v}_z}{\partial \tilde{z}} + \tilde{v}_r\frac{\partial \tilde{v}_z}{\partial \tilde{r}} + \frac{\partial \tilde{p}}{\partial \tilde{z}} - \frac{1}{Re}\left\{\frac{1}{\tilde{r}}\frac{\partial}{\partial \tilde{r}}\left(\tilde{r}\frac{\partial \tilde{v}_z}{\partial \tilde{r}}\right)\right\} = 0, \tag{9}$$

$$\frac{\partial \tilde{p}}{\partial \tilde{r}} = 0, \qquad \frac{\partial}{\partial \tilde{r}}(\tilde{r}\tilde{v}_r) + \frac{\partial}{\partial \tilde{z}}(\tilde{r}\tilde{v}_z) = 0, \tag{10}$$

where $\tilde{v}_r^0 = 0$ and

$$Sh := \frac{L\omega^\varepsilon}{V}, \ Re := \frac{\rho V R^2}{\mu L}; \quad \tilde{v}_r = \tilde{v}_r^1 + \varepsilon\tilde{v}_r^2, \ \tilde{v}_z = \tilde{v}_z^0 + \varepsilon\tilde{v}_z^1, \ \tilde{p} := \tilde{p}^0 + \varepsilon\tilde{p}^1. \tag{11}$$

Using our values we see that $Re = 35$ and so the viscous coefficient is of order $1/Re = 0.03 = \epsilon/2$. The Strouhal number is $Sh = 61$.

Using (2) the asymptotic form of the contact force becomes

$$\left((p^\varepsilon - p_{ref})I - 2\mu D(v^\varepsilon)\right)\mathbf{n}e_r = \rho V^2\left(\tilde{p} - \tilde{p}_{ref} + \mathcal{O}(\varepsilon^2)\right)\left(1 + \frac{\Xi}{R}\tilde{\eta}\right).$$

In non-dimensional variables the deformed interface is defined by the equation $\tilde{r} = 1 + \frac{\Xi}{R}\tilde{\eta}(\tilde{z},\tilde{t})$. The leading-order equation for the coupling across the deformed lateral boundary describing continuity of forces and the continuity of velocity become

$$\frac{\rho V^2}{\mathcal{P}}\left(\tilde{p} - \tilde{p}_{ref} + \mathcal{O}(\varepsilon^2)\right)\left(1 + \frac{\Xi}{R}\tilde{\eta}\right) = \tilde{\eta} + \mathcal{O}(\varepsilon^2)$$

$$\tilde{v}_r\left(\tilde{z}, 1 + \frac{\Xi}{R}\tilde{\eta}(z,t),\tilde{t}\right) = \frac{\partial\tilde{\eta}}{\partial\tilde{t}}, \quad \tilde{v}_z = 0.$$

3.2 The Reduced Two-Dimensional Coupled Problem

We summarize here the two-dimensional reduced coupled problem in non-dimensional variables. Define the scaled domain

$$\tilde{\Omega}(\tilde{t}) = \{(\tilde{z},\tilde{r}) \in \mathbb{R}^2 | \tilde{r} < 1 + \frac{\Xi}{R}\tilde{\eta}(\tilde{z},\tilde{t}), 0 < \tilde{z} < 1\},$$

and the lateral boundary $\tilde{\Sigma}(\tilde{t}) = \{\tilde{r} = 1 + \frac{\Xi}{R}\tilde{\eta}(\tilde{z},\tilde{t})\} \times (0,1)$. The problem consist of finding a $(\tilde{v}_z, \tilde{v}_r, \tilde{\eta})$ such that in $\tilde{\Omega}(\tilde{t}) \times \mathbb{R}^+$ the following is satisfied

$$Sh\frac{\partial \tilde{v}_z}{\partial \tilde{t}} + \tilde{v}_z\frac{\partial \tilde{v}_z}{\partial \tilde{z}} + \tilde{v}_r\frac{\partial \tilde{v}_z}{\partial \tilde{r}} + \frac{\partial \tilde{p}}{\partial \tilde{z}} = \frac{1}{Re}\left\{\frac{1}{\tilde{r}}\frac{\partial}{\partial \tilde{r}}\left(\tilde{r}\frac{\partial \tilde{v}_z}{\partial \tilde{r}}\right)\right\}, \tag{12}$$

$$\frac{\partial}{\partial \tilde{r}}(\tilde{r}\tilde{v}_r) + \frac{\partial}{\partial \tilde{z}}(\tilde{r}\tilde{v}_z) = 0, \tag{13}$$

$$\tilde{p}(\tilde{z},\tilde{t}) - \tilde{p}_{ref} = \frac{\mathcal{P}}{\rho V^2}\frac{1}{\left(1 + \frac{\Xi}{R}\tilde{\eta}\right)}\tilde{\eta}, \tag{14}$$

$$\tilde{v}_r\left(\tilde{z}, 1 + \frac{\Xi}{R}\tilde{\eta}(z,t),\tilde{t}\right) = \frac{\partial\tilde{\eta}}{\partial\tilde{t}}, \quad \tilde{v}_z\left(\tilde{z}, 1 + \frac{\Xi}{R}\tilde{\eta}(z,t),\tilde{t}\right) = 0, \tag{15}$$

with the initial and boundary conditions given by

$$\tilde{v}_r = 0 \quad \text{and} \quad \tilde{p} = (P_1(\tilde{t}) + p_{ref})/(\rho V^2) \quad \text{on} \quad (\partial\tilde{\Omega}(\tilde{t}) \cap \{\tilde{z} = 0\}) \times \mathbb{R}_+, \quad (16)$$

$$\tilde{v}_r = 0 \quad \text{and} \quad \tilde{p} = (P_2(\tilde{t}) + p_{ref})/(\rho V^2) \quad \text{on} \quad (\partial\tilde{\Omega}(\tilde{t}) \cap \{\tilde{z} = 1\}) \times \mathbb{R}_+, \quad (17)$$

$$\tilde{\eta}|_{\tilde{t}=0} = \frac{\partial\tilde{\eta}}{\partial\tilde{t}}|_{\tilde{t}=0} = 0; \quad \tilde{\eta}|_{\tilde{z}=0} = 0, \quad \text{and} \quad \tilde{\eta}|_{\tilde{z}=1} = 0, \, \forall \tilde{t} \in \mathbb{R}_+. \quad (18)$$

This is a closed, free-boundary problem for a two-dimensional degenerate hyperbolic system with a parabolic regularization. As in the simpler case of the rigid walls (see [3]) we see that $\tilde{v}_r$ depends non-locally on $\tilde{v}_z$ and solving system (12)-(18) is difficult both theoretically and numerically. Since our system generalizes the shallow water equations, it is customary to use a similar approach.

3.3 The Reduced Equations with the Closure Hypothesis

To simplify the problem even further and obtain the effective equations in one space dimension we use a typical approach of averaging the two-dimensional equations across the vessel cross-section. Introduce

$$\tilde{U} = \frac{2}{(1 + \frac{\Xi}{R}\tilde{\eta})^2} \int_0^{1+\frac{\Xi}{R}\tilde{\eta}} \tilde{v}_z \tilde{r} d\tilde{r}, \quad \tilde{\alpha} = \frac{2}{(1 + \frac{\Xi}{R}\tilde{\eta})^2 \tilde{U}^2} \int_0^{1+\frac{\Xi}{R}\tilde{\eta}} \tilde{v}_z^2 \tilde{r} d\tilde{r},$$

$$\tilde{A} = (1 + \frac{\Xi}{R}\tilde{\eta})^2, \quad \tilde{m} = \tilde{A}\tilde{U}.$$

We integrate the incompressibility condition and the axial momentum equations with respect to $\tilde{r}$ from 0 to $1 + \frac{\Xi}{R}\tilde{\eta}$ and obtain, after taking into account the no-slip condition at the lateral boundary,

$$\frac{\partial\tilde{A}}{\partial\tilde{t}} + \frac{\Xi}{R}\frac{\partial\tilde{m}}{\partial\tilde{z}} = 0, \quad Sh\frac{\partial\tilde{m}}{\partial\tilde{t}} + \frac{\partial}{\partial\tilde{z}}\left(\tilde{\alpha}\frac{\tilde{m}^2}{\tilde{A}}\right) + \tilde{A}\frac{\partial\tilde{p}}{\partial\tilde{z}} = \frac{2}{Re}\sqrt{\tilde{A}}\left[\frac{\partial\tilde{v}_z}{\partial\tilde{r}}\right]_{\tilde{\Sigma}}.$$

In the above system the Coriolis factor $\tilde{\alpha}$ depends on v_z and the interface shear stress $\left[\frac{\partial\tilde{v}_z}{\partial\tilde{r}}\right]_{\tilde{\Sigma}}$ is unknown. A typical way of handling this problem in the theory of shallow water equation is to choose a closure, giving the dependence of $\tilde{\alpha}$ and $\left[\frac{\partial\tilde{v}_z}{\partial\tilde{r}}\right]_{\tilde{\Sigma}}$ on $\tilde{A}$ and $\tilde{m}$. The usual choice in the literature is

$$\tilde{v}_z = \frac{\gamma + 2}{\gamma}\tilde{U}\left(1 - \left(\frac{\tilde{r}}{1 + \frac{\Xi}{R}\tilde{\eta}}\right)^\gamma\right). \quad (19)$$

(see [12]), with $\gamma = 9$. We refer to [11] for the review of the closure formulas for the axial velocity $\tilde{v}_z$. Now the term on the right hand-side of the momentum equation becomes $-\frac{2}{Re}(\gamma + 2)\frac{\tilde{m}}{\tilde{A}}$. After inserting the expression (14) for the pressure and returning to dimensional variables, we obtain the following quasilinear hyperbolic system

$$\frac{\partial A}{\partial t} + \frac{\partial m}{\partial z} = 0, \tag{20}$$

$$\frac{\partial m}{\partial t} + \frac{\partial}{\partial z}\left(\alpha \frac{m^2}{A}\right) + \frac{A}{\rho}\frac{\partial}{\partial z}\left(RC\sqrt{\frac{A_0}{A}}\left(\sqrt{\frac{A}{A_0}} - 1\right)\right) = -\frac{2\mu}{\rho}(\gamma + 2)\frac{m}{A}, \tag{21}$$

where $A_0 = R^2$. It is known that shocks do not form in system (20)-(21) for the realistic physiological parameters corresponding to a healthy human (see [4]). Nevertheless, the weak point of the model is the closure hypothesis (19). It **could introduce an error of order** $\mathcal{O}(1)$ in the approximation and the parameter γ is chosen to fit the experimental data. Moreover, the important Womersley flow could not be handled through (19). Our conclusion is that it would be of **importance to get a closed model giving an approximation of order** $\mathcal{O}(\varepsilon^2)$.

4 An ε^2-Approximation without the ad hoc Closure Assumption

In order to find a closure for the reduced problem, we are going to use homogenization theory. Homogenization theory is used to find effective equations for non-homogeneous flows. For porous media problems it can be applied when (a) the pore size (characteristic size of the fluid region free of another phase) is smaller than a characteristic length of the macroscopic problem (here, vessel diameter) and (b) the pore includes a large number of molecules to be considered as continuum.

At a first glance using it in our setting is pointless. One should rather do a simple averaging of the equations for the fluid phase over the cross-section of the vessel. This approach is classical and we presented it in Section 3. It leads to an $\mathcal{O}(\varepsilon^2)$ approximation, but the resulting system (12)-(18) is very difficult to solve and its complexity was the reason for imposing an **ad hoc** velocity profile for the effective axial velocity.

But we know how to obtain nonlinear filtration laws in rigid periodic porous media by homogenization. In rigid periodic porous media the expansions are of lower order of precision, but we got a closed system. In this case it was possible to link the homogenized equations with the nonlinear algebraic relations between the pressure gradient and the velocity (Forchheimer's filtration law), found in experiments. For more details we refer to [9] and [10]. We note that, in a similar way in [11], the equation (21) is replaced by a variant of Forchheimer's law linking $\dfrac{\partial \tilde{p}}{\partial \tilde{z}}$ with $\tilde{m}$, $\tilde{m}^2$ and $\dfrac{\partial \tilde{m}}{\partial \tilde{t}}$, and optimal approximations are derived for the case of rigid walls.

How to link the artery flow with the filtration through porous media ? Due to the uniform bound on the maximal value of the radial displacement, our artery could be placed into a rectangle with the length of order 1 and of the small width. By repeating periodically the geometry in the radial direction, we get a network of parallel, long and narrow tubes. This is one of the simplest porous media which one can imagine.

It is not a rigid but a **deformable** porous medium, as in Biot's theories of deformable porous media. All results which we could obtain for deformable porous media are also valid in our situation.

Motivated by the results from [9] and [10], where closed effective porous medium equations were obtained using homogenization techniques, we would like to set up a problem that would mimic a similar scenario. In this vein, we introduce $y = \dfrac{1}{\varepsilon}\tilde{z}$ and assume periodicity in y of the domain and of the velocity and the pressure. Furthermore, recalling that we have a "thin" long tube with $\tilde{r} = \frac{1}{R}r = \frac{1}{\varepsilon}\frac{r}{L}$, we can assume periodicity in the radial direction thereby forming a network of a large number of strictly separated, parallel tubes. This now resembles a porous medium problem but with no flow from one horizontal tube to another. See Figure 2. We homogenize with respect

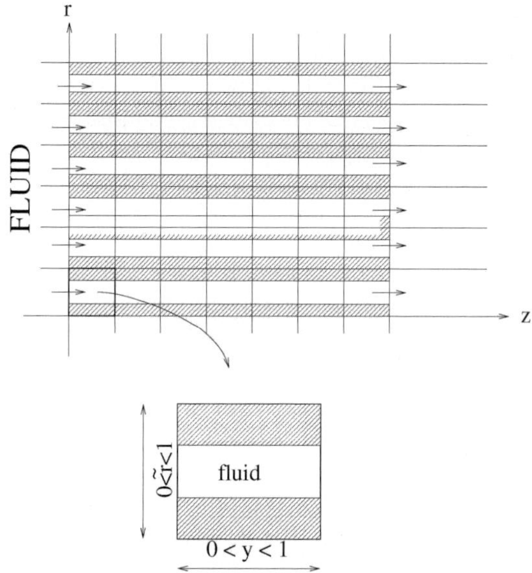

Fig. 2: Domain for a porous medium problem whitout flow from one horizontal tube to another.

to all directions. Since there is nothing in the physics of the problem that depends periodically on y we expect to get the effective equations and the solution independent of y.

More precisely, we start with the following relations between the "slow" variables (r and z (or $\tilde{z}$)) and "fast" variables ($\tilde{r}$ and y)

$$z = L\tilde{z} := L\varepsilon y = Ry, \ r = R\tilde{r}.$$

The equations at zero order read

$$Sh_0 \frac{\partial \tilde{v}_z^0}{\partial \tilde{t}} + (\tilde{v}^0 \nabla_{\tilde{r},y})\tilde{v}_z^0 + \frac{\partial \tilde{p}^0}{\partial \tilde{z}} + \frac{\partial \tilde{p}^1}{\partial y} - \frac{1}{Re_0}\left\{\frac{1}{\tilde{r}}\frac{\partial}{\partial \tilde{r}}\left(\tilde{r}\frac{\partial \tilde{v}_z^0}{\partial \tilde{r}}\right) + \frac{\partial^2 \tilde{v}_z^0}{\partial y^2}\right\} = 0,$$

$$\tag{22}$$

$$Sh_0 \frac{\partial \tilde{v}_r^0}{\partial \tilde{t}} + (\tilde{v}^0 \nabla_{\tilde{r},y})\tilde{v}_r^0 + \frac{\partial \tilde{p}^0}{\partial r} + \frac{\partial \tilde{p}^1}{\partial \tilde{r}} - \frac{1}{Re_0}\left\{\frac{1}{\tilde{r}}\frac{\partial}{\partial \tilde{r}}\left(\tilde{r}\frac{\partial \tilde{v}_r^0}{\partial \tilde{r}}\right) + \frac{\partial^2 \tilde{v}_r^0}{\partial y^2}\right\} = 0,$$

$$\tag{23}$$

$$\nabla_{\tilde{r},y}\tilde{p}^0 = 0, \tag{24}$$

$$\frac{\partial}{\partial \tilde{r}}\left(\tilde{r}\tilde{v}_r^0\right) + \frac{\partial}{\partial y}\left(\tilde{r}\tilde{v}_z^0\right) = 0, \tag{25}$$

$$\tilde{v}_r^0, \tilde{v}_z^0 \ \text{and} \ \tilde{p}^1 \ \text{are 1-periodic in} \ y \ \text{and} \ \tilde{v}_r^0 = \tilde{v}_z^0 = 0 \ \text{at} \ \tilde{r} = 1 + \frac{\Xi}{R}\tilde{\eta}, \tag{26}$$

where

$$Sh_0 := \frac{\varepsilon L\omega^\varepsilon}{V}, \quad Re_0 := \frac{\rho RV}{\mu}.$$

Notice $Sh_0 = \varepsilon Sh$ and $Re = \varepsilon Re_0$. For our values, Sh_0 is of order 1 ($Sh_0 \in (3,4)$) and Re_0 is around 600. We remark that equation (24) corresponds to the ε^{-1} term. Here, a new scaling for the pressure was used to obtain equations (22)-(24). This "z-blown up" pressure scaling reads

$$p = \frac{\rho LV^2}{R}\tilde{\tilde{p}} = \rho V^2 \frac{1}{\varepsilon}\tilde{\tilde{p}} = \rho V^2 \tilde{p}, \quad \text{so} \quad \tilde{\tilde{p}} = \varepsilon\tilde{p}.$$

The leading order Navier equations for the membrane force are unchanged.

We now focus on the case corresponding to the magnitude of the parameters Sh_0 and Re_0 which is of interest to us.

4.1   Case with $Sh > 0$ and Moderate Re

In this case, for a given pressure gradient $\frac{\partial \tilde{p}^0}{\partial \tilde{z}}$, the non-stationary, axially symmetric system (22)-(26) admits a unique unidirectional, but strongly non-stationary solution. The unidirectional solution refers to the y direction. We will write the solution of system (22)-(26) as a sum of this y-unidirectional solution and a small perturbation of it. This perturbation satisfies a linearized system, see (22)-(26), where the linearization is calculated around the unidirectional solution. This system is *closed*.

The zero-th order approximation: the y-unidirectional flow

For every given smooth $\tilde{p}^0$, system (22)-(26) has a unique strong solution

$$\tilde{v}_z^0 = w(\tilde{r}, \tilde{z}, t), \quad \tilde{v}_r^0 = 0,$$

where w satisfies

$$Sh_0 \frac{\partial w}{\partial \tilde{t}} - \frac{1}{Re_0} \frac{1}{\tilde{r}} \frac{\partial}{\partial \tilde{r}} \left(\tilde{r} \frac{\partial w}{\partial \tilde{r}} \right) = -\frac{\partial \tilde{p}^0}{\partial \tilde{z}}(\tilde{z}, \tilde{t}) = -\frac{RC}{\mathcal{P}} \frac{\partial \tilde{\eta}^0}{\partial \tilde{z}}$$

$$w(0, \tilde{z}, \tilde{t}) \text{ bounded}, \ w(1 + \Xi \tilde{\eta}^0(\tilde{z}, \tilde{t})/R, \tilde{z}, \tilde{t}) = 0 \quad \text{and} \quad w(\tilde{r}, \tilde{z}, 0) = 0.$$

Furthermore, solution $\tilde{p}^1$ is a linear function of y, independent of $\tilde{r}$. Due to 1-periodicity with respect to y we get $\tilde{p}^1 = \tilde{p}^1(\tilde{z}, \tilde{t})$. Then the next order in Laplace's law implies $\tilde{p}^1 = 0$. This is a free-boundary problem because the condition at the lateral boundary depends on the solution. For a known pressure or the radial displacement (or the cross-sectional area) this problem is well-posed. We can eliminate $\tilde{p}^0$, and use the definitions of $\tilde{A}$ and $\tilde{m}$ to write this in terms of w and $\tilde{A}$ as

$$\frac{\partial \tilde{A}}{\partial \tilde{t}} + \frac{\Xi}{R} \frac{\partial}{\partial \tilde{z}} \int_0^{\sqrt{\tilde{A}}} 2\tilde{r} w \, d\tilde{r} = 0,$$

$$Sh_0 \frac{\partial w}{\partial \tilde{t}} + \left(\frac{R}{\Xi} \right)^2 \frac{R}{L} \frac{\partial \sqrt{\tilde{A}}}{\partial \tilde{z}} = \frac{1}{Re_0} \frac{1}{\tilde{r}} \frac{\partial}{\partial \tilde{r}} \left(\tilde{r} \frac{\partial w}{\partial \tilde{r}} \right),$$

$$w(0, \tilde{z}, \tilde{t}) \text{ bounded}, \ w(\sqrt{\tilde{A}}, \tilde{z}, \tilde{t}) = 0, \ \tilde{A}(\tilde{z}, 0) = 0, \ w(\tilde{r}, \tilde{z}, 0) = 0$$

$$\tilde{A}(0, \tilde{t}) = \tilde{A}(L, \tilde{t}) = 0 \ w(\tilde{r}, 0, \tilde{t}) = w_0(t), \ w(\tilde{r}, L, \tilde{t}) = w_L(t).$$

This is a two-dimensional, free-boundary problem of mixed, hyperbolic-parabolic type. It has a simpler form than system (9)-(10).

The first-order correction: perturbation of the y-unidirectional flow

We will be using the zero-th order approximation to the solution consisting of the velocity $(w, 0)$ and displacement $\tilde{\eta}^0$ (or, equivalently, the pressure $\tilde{p}^0$) to find an ε-correction by solving (9)-(10), linearized around the zero-th order approximation:

$$Sh_0 \frac{\partial \tilde{v}_z^1}{\partial \tilde{t}} + \tilde{v}_z^0 \left\{ \frac{\partial \tilde{v}_z^1}{\partial y} + \frac{\partial \tilde{v}_z^0}{\partial \tilde{z}} \right\} + \tilde{v}_r^1 \frac{\partial \tilde{v}_z^0}{\partial \tilde{r}} + \frac{\partial \tilde{p}^2}{\partial y} = \frac{1}{Re_0} \left\{ \frac{1}{\tilde{r}} \frac{\partial}{\partial \tilde{r}} \left(\tilde{r} \frac{\partial \tilde{v}_z^1}{\partial \tilde{r}} \right) + \frac{\partial^2 \tilde{v}_z^1}{\partial y^2} \right\}$$

$$Sh_0 \frac{\partial \tilde{v}_r^1}{\partial \tilde{t}} + \tilde{v}_z^0 \frac{\partial \tilde{v}_r^1}{\partial y} + \frac{\partial \tilde{p}^2}{\partial \tilde{r}} = \frac{1}{Re_0} \left\{ \frac{1}{\tilde{r}} \frac{\partial}{\partial \tilde{r}} \left(\tilde{r} \frac{\partial \tilde{v}_r^1}{\partial \tilde{r}} \right) + \frac{\partial^2 \tilde{v}_r^1}{\partial y^2} \right\}$$

$$\frac{\partial}{\partial \tilde{r}} \left(\tilde{r} \tilde{v}_r^1 \right) + \frac{\partial}{\partial y} \left(\tilde{r} \tilde{v}_z^1 \right) + \frac{\partial \tilde{v}_z^0}{\partial \tilde{z}} = 0,$$

$$\tilde{v}_r^1, \tilde{v}_z^1, \tilde{p}^2 \text{ are 1-periodic in } y; \ \tilde{v}_r^1 = \frac{\partial \tilde{\eta}^0}{\partial \tilde{t}}, \ \tilde{v}_z^0 = 0 \text{ at } \tilde{r} = 1 + \frac{\Xi}{R} \tilde{\eta}^0.$$

This is an Oseen's system and it has a $\tilde{v}^1$ being uniquely determined. We search $\tilde{v}_z^1 = \tilde{v}_z^1(\tilde{r}, \tilde{z}, \tilde{t})$. Then

$$\tilde{r}\tilde{v}_r^1(\tilde{r}, \tilde{z}, \tilde{t}) = (1 + \Xi\tilde{\eta}^0/R)\frac{\partial\tilde{\eta}^0}{\partial\tilde{t}} + \int_{\tilde{r}}^{1+\Xi\tilde{\eta}^0/R} \frac{\partial\tilde{v}_z^0}{\partial\tilde{z}}(\xi, \tilde{z}, \tilde{t})\, \xi\, d\xi.$$

Furthermore

$$Sh_0\frac{\partial\tilde{v}_z^1}{\partial\tilde{t}} - \frac{1}{Re_0}\frac{1}{\tilde{r}}\frac{\partial}{\partial\tilde{r}}\left(\tilde{r}\frac{\partial\tilde{v}_z^1}{\partial\tilde{r}}\right) + \frac{\partial\varphi}{\partial y}(y, \tilde{z}, \tilde{t}) = -\tilde{v}_r^1\frac{\partial\tilde{v}_z^0}{\partial\tilde{r}} - \frac{\partial}{\partial\tilde{z}}\left(\frac{(\tilde{v}_z^0)^2}{2} + \tilde{p}^1\right)$$

$$\tilde{v}_z^1(0, \tilde{z}, \tilde{t}) \text{ is bounded}, \quad \tilde{v}_z^1(1 + \Xi\tilde{\eta}^0(\tilde{z}, \tilde{t})/R, \tilde{z}, \tilde{t}) = 0$$

$$\tilde{v}_z^1(\tilde{r}, \tilde{z}, 0) = 0 \quad \text{and} \quad \tilde{\tilde{p}}^2 = \tilde{\tilde{p}}^2(\tilde{r}, \tilde{z}, \tilde{t})$$

This solution also satisfies problem (12)-(48) to ε^2-order. More precisely, since $\tilde{\tilde{p}}^0 = \varepsilon\tilde{p}$ and due to the boundary conditions for the pressure, we have that $\tilde{\tilde{p}}^0$ is of order ε. Consequently, both $\tilde{v}_z^0$ and $\tilde{v}_r^1$ are of order ε. We have

Proposition 2. *The velocity field $(\tilde{v}_z^0 + \varepsilon\tilde{v}_z^1)$ and the pressure field $\frac{1}{\varepsilon}\tilde{\tilde{p}}^0$ satisfy equations (12)-(14) to $\mathcal{O}(\varepsilon^2)$.*

5 Conclusion: the Problem with Nonlinear Coupling in Dimensional Form

Using the homogenization approach we obtained a closed "one-and-a-half-dimensional" effective model, which approximates the system (1)-(3), in the limit $\varepsilon \to 0$. We did not need any **ad hoc** closure assumptions. Our limit system could be classified as a special case of the diphasic Biot's system (see [2]. Its numerical solution is much simpler than that of the shallow water systems. For detailed presentation of the numerical simulations we refer to [5] and to [6]. We repeat once more our construction, but this time in dimensional form.

The zero-th order approximation

Look for $v_z^0 = v_z^0(r, z, t)$ and $\eta^0 = \eta^0(z, t)$ and then recover $p^0 = p^0(z, t)$ by solving the following free-boundary problem defined on the domain $0 < z < L$, $0 < r < R + \eta^0(z, t)$

$$\frac{\partial(R + \eta^0)^2}{\partial t} + \frac{\partial}{\partial z}\int_0^{R+\eta^0} 2rv_z^0 dr = 0, \tag{27}$$

$$\rho\frac{\partial v_z^0}{\partial t} + \frac{\partial p}{\partial z} = \mu\frac{1}{r}\frac{\partial}{\partial r}\left(r\frac{\partial v_z^0}{\partial r}\right), \tag{28}$$

$$v_z^0(0, z, t) \text{ bounded}, \quad v_z^0(R + \eta^0(z, t), z, t) = 0, \quad v_z^0(r, z, 0) = 0 \tag{29}$$

with the following inlet and outlet boundary conditions $\forall t \in \mathbb{R}_+$

$$\eta^0 = 0 \ \text{ for } \ z = 0, \ \eta^0 = 0 \ \text{ for } \ z = L,$$
$$p = P_1(t) + p_{ref} \ \text{ for } \ z = 0, \ 0 \le r \le R,$$
$$p = P_2(t) + p_{ref} \ \text{ for } \ z = L, \ 0 \le r \le R,$$

with the pressure

$$p(z,t) = p_{ref} + RC\frac{\eta^0}{R + \eta^0}. \tag{30}$$

The ε-correction for the velocity

Solve for $v_z^1 = v_z^1(r,z,t)$ and $v_r^1 = v_r^1(r,z,t)$ by first recovering v_r^1 via

$$rv_r^1(r,z,t) = (R + \eta^0)\frac{\partial \eta^0}{\partial t} + \int_r^{R+\eta^0} \frac{\partial v_z^0}{\partial z}(\xi,z,t)\, \xi \, d\xi$$

and then solve the following linear *fixed* boundary problem for v_z^1, defined on the domain $0 < z < L$, $0 < r < R + \eta^0(z,t)$

$$\frac{\partial v_z^1}{\partial t} - \nu\frac{1}{r}\frac{\partial}{\partial r}\left(r\frac{\partial v_z^1}{\partial r}\right) = -S_{v_z^1}(r,z,t)$$
$$v_z^1(0,z,t) \ \text{bounded}, \ v_z^1(R + \eta^0(z,t),z,t) = 0$$
$$v_z^1(r,0,t) = v_z^1(r,L,t) = 0 \quad v_z^1(r,z,0) = 0$$

where $S_{v_z^1}(r,z,t)$ contains the already calculated functions and is defined by

$$S_{v_z^1}(r,z,t) = v_r^1\frac{\partial v_z^0}{\partial r} + v_z^0\frac{\partial v_z^0}{\partial z}.$$

The result of Proposition 2 implies that the velocity field $(v_z^0 + \varepsilon v_z^1)$ and the pressure field p represent a second order approximation for the solutions of the equations (1)-(3).

The mathematical theory for the system (27)-(30) is developed only for the linearized system (see [5] and [6] for details). Proving the global existence of a solution to this system is an open challenging problem.

Acknowledgements

The research of Andro Mikelić is supported by the NSF and NIH under grant DMS-0443826. The reasearch of Sunčica Čanić is supported by the NSF under grants DMS0245513 and DMS-0337355, and by the NSF and NIH under grant DMS-0443826.

References

1. H. Beirao da Veiga: On the existence of a strong solution to a coupled fluid-structure evolution problem, Journal of Mathematical Fluid Mechanics, Vol. **6** (2004), p. 21–52.
2. M.A. Biot: Theory of propagation of elastic waves in a fluid-saturated porous solid. I. Lower frequency range, and II. Higher frequency range, J. Acoust. Soc. Am. **28** (1956), 168–178 and 179–191.
3. Y. Brenier: Homogeneous hydrostatic flows with convex velocity profiles. Non-linearity, Vol. **12**, 495–512 (1999).
4. S. Čanić and E.-H. Kim: Mathematical analysis of the quasilinear effects in a hyperbolic model of blood flow through compliant axi-symmetric vessels. Mathematical Methods in the Applied Sciences, **26**, 1161–1186 (2003).
5. S. Čanić, D. Lamponi, A. Mikelić , J. Tambača : Self-Consistent Effective Equations Modeling Blood Flow in Medium-to-Large Compliant Arteries, SIAM Journal on Multiscale Analysis and Simulation, Vol. **3**, 559–596 (2005).
6. S. Čanić, A. Mikelić , J. Tambača : A Two-Dimensional Effective Model Describing Fluid-Structure Interaction in Blood Flow: Analysis, Numerical Simulation and Experimental Validation, Comptes Rendus Mécanique, **333**, 867–883 (2005).
7. B. Desjardins, M.J. Esteban, C. Grandmont, P. Le Tallec: Weak solutions for a fluid-structure interaction model, Rev. Mat. Complut. **14**, 523–538 (2001).
8. Y.C. Fung. Biomechanics: Circulation. Springer New York (1993). Second Edition.
9. E. Marušić-Paloka and A. Mikelić: The derivation of a nonlinear filtration law including the inertia effects via homogenization. Nonlinear Analysis **42**, 97–137 (2000).
10. A. Mikelić: Homogenization theory and applications to filtration through porous media, chapter in "Filtration in Porous Media and Industrial Applications," by M. Espedal, A. Fasano and A. Mikelić, Lecture Notes in Mathematics Vol. **1734**, Springer, 127–214 (2000).
11. A.M. Robertson, A. Sequeira: A director theory approach for modeling blood flow in the arterial system: an alternative to classical 1D models, M^3 AS : Math. Models Methods Appl. Sci., Vol. **15**, 871–906 (2005).
12. A. Quarteroni, M. Tuveri and A. Veneziani: Computational vascular fluid dynamics: problems, models and methods. Survey article, Comput. Visual. Sci. **2**, 163–197 (2000).

Pattern Formation in Butterfly Wings: Experiments and Models

Toshio Sekimura

Department of Biological Chemistry, College of Bioscience and Biotechnology,
Chubu University, Kasugai, Aichi 487-8501, Japan
sekimura@isc.chubu.ac.jp

Summary. Butterfly wings are covered with a large number of colored scale cells.
It is well known that there exist two different kinds of patterns in butterfly wings -
the spacing pattern of scale cells and color pattern. The spacing pattern is cellular
pattern in which scale cells form nearly parallel rows along the anteroposterior axis
of the wing. On the other hand, the color pattern is mainly pigmentation pattern
which is constructed as a finely-tiled mosaic of colored scale cells. In this paper,
I present mathematical models together with numerical simulations for both the
cellular spacing pattern and color pattern with experimental evidences. The relationship between color patterns of fore- and hind-wing are also discussed within the
framework of the model.

1 Introduction

Butterfly wing markings are one of the most colorful examples of pattern formation in nature. Thousands of scale cells cover the wing in a highly ordered
pattern and these scale cells can be easily seen through a simple magnify-
ing glass. Two different kinds of patterns are associated with these scales –
the spacing pattern of scale cells and color pattern. The colors on wings are
due to the colors of scale cells which is mainly due to the presence of chemical pigments. The color patterns of wings are, in general, finely-tiled mosaic
patterns produced by monochromatic scales and are characteristic of each
butterfly species. On the other hand, the spacing pattern of scale cells do
not show species-specific patterns, but they are, in general, common to all
lepidopteran wings (Fig. 1).

In the following sections, we first summarize mechanisms for the spacing
pattern and present a mathematical model for the parallel row formation
with simulation results. We then discuss about what color pattern is and
present a reaction diffusion model for color pattern formation. Finally, we show
numerical simulations and discuss the relationship between color patterns of
fore- and hind-wing from mathematical modeling point of view.

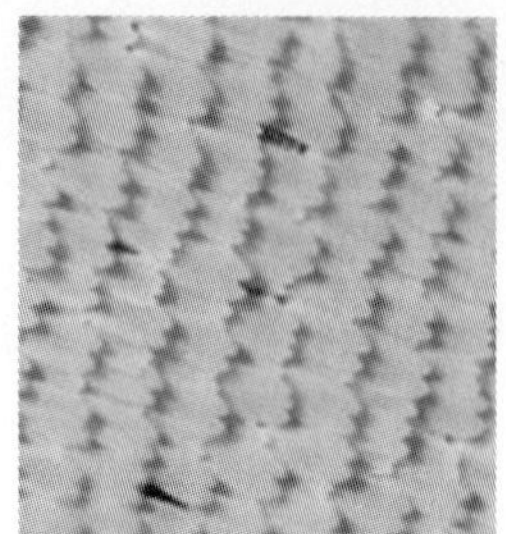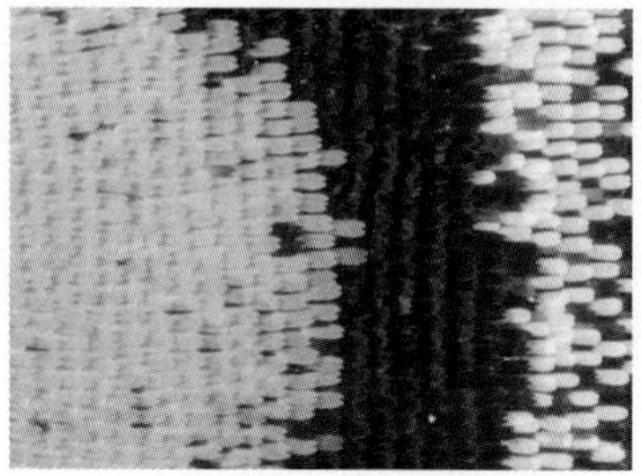

Fig. 1: Parallel rows of scale cells (left) and color pattern (right). The color pattern is a finely-tiled mosaic pattern produced by regularly arranged monochromatic scale cells. See also Plate 2 on page 338

2 Parallel Row Formation of Scale Cells

2.1 Mechanisms for Parallel Row Formation

Immediately after pupation, the epithelial cells of the wing are not differentiated and they are morphologically homogeneous. About one to three days after pupation, two cell types can be readily distinguished. The smaller cells are generalized epithelial cells (GECs) of the wing, and the larger cells are scale precursor cells (SPCs) that differentiate from GECs at the inception of adult development. SPCs are arranged in space such that they are separated from each other by GECs. Within a few hours of differentiation of the isotropically arranged SPCs, these cells become polarized along the proximodistal axis of the wing and begin to align into rows parallel to the anteroposterior axis of the wing. This row formation continues until a stable spatial periodicity of rows is established. These parallel rows of SPCs maintain their arrangement throughout adult development and represent the same rows of scales that appear on the surface of the adult wing(Fig. 2(a) [7]).

We next summarize what is known about the cellular and molecular processes involved in the spacing pattern formation [15].

(1) Cell rearrangement occurs in a monolayer.

(2) Lateral inhibition probably forms the uniform pattern of SPCs.

(3) Long-range interaction mediated by basal processes.

As the alignment of SPCs into rows proceeds, extension of processes from the basal surfaces of the epithelial cells simultaneously occurs. These processes can extend for distances of several cell diameters and can establish contacts not only with adjacent cells but with cells that are four or five cell diameters away.

(4) Origin-dependent cell adhesion.

Grafting experiments within the pupal wing monolayer of *Manduca* have shown that differences in adhesive properties of epithelial cells exist along the proximodistal axis of the wing [6].

(5) Short-range interaction mediated by cell adhesion proteins.

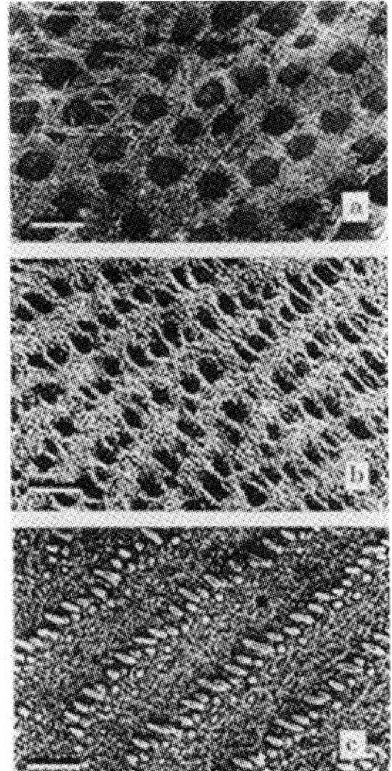 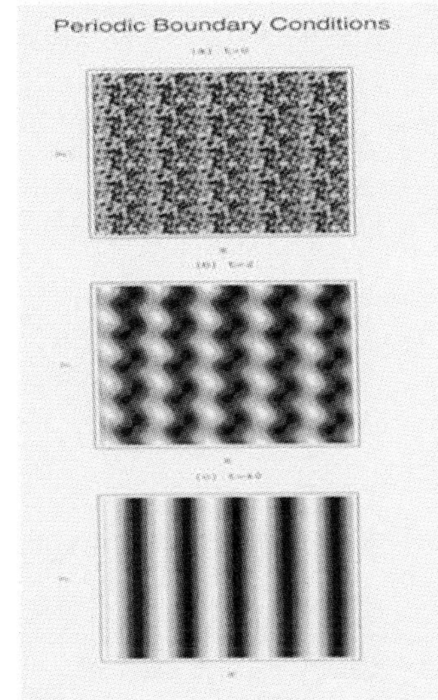

Fig. 2: (a) (left) Parallel row formation of scale cells on the moth *Mandusa* wing [7]. bar in the figures $= 50\mu m$. (b) (right) Results of numerical simulation by the model. The lighter color represents high cell density while the darker color represents low cell density. We use a random cell distribution as our initial condition and impose periodic boundary conditions.

2.2 A Model for Parallel Row Formation of SPCs with Origin-Dependent Cell Adhesivity [16]

Integral representation

In this model we assume that there is only one cell type of importance (SPCs) and that two cells interact with each other according to the distance between their original locations (as well as the distance between their current locations). Since cells can respond to non-adjacent neighbours during the row formation, we use averages to represent the local average adhesivity to which a cell responds.

Let $n(\mathbf{x}, a, t)$ signify the cell density at position $\mathbf{x} = (x,y)$ at time t for the cells of a given adhesivity a that originate from a position that is a units of distance away from the body axis (the base of the wing). Suppose that cell movement is due to two processes, diffusion and advection (directed movement) in response to gradients of adhesivity. Due to the evidence for long-range interactions noted in the previous section, we consider a cell to respond to gradients in a spatially averaged adhesivity. As an evolution equation for cell density in space we write

$$n_t = D \, \nabla^2 n - \nabla \cdot [n\mathbf{c}] \tag{1}$$

where D is the diffusion coefficient. The advection velocity, $\mathbf{c}$, is given by

$$\mathbf{c} = C \nabla \left[\int n(\mathbf{x} - \mathbf{y}, a - s) w(\mathbf{y}, s) ds dy_1 dy_2 \right], \tag{2}$$

where $\mathbf{x} = (x, y)$ and $\mathbf{y} = (y_1, y_2)$ are position variables, and C is a positive constant. The integral represents the spatially averaged adhesivity. The degree of adhesivity as a function of distance, $\mathbf{y}$, and adhesivity distance (distance in adhesivity space), s, are incorporated in the kernel $w(\mathbf{y}, s)$. For simplicity, we suppose that this is separable. We therefore write

$$w(\mathbf{y}, s) = g(\mathbf{y}) h(s) \tag{3}$$

We assume that g displays rotational symmetry in the two spatial dimensions, and h is symmetric in the adhesivity difference. One example is shown in Figure 3.

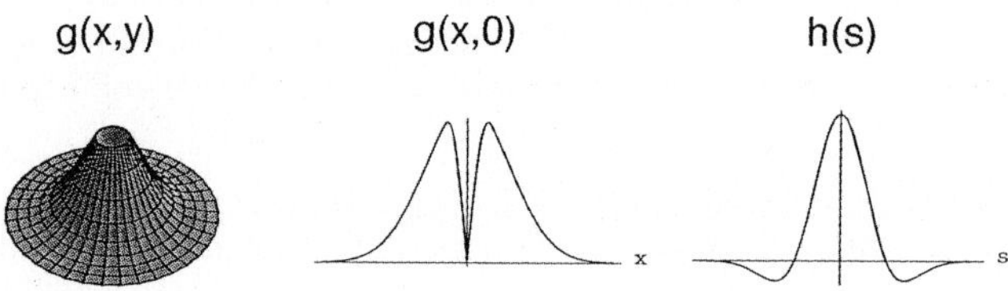

Fig. 3: (left and middle) The spatial kernel g. Adjacent cells are relatively unadhesive (diffusion dominates); for large distances adhesivity effects fall with distance between cells. (right) The adhesivity kernel h. Cells originally from nearby points attract each other. Cells of vastly different adhesivity repel each other.

Mathematical Discussion of the Model and Numerical Simulations

Using the assumption that $|\mathbf{y}| \ll 1$ and $|s| \ll 1$, we can simplify Eq. (1) by Taylor expanding Eq. (2):

$$n_t = D \nabla^2 n - C \nabla \cdot [n \nabla (n + \gamma \nabla^2 n + \beta n_{aa})] + O(s^4 + |\mathbf{y}|^4), \tag{4}$$

where

$$\beta = \frac{1}{2} \int s^2 h(s) ds, \tag{5}$$

$$\gamma = \frac{1}{2} \int y_1^2 g(\mathbf{y}) dy_1 dy_2. \tag{6}$$

The parameters β and γ are related directly to the effects of cell adhesion and distance, respectively. This procedure reduces the integro-partial differential equation (1) to a partial differential equation.

The Effect of Origin-Dependent Cell Adhesivity

Here we investigate the effect of including origin-dependent adhesivity in the model. We neglect the $O(s^4, |\mathbf{y}|^4)$ terms. With the origin-dependent adhesivity term the model equation becomes

$$n_t = D \nabla^2 n - C \nabla \cdot [n \nabla (n + \gamma \nabla^2 n + \beta n_{aa})]. \tag{7}$$

We assume that $n_{aa} = E n_{xx}$, where E is a proportionality constant. The motivation for making this assumption is as follows: Note that $\gamma \nabla^2 n = \gamma(n_{xx} + n_{yy})$ is a long range diffusion term. With the origin-dependent effect, cells are less likely to diffuse in the x-direction (i.e., perpendicular to the body axis), so βn_{aa} is acting as a negative diffusion term in the x-direction and reduces the net diffusion in the x-direction. Therefore, Eq. (7) becomes

$$n_t = D \nabla^2 n - C \nabla \cdot [n \nabla (n + \gamma \nabla^2 n + \beta^* n_{xx})], \tag{8}$$

where $\beta^* = E\beta$. Note that although β^* is negative, we assume that $\gamma + \beta^* \geq 0$, i.e., the effective diffusion in the x-direction is still positive.

A weakly non-linear analysis shows that rows predominate in a large region of parameter space. More importantly, the rows are predictably aligned, that is, stripes can only lie parallel to the body axis under the effect of origin-dependent adhesivity. We also note that as long as the effect of origin-dependent adhesivity is sufficiently strong, spotted patterns can not be generated (see [16] for details).

3 Color Pattern Formation

The colors on butterfly wings are due to the colors of regularly-arranged scale cells. The overall color pattern is constructed as a fine-tiled mosaic of colored scales. One of the central problems of color pattern formation is thus how a particular scale cell is induced to synthesize the right pigment for its particular location on the wing.

3.1 Color Pattern and the Cellular Spacing Pattern

It is known that the formation of the color pattern is independent of the spacing pattern of scale cells. The timescales on which these two patterns are generated are different from each other. The spacing pattern occurs in the early stages of pupation, while color patterns appear in the last stage of pupation after completion of parallel row formation. In addition, the length scale of color pattern extends from tens to several hundreds of cell diameters (Fig. 1), and no cell migration occurs during the period of color pattern determination. On the other hand, direct cell-cell interactions through filopodia during the period of the spacing pattern formation can only extend several cell diameters at most, which is very short relative to the scale of the color pattern. Diffusion of small molecules through gap junctions is assumed to be a feasible mechanism for long distance cell-to-cell communication to form color patterns [8].

3.2 Global Color Pattern and Ground Plan

Currently, there exist two different research directions on color pattern formation The first one is that of localized patterns such as eyespot patterns. The second one is of global patterns which cover the whole dorsal or ventral wing monolayer. The best understood mechanism is that of local eyespot patterns in which the spatial pattern of expressions of the gene *Distal-less* and several other genes have been detected and examined [1]. On the other hand, little is known about genes for global patterns except for a few cases such as the butterfly *Papilio dardanus* [2]. Global patterns look like very complicated in structure and they are sometimes used for identification of butterfly species. However, owing to the pioneering work of Schwanwitsch [11] and Süffert [17] on the Nymphalid ground plan, the complicated global patterns can be understood as a composite of a small number of pattern elements. The ground plan is not a really existing pattern in nature, but a hypothetical one from which a large number of real wing patterns could be generated by some organizing principles such as dislocation of pattern elements along the veins [8].

In spite of these simplifications, the problem of color pattern fomation in wings is not sufficiently resolved. A few mathematical models for color pattern formation have been proposed so far to account for specific features of the pattern.

3.3 Reaction Diffusion Model for Global Color Pattern Formation

We proposed a reaction diffusion model for formation of global pigmentation patterns in the butterfly wing of *Papilio dardanus* [14]. The model is based on the idea of the so-called diffusion driven instability [18]. By mathematical analysis and computer simulations of the model equations on a geometrically accurate wing domain, we showed that the global wing coloration is essentially due to underlying stripe-like patterns of some pigment inducing morphogen.

We also stressed the importance of some key factors to have realistic patterns in computer simulations such as parameter values for mode selection, threshold values which determine color, wing shape and boundary conditions.

In the next section, I introduce our reaction diffusion model and present computational results.

Model Equations

We solve the non–dimensionalised reaction–diffusion system with Gierer–Meinhardt reaction kinetics [3]

$$u_t = \gamma \left(a - b\,u + \frac{u^2}{v\,(1 + k\,u^2)} \right) + \nabla^2 u,$$

$$v_t = \gamma \left(u^2 - v \right) + d\,\nabla^2 v$$

using the finite element method on fixed two-dimensional wing domains [4]. Here $u(\underline{x}, t)$ and $v(\underline{x}, t)$ represent chemical(morphogen) concentrations at spatial position $\underline{x}$ and time t; a, b, d, k and γ are positive parameters.

Numerical Results

(1) Mimetic patterns in females of *Papilio dardanus*

A species of butterfly, *Papilio dardanus*, is widely distributed across sub-Saharan Africa, and well-known for the spectacular phenotypic polymorphism in females that has evolved as different geographic races have simultaneously come to mimic an array of different species in their specific regions. The females have evolved more than a dozen different wing color patterns, of which several mimic different species of unplatable danaids. The males, on the other hand, are monomorphic and strikingly different from the females, exhibiting a characteristic yellow and black color pattern and tailed hind-wing. In previous papers [14, 5, 9, 12], we demonstrated that our model could account well for pigmentation patterning in the wing of *Papilio dardanus*. Fig. 4 (a), (b) show some mimetic female forms of *Papilio dardanus*, and our numerical simulation results by the model, respectively. We have emphasized that different color patterns in female forms are similar to each other and they can be obtained under tight control of only a few key factors such as parameter values for mode selection, threshold values that determine color, wing shape and boundary conditions. This result could be important from the genetic point of view because it agrees with the result that most of the different female forms are controlled by a single genetic H locus [2].

(2) Patterns of the mimetic butterfly *Papilio polytes*

A species of butterfly, *Papilio polytes*, is widely distributed across India and Southeast Asia including the Southern Islands of Japan. *Papilio polytes* has monomorphic males and several female forms. The male-like female

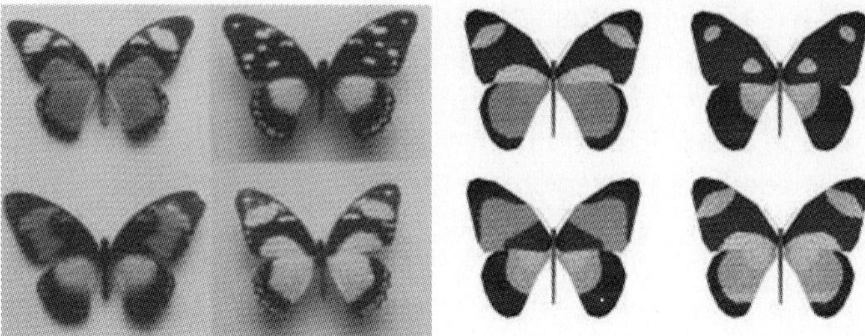

Fig. 4: (a)(left) Polymorphism in mimetic females of *Papilio dardanus. trophonius*(top left), *cenea*(top right),*planemoides*(bottom left),*hippocoon*(bottom right). (b)(right) Numerical simulation results by the model illustrating global color patterns for *trophonius*(top left), *cenea*(top right),*planemoides*(bottom left),*hippocoon*(bottom right). See also Plate 3 on page 338

is nonmimetic and resembles the male. Other female forms are mimetic and mimic different species of unpalatable *Aristolochia*-feeding swallowtail butterflies. The fore-wing pattern of the male has a white band along the distal wing margin in the entire black-colored wing. The hind-wing pattern has a white band passing through the middle of the wing in the anterior-posterior direction which looks like linking continuously to the forewing white band when both wings are held at rest. Computer simulations are carried out seperately for fore- and hind-wings. The close match between color patterns on fore- and hind-wings is logically reasonable from mathematical modeling point of view. Fig. 5 (a), (b) show a male of *Papilio polytes* and our simulation results by the model, respectively [13].

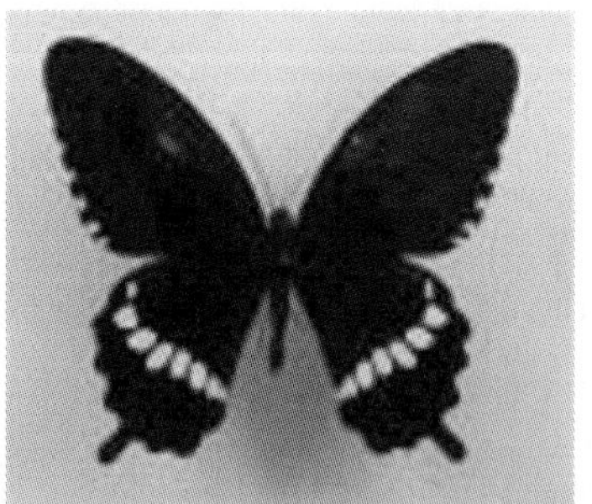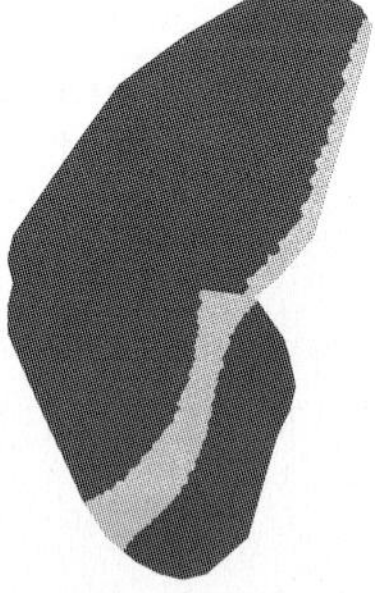

Fig. 5: (a) (left) A male of *Papilio polytes*. (b) (right) Numerical simulation results by the model.

4 Conclusions and Discussion

There exist two different kinds of patterns in butterfly wings *the cellular spacing pattern of scale cells and color pattern.* In this paper, I dealt with these patterns from both mathematical modeling and experimental points of view. Our main results are as follows.

The Spacing Pattern of Scale Cells

Based on a number of key biological observations, we have developed a novel model for pattern formation consisting of only one equation, of integro-partial differential type. We have shown that if we incorporate the origin-dependent adhesivity property in the equation, the model can exhibit only stripes of a specific orientation that is consistent with biological observations. This result implies that with the origin-dependent effect, cells are less likely to diffuse in the direction perpendicular to the body axis and the origin-dependent property is acting as a negative diffusion property to reduce the net diffusion in the proximal-distal direction of the wing.

Global Color Pattern

By mathematical analysis and computer simulations of the Turing-type reaction diffusion equations on a geometrically accurate wing domain, we showed that the global wing coloration is essentially due to underlying stripe-like patterns of some pigment inducing morphogen. We also emphasized the importance of some key factors to have realistic patterns in computer simulations such as parameter values for mode selection, threshold values which determine color, wing shape and boundary conditions. These results are consistent with experimental results on the gene regulation done by Clarke and Sheppard using the mimetic butterfly *Papilio dardanus* [2].

One of the most striking phenomena about wing color patterns is the close match between patterns of fore- and hind-wings. The close match between both patterns when wings are held at rest occurs on the dorsal sides of many species. This phenomenon is, in general, known as Oudemans' principle [10]. The integrated pattern of both fore-wing and hind-wing is often suggested to show an unified adaptive pattern just like as we see in the butterfly *Kallima inachus*. In section 3.3, we have chosen *Papilio polytes* as a model butterfly to test the relationship mathematically and computationally. Computations on the fore- and hind-wing shapes are carried out separately as usual. Except for a small change in a parameter value of the threshold function, we used the same parameter values to obtain a close match between fore- and hind-wing patterns. This means that from a mathematical modeling point of view, global color patterns of fore- and hind-wing are independent with each other in the sense that they are produced or controlled by the same formation mechanism.

Acknowledgments

I am grateful to Prof. V. Capasso for giving me the opportunity to talk about the topic. This work is based on joint researches with Prof. P. K. Maini of Centre for Mathematical Biology, University of Oxford.

References

1. Beldade, P. and Brakefield, P.M. (2002). The genetics and evo-devo of butterfly wing patterns, *Nature Rev Genet*, **3**, 442–452.
2. Clarke, C.A. and Sheppard, P.M. (1963). Interactions between major genes and polygenes in the determination of the mimetic pattern of *Papilio dardanus*, *Evolution*, **17**, 404–413.
3. Geirer, A. and Meinhardt, H. (1972). A theory of biological pattern formation. *Kybernetik*, **12**, 30–39.
4. Madzvamuse, A. (2000). A numerical approach to the study of spatial pattern formation. *D. Phil. Thesis*, University of Oxford.
5. Madzvamuse, A., Maini, P.K., Wathen, A.J., and Sekimura, T. (2002). A predictive model for color pattern formation in the butterfly wing of *Papilio dardanus*, *Hiroshima Mathematical Journal*, **32**, No.2, 325–336.
6. Nardi, J.B. (1988). Establishment of a two-dimensional neural network in an insect wing. *Current Issues in Neural Regeneration Research*, (ed. Reier, P.J.). New York: Alan R. Liss, 127–136.
7. Nardi, J.B. and Magee-Adams, S.M. (1986). Formation of scale spacing patterns in a moth wing. I. Epithelial feet may mediate cell rearrangement. *Dev. Biol.*, **116**, 278–290.
8. Nijhout, H.F. (1991). The development and evolution of butterfly wing patterns. Smithonian Institution Press, Washington and London.
9. Nijhout, H.F. , Maini, P.K., Madzvamuse, A., Wathen, J.W., and Sekimura, T. (2003). Pigmentation pattern formation in butterflies: experiments and models. *C. R. Biologies* **326**, 717–727.
10. Oudemans, J.T. (1903). Etudes sur la position de repos chez les Lepidopteres, *Verhandelingen der Koning-klijke Akademie van Wetenschappen*,**10**, 1–90.
11. Schwanwitsch, B.N. (1924). On the ground plan ofwing-pattern in nymphalids and certain other families ofrhopalocerous Lepidoptera. *Proc. Zool. Soc. Lond.*, ser B **34**, 509–528.
12. Sekimura, T. (2005). Patterns in butterfly wings and their evolution - experiments and models -, In Patterns Seen in Biological Systems and Their Origin,(eds. Matsushita, M.), University of Tokyo Press, 49–110.
13. Sekimura, T., Madzvamuse, A., and Maini, P.K. (2006). Pigmentation pattern formation in butterfly wings: Global patterns on fore- and hind-wing. In series: Modeling and Simulation in Science, Engineering and Technology (ed.Bellomo, N.), Birkhauser Boston and Basel (in press).
14. Sekimura, T., Madzvamuse, A., Wathen, A.J., and Maini, P.K. (2000). A model for colour pattern formation in the butterfly wing of *Papilio dardanus*, *Proc. R. Soc. Lond.*, B **267**, 851–859.
15. Sekimura, T., Maini, P.K., Nardi, J.B., Zhu M., and Murray, J.D. (1998). Pattern formation in lepidopteran wings. *Comments Theor. Biol.*, **5**, No.2–4, 69–87.

16. Sekimura, T., Zhu, M., Cook, J., Maini, P.K., and Murray, J.D. (1999). Pattern formation of scale cells in lepidoptera by differential origin-dependent cell adhesion. *Bull. Math. Biol.*, **61**, 807–827.

17. Süffert, F. (1927). Zur vergleichende analyse der schmetterlingszeichung. *Biologisches zentralblatt* **47**, 385–413.

18. Turing, A.M. (1952). The chemical basis of morphogenesis, *Phil. Trans. Roy. Soc. Lond.* B**237**, 37–72.

Stabilization for a Reaction-Diffusion System in Epidemiology

Sebastian Aniţa

Faculty of Mathematics, University "Al.I. Cuza"and Institute of Mathematics, Romanian Academy, Iaşi 700506, Romania
`sanita@uaic.ro`

Summary. The internal stabilization for a spatially structured epidemic system describing the spatial spread of epidemic diseases mediated by environmental pollution is investigated. The control acts on the pollutant in a subdomain. We provide in the affirmative case a simple stabilizing feedback control.

1 Introduction

We shall investigate the internal stabilization in a reaction-diffusion system modelling the evolution of an infectious disease with indirect transmission. The indirect transmission appears for infectious diseases transmitted via the pollution of the environment due to the infected population (typhoid fever, malaria, etc.).

The force of infection at time $t \geq 0$ and location x of the habitat $\overline{\Omega}$ depends on the concentration of the pollutant (etiological agent) available at time t and location x. Here, $\Omega \subset \mathbb{R}^n$ ($n \in \{1, 2, 3\}$) is a nonempty domain with a smooth boundary $\partial\Omega$. Denote by $u(x,t)$ the concentration of the pollutant at position $x \in \overline{\Omega}$ and moment $t \geq 0$ and by $v(x,t)$ the concentration of infective population at position $x \in \overline{\Omega}$ and moment $t \geq 0$.

The model which describes the dynamics of u and v has been proposed and investigated by V. Capasso [7], [9]:

$$\begin{cases} \dfrac{\partial u}{\partial t}(x,t) - D\Delta u(x,t) + a_{11}u(x,t) = \displaystyle\int_\Omega k(x,x')v(x',t)dx', & x \in \Omega, \ t > 0 \\[2ex] \dfrac{\partial v}{\partial t}(x,t) + a_{22}v(x,t) = g(u(x,t)), & x \in \Omega, \ t > 0 \\[2ex] \dfrac{\partial u}{\partial \nu}(x,t) + \alpha u(x,t) = 0, & x \in \partial\Omega, \ t > 0 \\[2ex] u(x,0) = u_0(x), & x \in \Omega \\[1ex] v(x,0) = v_0(x), & x \in \Omega, \end{cases} \tag{1}$$

where a_{11}, $\alpha \geq 0$ and D, $a_{22} > 0$. $\int_\Omega k(x,x')v(x',t)dx'$ gives the pollution production term at position x and moment t; k is the transfer kernel of pollutant produced by the infected population. $g(u(x,t))$ gives the local incidence rate (it has been assumed that the susceptible population is large with respect to the infected population and constant). Further generalizations are given in [8].

Our goal is to precise if we can diminish exponentially the epidemic in the whole habitat based on the elimination of the pollutant in a subregion $\omega \subset\subset \Omega$. In other words, is there any control $w \in L^2_{loc}(\overline{\omega} \times [0, +\infty))$ such that the solution (u,v) of

$$\begin{cases} \dfrac{\partial u}{\partial t}(x,t) - D\Delta u(x,t) + a_{11}u(x,t) = \displaystyle\int_\Omega k(x,x')v(x',t)dx' \\ \qquad\qquad\qquad\qquad\qquad\qquad +m(x)w(x,t), \quad x \in \Omega,\ t > 0 \\[2mm] \dfrac{\partial v}{\partial t}(x,t) + a_{22}v(x,t) = g(u(x,t)), \quad x \in \Omega,\ t > 0 \\[2mm] \dfrac{\partial u}{\partial \nu}(x,t) + \alpha u(x,t) = 0, \qquad\qquad x \in \partial\Omega,\ t > 0 \\[2mm] u(x,0) = u_0(x), \qquad\qquad\qquad x \in \Omega \\[2mm] v(x,0) = v_0(x), \qquad\qquad\qquad x \in \Omega, \end{cases} \tag{2}$$

satisfies

$$\lim_{t\to+\infty} \|u(t)\|_{L^2(\Omega)} = \lim_{t\to+\infty} \|v(t)\|_{L^2(\Omega)} = 0 \tag{3}$$

and

$$u(x,t) \geq 0, \quad v(x,t) \geq 0 \quad a.e.\ x \in \Omega,\ \forall t \geq 0 \quad ?'' \tag{4}$$

If the answer to the above mentioned question is affirmative, we say that (2) is internally zero stabilizable. We have to notice that we deal with a stabilization problem with state constraints (because $u(x,t)$, $v(x,t) \geq 0$).

Here, $\omega \subset\subset \Omega$ is a nonempty open subdomain with a smooth boundary $\partial\omega$ and m is the characteristic function of $\overline{\omega}$.

We work under the following assumptions:

- $g : \mathbb{R} \to [0,+\infty)$ is a function satisfying
  $g(x) = 0,\ \forall x \in (-\infty, 0]$,
  g is Lipschitz continuous and increasing and
  $\exists a_{12} \geq 0 \colon g(x) \leq a_{12}x,\ \forall x \in \mathbb{R}_+$
- $k \in L^\infty(\Omega \times \Omega),\ k(x,y) \geq 0\ a.e.\ (x,y) \in \Omega \times \Omega$
- $u_0,\ v_0 \in L^\infty(\Omega),\ u_0(x) \geq 0,\ v_0(x) \geq 0\ a.e.\ x \in \Omega.$

All the assumptions are in accordance to real situations. For detailed discussion of models (1) and (2) we refer to [5], [7], [8].

The importance of the stabilization problem from public health point is obvious. The study will show that it could be sufficient to act on the pollutant by environmental sanitation programs (in the subregion $\overline{\omega}$) in order to exponentially diminish the epidemic. Some stabilization results for (2) have been obtained in a joint paper with V. Capasso (see [5]) and in [4]. Related stabilizability results for nonnegative solutions to some parabolic equations have been established in [1], [2], [3]. For basic results concerning stabilization we refer to [11]. Denote by $\lambda_1(\omega)$ the principal eigenvalue for

$$\begin{cases} -D\Delta\varphi = \lambda\varphi, & x \in \Omega \setminus \overline{\omega} \\ \dfrac{\partial\varphi}{\partial\nu} + \alpha\varphi = 0, & x \in \partial\Omega \\ \varphi = 0, & x \in \partial\omega. \end{cases} \tag{5}$$

The main result of this paper amounts to saying that if $\lambda_1(\omega)$ is large enough, then (2) is internally zero stabilizable (by a simple feedback control). Moreover, for a larger value of $\lambda_1(\omega)$ we get a faster stabilization rate.

Here is the plan of this paper. In section 2 we shall review the main result in [4]. In section 3 we shall investigate the derivative of $\lambda_1(\omega)$ with respect to the translations of ω. Some final remarks will be made in the fourth section.

2 A Stabilization Result

In this section we review the main result in [4].

Theorem 1. *If*

$$\lambda_1(\omega) > \frac{(\|k\|_{L^2(\Omega\times\Omega)} + a_{12})^2}{4a_{22}} - a_{11},$$

then the feedback control $w := -\gamma \cdot u$ (where $\gamma > 0$ is large enough), stabilizes (2), i.e. the solution (u, v) of

$$\begin{cases} \dfrac{\partial u}{\partial t}(x,t) - D\Delta u(x,t) + a_{11}u(x,t) = \displaystyle\int_\Omega k(x,x')v(x',t)dx' \\ \qquad\qquad\qquad - m(x)\gamma u(x,t), & x \in \Omega,\ t > 0 \\ \dfrac{\partial v}{\partial t}(x,t) + a_{22}v(x,t) = g(u(x,t)), & x \in \Omega,\ t > 0 \\ \dfrac{\partial u}{\partial\nu}(x,t) + \alpha u(x,t) = 0, & x \in \partial\Omega,\ t > 0 \\ u(x,0) = u_0(x), & x \in \Omega \\ v(x,0) = v_0(x), & x \in \Omega, \end{cases} \tag{6}$$

satisfies (3) and (4).

Proof. The existence of a unique (and nonnegative) solution (u, v) for (6) follows via a fixed point argument.

For any $\gamma > 0$ we define $\lambda_{1\gamma}$ as the principal eigenvalue of

$$\begin{cases} -D\Delta\varphi + m(x)\gamma\varphi = \lambda\varphi, & x \in \Omega \\ \dfrac{\partial\varphi}{\partial\nu} + \alpha\varphi = 0, & x \in \partial\Omega. \end{cases} \tag{7}$$

It has been proved in [4] that

$$\lim_{\gamma\to+\infty} \lambda_{1\gamma} = \lambda_1(\omega).$$

Consider an arbitrary but fixed $\gamma > 0$. Multiplying $(6)_1$ by u and $(6)_2$ by v and integrating over Ω, we obtain

$$\left(\frac{1}{2}\|u(t)\|_{L^2(\Omega)}^2 + \frac{1}{2}\|v(t)\|_{L^2(\Omega)}^2\right)' \leq -\lambda_{1\gamma}\|u(t)\|_{L^2(\Omega)}^2 - a_{11}\|u(t)\|_{L^2(\Omega)}^2$$

$$+ \int_\Omega u(x,t)\int_\Omega k(x,x')v(x',t)dx'dx - a_{22}\|v(t)\|_{L^2(\Omega)}^2$$

$$+ a_{12}\|u(t)\|_{L^2(\Omega)}\|v(t)\|_{L^2(\Omega)}$$

$$\leq (-\lambda_{1\gamma} - a_{11})\|u(t)\|_{L^2(\Omega)}^2 - a_{22}\|v(t)\|_{L^2(\Omega)}^2$$

$$+ (a_{22} - \delta)\|v(t)\|_{L^2(\Omega)}^2 + \frac{(\|k\|_{L^2(\Omega\times\Omega)} + a_{12})^2}{4(a_{22} - \delta)}\|u(t)\|_{L^2(\Omega)}^2, \ \forall t > 0$$

(where $\delta > 0$ is a small enough constant).
Since

$$\lambda_1(\omega) > \frac{(\|k\|_{L^2(\Omega\times\Omega)} + a_{12})^2}{4a_{22}} - a_{11},$$

it follows that for $\gamma > 0$ large enough and for $\delta > \varepsilon > 0$ small enough we get

$$-\lambda_{1\gamma} - a_{11} + \frac{(\|k\|_{L^2(\Omega\times\Omega)} + a_{12})^2}{4(a_{22} - \delta)} < -\varepsilon$$

and consequently

$$\left(\frac{1}{2}\|u(t)\|_{L^2(\Omega)}^2 + \frac{1}{2}\|v(t)\|_{L^2(\Omega)}^2\right)' \leq -\varepsilon(\|u(t)\|_{L^2(\Omega)}^2 + \|v(t)\|_{L^2(\Omega)}^2), \ \forall t > 0 \ .$$

It follows that

$$\|u(t)\|_{L^2(\Omega)}^2 + \|v(t)\|_{L^2(\Omega)}^2 \leq e^{-2\varepsilon t}(\|u_0\|_{L^2(\Omega)}^2 + \|v_0\|_{L^2(\Omega)}^2), \ \forall t \geq 0$$

and we get the conclusion. $\quad\square$

Remark 1. Under the conditions of theorem 1, the feedback control $w := -\gamma u$ (where $\gamma > 0$ is large enough) achieves an exponential stabilization of (2).

The proof of theorem 1 shows that $\lambda_{1\gamma}$, the principal eigenvalue for (7) dictates the asymptotic behaviour of the solution (u, v) to (6). As a consequence this shows how important is to find a position for ω for which $\lambda_1(\omega)$ to be large.

3 The Derivative of $\lambda_1(\omega)$ with Respect to Translations of ω

Assume that $n \in \{2,3\}$. Let ω^* be a nonempty subdomain of $\mathbb{R}^n$ with a smooth boundary and consider

$$\mathcal{O} = \{\omega \subset \mathbb{R}^n;\ \omega \subset\subset \Omega \text{ and } \exists V \in \mathbb{R}^n : \omega = V + \omega^*\},$$

the set of all translations $\omega \subset\subset \Omega$ of ω^*.

For any $\omega \in \mathcal{O}$ and $V \in \mathbb{R}^n$ we define the derivative $d\lambda_1(\omega)(V)$:

$$d\lambda_1(\omega)(V) = \lim_{\varepsilon \to 0} \frac{\lambda_1(\varepsilon V + \omega) - \lambda_1(\omega)}{\varepsilon}.$$

Since we wish to find a sufficiently large value of $\lambda_1(\omega)$, subject to $\omega \in \mathcal{O}$, it is obvious that the evaluation of the derivative $d\lambda_1(\omega)(V)$ would be of great importance.

So, in this section we shall investigate the derivative of $\lambda_1(\omega)$ with respect to the translations of ω.

Namely, the following result holds:

Theorem 2. *For any $\omega \in \mathcal{O}$ (arbitrary but fixed) and $V^0 = (V_1^0, V_2^0, ..., V_n^0) \in \mathbb{R}^n$ we have*

$$d\lambda_1(\omega)(V^0) = -D \int_{\partial\omega} |\nabla\varphi(x)|^2 (V^0 \cdot \nu(x)) d\sigma,$$

where φ is the eigenfunction of (5) corresponding to $\lambda := \lambda_1(\omega)$ and satisfying $\|\varphi\|_{L^2(\Omega\setminus\overline{\omega})} = 1$, $\varphi(x) > 0$ a.e. $x \in \Omega \setminus \overline{\omega}$.

Proof. Let us prove for the beginning that

$$\limsup_{\varepsilon \searrow 0} \frac{\lambda_1(\varepsilon V^0 + \omega) - \lambda_1(\omega)}{\varepsilon} \leq -D \int_{\partial\omega} |\nabla\varphi(x)|^2 (V^0 \cdot \nu(x)) d\sigma.$$

Consider $\psi \in C_0^\infty(\Omega)$ such that

$$\begin{cases} \psi(x) = 1, & \forall x \in \overline{\omega} \\ \psi(x) \leq 1, & \forall x \in \mathbb{R}^n \end{cases}$$

and let

$$V(x) = (V_1(x), V_2(x), ..., V_n(x)) = \psi(x)V^0 = (V_1^0\psi(x), V_2^0\psi(x), ..., V_n^0\psi(x)).$$

It is obvious that

$$V(x) = \begin{cases} 0, & x \in \partial\Omega \\ V^0, & x \in \partial\omega. \end{cases}$$

For any $\varepsilon > 0$ small enough, we define φ_ε by

$$\varphi_\varepsilon(x + \varepsilon V(x)) = \varphi(x), \quad \forall x \in \overline{\Omega}.$$

It is obvious that for $\varepsilon > 0$ small enough, $I_n + \varepsilon V$ is a diffeomorphism from $\mathbb{R}^n$ to $\mathbb{R}^n$ and from $\overline{\Omega} \setminus \omega$ to $\overline{\Omega} \setminus (I_n + \varepsilon V)\omega$. By Rayleigh's principle (see [6]) we get that for $\varepsilon > 0$ small enough:

$$\lambda_1(\varepsilon V^0 + \omega) - \lambda_1(\omega) = \lambda_1((I_n + \varepsilon V)\omega) - \lambda_1(\omega)$$

$$\leq D \frac{\int_{\Omega \setminus (I_n + \varepsilon V)\overline{\omega}} |\nabla \varphi_\varepsilon(\tilde{x})|^2 d\tilde{x} + \alpha \int_{\partial\Omega} |\varphi_\varepsilon(\tilde{x})|^2 d\sigma_{\tilde{x}}}{\int_{\Omega \setminus (I_n + \varepsilon V)\overline{\omega}} |\varphi_\varepsilon(\tilde{x})|^2 d\tilde{x}}$$

$$- D \Big(\int_{\Omega \setminus \overline{\omega}} |\nabla \varphi(x)|^2 dx + \alpha \int_{\partial\Omega} |\varphi(x)|^2 d\sigma_x \Big).$$

Denote by

$$\begin{cases} A_1(\varepsilon) &= \int_{\Omega \setminus (I_n + \varepsilon V)\overline{\omega}} |\nabla \varphi_\varepsilon(\tilde{x})|^2 d\tilde{x}, \\ A_2(\varepsilon) &= \alpha \int_{\partial\Omega} |\varphi_\varepsilon(\tilde{x})|^2 d\sigma_{\tilde{x}} = \alpha \int_{\partial\Omega} |\varphi(x)|^2 d\sigma_x = C, \\ (because \ \ x + \varepsilon V(x) = x, \ \forall x \in \partial\Omega) \\ A_3(\varepsilon) &= \int_{\Omega \setminus (I_n + \varepsilon V)\overline{\omega}} |\varphi_\varepsilon(\tilde{x})|^2 d\tilde{x}. \end{cases}$$

We conclude that

$$\limsup_{\varepsilon \searrow 0} \frac{\lambda_1(\varepsilon V^0 + \omega) - \lambda_1(\omega)}{\varepsilon} \leq D \frac{A_1'(0)A_3(0) - (A_1(0) + C)A_3'(0)}{A_3(0)^2}. \tag{8}$$

Let us calculate $A_1'(0)$, $A_3'(0)$, $A_1(0)$, $A_3(0)$, C. Making the change of variables $\tilde{x} = x + \varepsilon V(x)$ we get

$$\begin{cases} \varphi_\varepsilon(x + \varepsilon V(x)) = \varphi(x), \quad \forall x \in \Omega \setminus \overline{\omega} \\ \det \dfrac{D(x + \varepsilon V(x))}{Dx} = 1 + \varepsilon \cdot divV(x) + O(\varepsilon^2) \\ \nabla \varphi(x) = (I_n + \varepsilon \dfrac{DV}{Dx}) \nabla \varphi_\varepsilon(x + \varepsilon V(x)). \end{cases}$$

These yield

$$A_1(\varepsilon) = \int_{\Omega \setminus \overline{\omega}} |(I_n + \varepsilon \frac{DV}{Dx})^{-1} \nabla \varphi(x)|^2 (1 + \varepsilon \cdot divV(x) + O(\varepsilon^2)) dx,$$

$$A_3(\varepsilon) = \int_{\Omega \setminus (I_n + \varepsilon V)\overline{\omega}} |\varphi_\varepsilon(\tilde{x})|^2 d\tilde{x}$$

$$= \int_{\Omega \setminus \overline{\omega}} |\varphi(x)|^2 \det \frac{D(x + \varepsilon V(x))}{Dx} dx$$

$$= \int_{\Omega \setminus \overline{\omega}} |\varphi(x)|^2 (1 + \varepsilon divV(x) + O(\varepsilon^2)) dx.$$

It follows immediately that

$$A_3(0) = \int_{\Omega\setminus\overline{\omega}} |\varphi(x)|^2 dx = 1$$

and (by (8))

$$\limsup_{\varepsilon\searrow 0} \frac{\lambda_1(\varepsilon V^0 + \omega) - \lambda_1(\omega)}{\varepsilon} \leq D[A_1'(0) - (A_1(0) + C)A_3'(0)]. \qquad (9)$$

Moreover,

$$A_3'(0) = \int_{\Omega\setminus\overline{\omega}} |\varphi(x)|^2 div V(x) dx.$$

Since

$$|\varphi(x)|^2 div V(x) = div(|\varphi(x)|^2 V(x)) - 2\varphi(x)(\nabla\varphi(x) \cdot V(x)), \quad \forall x \in \Omega\setminus\overline{\omega},$$

we conclude that

$$\begin{aligned}
A_3'(0) &= \int_{\Omega\setminus\overline{\omega}} div(|\varphi(x)|^2 V(x)) dx - 2\int_{\Omega\setminus\overline{\omega}} \varphi(x)(\nabla\varphi(x) \cdot V(x)) dx \\
&= \int_{\partial\Omega} |\varphi(x)|^2 (V(x) \cdot \nu(x)) d\sigma + \int_{\partial\omega} |\varphi(x)|^2 (V(x) \cdot \nu(x)) d\sigma \\
&\quad - 2\int_{\Omega\setminus\overline{\omega}} \varphi(x)(\nabla\varphi(x) \cdot V(x)) dx \\
&\quad \text{(we have used Gauss-Ostrogradski's formula - see [6])} \\
&= -2\int_{\Omega\setminus\overline{\omega}} \varphi(x)(\nabla\varphi(x) \cdot V(x)) dx
\end{aligned}$$

(because $V(x) = 0$ on $\partial\Omega$ and $\varphi(x) = 0$ on $\partial\omega$). In conclusion we get that

$$\begin{aligned}
A_3'(0) &= -2\int_{\Omega\setminus\overline{\omega}} \varphi(x)(\nabla\varphi(x) \cdot V(x)) dx \\
&= -2\int_{\Omega\setminus\overline{\omega}} \varphi(x)(\nabla\varphi(x) \cdot V^0)\psi(x) dx.
\end{aligned} \qquad (10)$$

Analyzing $A_1(\varepsilon)$ we obtain:

$$\left\{ \begin{aligned}
A_1(0) &= \int_{\Omega\setminus\overline{\omega}} |\nabla\varphi(x)|^2 dx \\
&\text{and} \\
A_1'(0) &= \int_{\Omega\setminus\overline{\omega}} (\nabla I_n(x) \cdot V(x))\nabla\varphi(x) \cdot \nabla\varphi(x) dx \\
&\quad - 2\int_{\Omega\setminus\overline{\omega}} (I_n(x)\frac{DV}{Dx}(x)\nabla\varphi(x)) \cdot \nabla\varphi(x) dx \\
&\quad + \int_{\Omega\setminus\overline{\omega}} (I_n(x)\nabla\varphi(x)) \cdot \nabla\varphi(x) div V(x) dx.
\end{aligned} \right. \qquad (11)$$

Making now ψ tend to ψ^* in $L^2(\mathbb{R}^n)$, i.e.

$$\psi \to \psi^* \quad \text{in } L^2(\mathbb{R}^n),$$

where

$$\psi^*(x) = \begin{cases} 1, & x \in \overline{\omega} \\ 0, & x \in \mathbb{R}^n \setminus \overline{\omega}, \end{cases}$$

and using (10) and (11) we obtain after some calculation that

$$A_3'(0) \to 0 \tag{12}$$

and

$$A_1'(0) \to -\int_{\partial\omega} |\nabla\varphi(x)|^2 (V^0 \cdot \nu(x))d\sigma, \tag{13}$$

(for details see [2])

By (9), (12) and (13) we may conclude that

$$\limsup_{\varepsilon\searrow 0} \frac{\lambda_1(\varepsilon V^0 + \omega) - \lambda_1(\omega)}{\varepsilon} \le -D\int_{\partial\omega} |\nabla\varphi(x)|^2 (V^0 \cdot \nu(x))d\sigma.$$

Let $\varepsilon_0 > 0$ such that $\theta V^0 + \omega \in \mathcal{O}$, $\forall |\theta| \le \varepsilon_0$.

Denote by φ^θ an eigenfunction of (5) corresponding to $\omega := \theta V^0 + \omega$, $\lambda_1(\theta V^0 + \omega)$ and satisfying

$$\varphi^\theta(x) > 0 \quad a.e.\ x \in \Omega \setminus (\theta V^0 + \overline{\omega})$$

and

$$\|\varphi^\theta\|_{L^2(\Omega\setminus(\theta V^0 + \overline{\omega}))} = 1.$$

If we denote by f_{V^0} the function defined by

$$f_{V^0}(\theta) = -D\int_{\theta V^0 + \partial\omega} |\nabla\varphi^\theta(x)|^2 (V^0 \cdot \nu(x))d\sigma,$$

$f_{V^0} : [-\varepsilon_0, \varepsilon_0] \to \mathbb{R}$, it is possible to prove that f_{V^0} is continuous and also that the mapping $\theta \mapsto \lambda_1(\theta V^0 + \omega)$ is continuous on $[-\varepsilon_0, \varepsilon_0]$.

This yields

$$\limsup_{\varepsilon\searrow 0} \frac{\lambda_1((\theta + \varepsilon)V^0 + \omega) - \lambda_1(\theta V^0 + \omega)}{\varepsilon} \le f_{V^0}(\theta), \quad \forall\theta \in [-\varepsilon_0, \varepsilon_0]$$

and in conclusion we get that for any θ_1, θ_2 satisfying $-\varepsilon_0 \le \theta_1 \le \theta_2 \le \varepsilon_0$:

$$\lambda_1(\theta_2 V^0 + \omega) - \lambda_1(\theta_1 V^0 + \omega) \le \int_{\theta_1}^{\theta_2} f_{V^0}(\theta)d\theta.$$

If we take now $V^0 := -V^0$, we may conclude that

$$\lambda_1((-\theta_1)(-V^0)+\omega) - \lambda_1((-\theta_2)(-V^0)+\omega) \le \int_{-\theta_2}^{-\theta_1} f_{-V^0}(\tau)d\tau$$

and since $f_{-V^0}(\tau) = -f_{V^0}(-\tau)$, it follows that

$$\lambda_1(\theta_1 V^0 + \omega) - \lambda_1(\theta_2 V^0 + \omega) \le \int_{-\theta_2}^{-\theta_1} f_{-V^0}(\tau)d\tau$$

$$= \int_{\theta_2}^{\theta_1} -f_{V^0}(\theta)(-1)d\theta = -\int_{\theta_1}^{\theta_2} f_{V^0}(\theta)d\theta$$

(we have made the change of variables: $\tau = -\theta \Rightarrow d\tau = -d\theta$)
and consequently

$$\lambda_1(\theta_2 V^0 + \omega) - \lambda_1(\theta_1 V^0 + \omega) = \int_{\theta_1}^{\theta_2} f_{V^0}(\theta)d\theta, \quad \forall - \varepsilon_0 \le \theta_1 \le \theta_2 \le \varepsilon_0.$$

In conclusion, the function $\theta \mapsto \lambda_1(\theta V^0 + \omega)$ is continuously differentiable on $[-\varepsilon_0, \varepsilon_0]$ and satisfies

$$\frac{d}{d\theta}\lambda_1(\theta V^0 + \omega) = f_{V^0}(\theta), \quad \forall - \varepsilon_0 \le \theta \le \varepsilon_0.$$

For $\theta := 0$ we obtain that

$$\lim_{\varepsilon \to 0} \frac{\lambda_1(\varepsilon V^0 + \omega) - \lambda_1(\omega)}{\varepsilon} = -D \int_{\partial \omega} |\nabla\varphi(x)|^2 (V^0 \cdot \nu(x))d\sigma$$

and this ends the proof of theorem 2. $\square$

Remark 2. For general results on shape design we refer to [10].

Remark 3. Theorem 2 allows to obtain a gradient algorithm to maximize $\lambda_1(\omega)$ with respect to all translations of ω.

4 Further Remarks

Here we discuss several ways in which one can generalize theorem 1 and theorem 2.

(i) (variable coefficients) The Laplacian can be replaced by any second-order elliptic (and selfadjoint) operator with Lipschitz coefficients

$$P(x, \partial) = -a^{ij}\partial_i\partial_j + b^i\partial_i + c.$$

(ii) (boundary conditions) The boundary condition can be replaced by the Dirichlet boundary condition.

(iii) (the derivative of $\lambda_1(\omega)$) It is possible to investigate in the same manner the derivative of $\lambda_1(\omega)$ with respect to the rotations of ω.

Acknowledgments

This work was supported by the CNCSIS grant 1416/2005.

References

1. Ainseba, B., Aniţa, S.: Internal stabilizability for a reaction-diffusion problem modelling a predator-prey system. Nonlin. Anal.; Theory Meth. Appl., **61**, 491–501 (2005).
2. Ainseba, B., Aniţa, S.: Internal nonnegative stabilizability for some parabolic equations. To appear.
3. Ainseba, B., Aniţa, S., Langlais, M.: Internal stabilizability of some diffusive models. J. Math. Anal. Appl., **265**, 91–102 (2002).
4. Aniţa, L.-I., Aniţa, S.: Note on the stabilization of a reaction-diffusion model in epidemiology. Nonlin. Anal.; Real World Appl., **6**, 537–544 (2005).
5. Aniţa, S., Capasso, V.: A stabilizability problem for a reaction-diffusion system modelling a class of spatially structured epidemic model. Nonlin. Anal.; Real World Appl., **3**, 453–464 (2002).
6. Barbu, V.: Partial Differential Equations and Boundary Value Problems. Kluwer Acad. Publ., Dordrecht (1998).
7. Capasso, V.: Asymptotic stability for an integro-differential reaction-diffusion system. J. Math. Anal. Appl., **103**, 575–588 (1984).
8. Capasso, V.: Mathematical Structures of Epidemic Systems. Lecture Notes Biomath., Vol. 97, Springer-Verlag, Heidelberg (1993).
9. Capasso, V., Wilson, R.E.: Analysis of a reaction-diffusion system modelling man-environment-man epidemics. SIAM J. Appl. Math., **57**, 327–346 (1997).
10. Kawohl, B., Pironneau, O., Tartar, L., Zolesio, J.-P.: Optimal Shape Design. Springer-Verlag, Berlin (2001).
11. Lions, J.L.: Controlabilité exacte, stabilisation et perturbation de systemes distribués. RMA 8, Masson, Paris (1988).

Global Stability of Equilibria
for a Metapopulation S–I–S Model

Francesca Arrigoni and Andrea Pugliese

Dept. of Mathematics, University of Trento, via Sommarive, 14, 38050 Povo, Trento, Italy
{arrigoni,pugliese}@science.unitn.it

1 Introduction

Standard models for the dynamics of infection disease are based on the assumption of homogeneous mixing among individuals. However, individuals are generally aggregated in patches (pieces of woodland, farms, households, villages...) and transmission of infection is much easier within patches than from one patch to the other.

Different approaches have been used to handle the "patchy" structure of populations, that run from individual-based simulation models (see, for instance, [11] for avian flu in Thailand) to systems of differential equations for the infection classes at each patch (see, for instance, [2]). An interesting approach is the use of "spatially implicit metapopulation models": in these, the discrete nature of individual and patches is clearly retained, so that each patch has always an integer number of infectives; however, the spatial arrangement of patches is not considered, so that infection transmission is the same to any other patch.

Following a long tradition of stochastic models for infection transmission within and between households[5], Ball [4] has derived a deterministic system for an epidemic of SIS type spreading in a population distributed in an infinite number of households, each one of size N; mixing outside the households is assumed to be random. The system can be obtained [9] as the limit, as M goes to infinity, of a corresponding stochastic model with a finite number M of households. This system, which is the focus of this contribution, will be presented in detail in the next Section. Ball [4] obtains complete results on the stability of the endemic equilibrium for $N = 2$ and numerical simulations are given for $N \geq 3$. Arrigoni and Pugliese [3] compute the reproduction ratio R_0 for the limiting system, and study how this depends on the household size N. Ghoshal et al. [12] show that R_0 is indeed the usual threshold quantity for epidemic models: for $R_0 < 1$ the infection-free equilibrium is stable, and there are no endemic equilibria; for $R_0 > 1$, the infection-free equilibrium is unstable, and there is exactly one endemic equilibrium.

In this contribution, we extend the previous results, by showing that the endemic equilibrium is globally stable for $R_0 > 1$. The result is not unexpected, because S–I–S models have been proved to be stable in populations with spatial structure [8] or with age structure [7]. The key to these proofs has been to employ methods from the theory of monotone dynamical systems (see [15] for a general treatment), thanks to the monotone properties of S–I–S epidemic models.

Here, we exploit too the monotonicity of the dynamical system (albeit relative to an appropriate stochastic ordering), together with a probabilistic interpretation, suggested in [6], of the solutions of the deterministic system.

2 The Model

The main variable in the system under study will be the vector-valued function $\xi(t) = (\xi_0(t), \ldots, \xi_N(t))$: the j-th component $\xi_j(t)$ represents the fraction of households with j infectives at time t (j will be named the state of the household). The state space is $\Sigma = \left\{ \sum_{j=0}^{N} \xi_j = 1, \quad \xi_j \geq 0, \ j = 0, \ldots, N \right\}$.

When an infective recovers, her household moves from state j to $j - 1$; if γ is the recovery rate of infectives, the overall rate at which a household moves from state j to $j - 1$ is γj.

Conversely, a household moves from j to $j+1$ when a new infection occurs. Each susceptible can get infected from an infective in the same household (at a rate proportional to the fraction of infected individuals, j/N) or from an infective everywhere in the population (at a rate proportional to the fraction of infected individuals: $\frac{1}{N} \sum_{l=0}^{N} l\xi_l$). Overall (in a household at state j, there are $N - j$ susceptibles), the rate at which households move from state j to $j + 1$ is $(N - j) \left(c\frac{j}{N} + \frac{d}{N} \sum_{l=0}^{N} l\xi_l \right)$, where c is the rate of within-household infection, and d is the rate of between-household infection.

Hence:

$$
\begin{cases}
\dot{\xi}_j(t) = - \left[(N - j) \left(c\frac{j}{N} + \frac{d}{N} \sum_{l=0}^{N} l\xi_l \right) + \gamma j \right] \xi_j \\
\qquad + \gamma(j + 1)\xi_{j+1} + (N - j + 1) \left(c\frac{j - 1}{N} + \frac{d}{N} \sum_{l=0}^{N} l\xi_l \right) \\
\dot{\xi}_0(t) = \gamma \xi_1 - \xi_0 d \sum_{l=0}^{N} \xi_l l
\end{cases}
\tag{1}
$$

with initial value $\xi_j(0) = y_j$, $j = 0, \ldots, N$, a probability distribution, so that $\underline{y}$ is non-negative and satisfies $\sum_{j=0}^{N} y_j = 1$.

Note that system (1) is monotone not relatively to the usual ordering in $\mathbb{R}^{N+1}$ but to a natural ordering for probability distributions:

$$\xi \overset{s}{\leq} \eta \iff \sum_{i=0}^{N} g(i)\xi_i \leq \sum_{i=0}^{N} g(i)\eta_i \quad \text{for all non-decreasing functions } g.$$

Alternatively, one can introduce the variables $w_j(t) = \sum_{k=j}^{N} \xi_k(t)$ and notice that $\underline{w}$ satisfies the system of differential equations:

$$\dot{w}_i = \gamma i(w_{i+1} - w_i) + (N - i + 1)\left(c\frac{(i-1)}{N} + \frac{d}{N}\sum_{l=1}^{N} w_l \right)(w_{i-1} - w_i) \quad (2)$$

Since (2) has to be studied in the set $\{1 \geq w_1 \geq w_2 \cdots \geq w_N \geq 0\}$, which is invariant, it is easy to see that the Kamke condition [15] is satisfied; hence, (2) is monotone relatively to the standard order.

The overall structure of the model is similar to that studied in [6] where $p_j(t)$ represents the fraction of local populations (within a metapopulation) with j individuals. The system considered there is

$$\begin{cases} p_i' = -\left[(b_i + d_i + \lambda)i + \nu + \rho\lambda\sum_{j=0}^{\infty} jp_j \right] p_i \\[2mm] \quad + \left[b_{i-1}(i-1) + \rho\lambda\sum_{j=0}^{\infty} jp_j \right] p_{i-1} \\[2mm] \quad + [d_{i+1} + \lambda](i+1)\,p_{i+1}; \qquad\qquad i \geq 1 \\[2mm] p_0' = \nu\left(\sum_{j=0}^{\infty} p_j - p_0 \right) + (d_1 + \lambda)p_1 - \rho\lambda\left(\sum_{j=0}^{\infty} jp_j \right) p_0, \end{cases} \quad (3)$$

where b_i and d_i represent the *per capita* birth and death rates in a patch occupied by i individuals, ν is the catastrophe rate (i.e. the rate at which all individuals in a patch are destroyed), λ is the migration rate, and ρ is the probability of a migrant to successfully reach another patch.

Under the condition that ib_i is concave and non-decreasing, and id_i is convex and non-decreasing, plus some technical assumptions, it was proved [6] that there exists a threshold quantity R for (3): when $R \leq 1$, all solutions converge to the extinction equilibrium ($p_0 = 1$, $p_i \equiv 0$ for $i \geq 1$); when $R > 1$ all non trivial solutions converge to the unique positive equilibrium.

Although (1) could be seen as a special case of (3), it is not possible to directly apply the results of [6]. Hence, we show how the methods used in [6] can be modified to handle system (1) (and, indeed, any system with similar assumptions).

The main idea is to analyse system (1) assuming that the average proportion of infectives per household is known. By setting $s = \sum_{l=1}^{N} l\xi_l$ in (1), we obtain a family of linear systems, indexed by the parameter s,

$$\frac{d\underline{\xi}(t)}{dt} = A_s \underline{\xi}(t). \tag{4}$$

$$\text{with } (A_s)_{k,j} = \begin{cases} c(1 - \frac{j-1}{N})(j-1) + ds(1 - \frac{j-1}{N}) & k = j-1 \\ -c(1 - \frac{j}{N})j - ds(1 - \frac{j}{N}) - \gamma j & k = j \\ \gamma(j+1) & k = j+1 \end{cases}$$

and $(A_s)_{k,j} = 0$ for $|j - k| > 1$, where $j, k = 0, \ldots, N$.

3 Probabilistic Interpretation

We adopt a probabilistic interpretation of the functions $\xi_l(t)$, used by Barbour and Pugliese [6]. In this framework, the solution $\underline{\xi}$ of system (4) represents the distribution at time t of a birth and death Markov process with finite state-space $S = \{0, 1, \ldots, N\}$ and initial distribution $\underline{y}$. We will denote it by $X_t^{(s)}$, so that $\xi_i(t) = \mathbb{P}_{\underline{y}}[X_t^{(s)} = i] = \mathbb{P}[X_t^{(s)} = i | X_0^{(s)} \sim \underline{y}]$. Its transitions are

$$\begin{cases} j \to j+1 \text{ at rate} & cj(1 - \frac{j}{N}) + ds(1 - \frac{j}{N}) \\ j \to j-1 \text{ at rate} & \gamma j \end{cases}$$

$X_t^{(s)}$ has a stationary distribution $\pi^{(s)} = \{\pi_i^{(s)}\}_{j=0}^{N}$:

- if $s = 0$ then $\pi_0^{(s)} = 1$ and $\pi_j^{(s)} = 0$ for $j \geq 1$;

- if $s > 0$ then $\pi_j^{(s)} = \dfrac{\theta_j^{(s)}}{\sum_{j=0}^{N} \theta_j^{(s)}}$ where

$$\theta_0^{(s)} = 1, \quad \theta_j^{(s)} = \frac{\displaystyle\prod_{k=0}^{j-1} \left(1 - \frac{k}{N}\right)(ck + ds)}{\gamma^j j!}. \tag{5}$$

Moreover, we can apply to the process $X_t^{(s)}$ the following theorem (see [1]).

Theorem 1. *Let X_t be a birth-and-death process with finite state-space $S = \{0, 1, \ldots, m, \ldots, N\}$ such that $C = \{0, 1, \ldots, m\}$ is an ergodic class and $T = \{m+1, \ldots, N\}$ is a transient class, every state of which leads to all states in C. Then there exist non-negative numbers α and $\rho < 1$ such that*

$$|p_{ji}(t) - \pi_i| < \alpha\rho^t, \qquad \forall j \in S. \tag{6}$$

where $\pi_i > 0, i \in C$, $\pi_i = 0, i \in T$ and $\sum_{i \in C} \pi_i = 1$.

Using this theorem (with $m = 0$ for $s = 0$; with $m = N$ for $s > 0$), we see that the transition probabilities $p_{ji}^{(s)} = \mathbb{P}[X_t^{(s)} = i | X_0^{(s)} = j]$ of the process $X_t^{(s)}$ attain their limit $\pi_i^{(s)}$, at an exponential rate. The vector $(\pi_0^{(s)}, \pi_1^{(s)}, \ldots, \pi_N^{(s)})$ is the stationary solution of the system (4).

4 Properties of the Fixed Point Map

Our aim is to show the existence and uniqueness of a non-trivial equilibrium of the non-linear system (1), when the parameters satisfy the threshold condition shown below.

For every non-negative value of the parameter s, we have found the stationary solution $\pi^{(s)}$ of the system (4). Letting $\pi^{(s)}(f)$ be the mean of a function f relatively to the distribution $\pi^{(s)}$, we define the map G as

$$G(s) = \pi^{(s)}(e) = \sum_{i=1}^{N} i\pi_i^{(s)} \qquad (e \text{ the identity function})$$

Note that to every positive fixed point $s^\star$ of G (that is, $G(s^\star) = s^\star$) corresponds an endemic equilibrium solution of the non-linear system (1). The disease-free equilibrium, instead, corresponds to the null fixed point ($G(0) = 0$).

It can be shown that G is a continuous, increasing and concave function. From this, the uniqueness of a positive fixed point follows easily.

The properties of G are established in [6]. Here, we just state some intermediate steps, together with a sketch of the proofs that require small changes.

Proposition 1. $\qquad \dfrac{d}{ds}\pi^{(s)}(f) = -d\pi^{(s)}(R(f)) \qquad with$

$$R(f)(j) = (1 - \frac{j}{N})(\Theta^{(s)}(f)(j+1) - \Theta^{(s)}(f)(j))$$

$$\Theta^{(s)}(f)(j) = -\int_0^{+\infty} \{\mathbb{E}^{(j)} f(Z_t^{(s)}) - \pi^{(s)}(f)\}dt$$

Proof (sketch). Let $\mathcal{A}^{(s)}$ be the generator of the Markov process $Z^{(s)}$.

$$\mathcal{A}^{(s)} f(j) = (cj(1 - \tfrac{j}{N}) + ds(1 - \tfrac{j}{N}))[f(j+1) - f(j)]$$
$$+\gamma j[f(j-1) - f(j)].$$

By Dynkin's formula [13], $\pi^{(s)}(\mathcal{A}^{(s)}g) = 0$ for all g. Hence

$$0 = \pi^{(s+h)}(\mathcal{A}^{(s+h)}g) = \mathbb{E}^{\pi^{(s+h)}}\left(\mathcal{A}^{(s+h)}g(Z_0^{(s)})\right)$$

$$= \mathbb{E}^{\pi^{(s+h)}}\left\{\mathcal{A}^{(s)}g(Z_0^{(s)}) + dh(1 - \frac{Z_0^{(s)}}{N})\Delta g(Z_0^{(s)})\right\}$$

Set $g = \Theta^{(s)}(f)$ (as defined in the thesis, thanks to (6)) and note that $\Theta^{(s)}(f)$ satisfies the equation

$$\mathcal{A}^{(s)}(\Theta^{(s)}(f))(j) = f(j) - \pi^{(s)}(f).$$

Then

$$0 = \mathbb{E}^{\pi^{(s+h)}}\{f(Z_0^{(s)}) - \pi^{(s)}(f) + dh(1 - \frac{Z_0^{(s)}}{N})\Delta\Theta^{(s)}(f))(Z_0^{(s)})\}$$

so that

$$|\pi^{(s+h)}(f) - \pi^{(s)}(f) + dh\pi^{(s)}(R(f))| \le d|h|o(1)$$

and the thesis follows. $\square$

Applying the previous proposition to the identity function e, we obtain

$$G'(s) = d\pi^{(s)}(R(e)) = d\pi^{(s)}(g) \qquad \text{with}$$

$$g(j) = (1 - \frac{j}{N})\int_0^{+\infty}\{\mathbb{E}^{(j+1)}(Z_t^{(s)}) - \mathbb{E}^{(j)}(Z_t^{(s)})\}\,dt.$$

In the next Section we will prove, through coupling methods, the rather intuitive fact that $\mathbb{E}^{(j+1)}(Z_t^{(s)}) \ge \mathbb{E}^{(j)}(Z_t^{(s)})$. It will then follow that $G'(s) \ge 0$.

The quantity $G'(0) = d\int_0^{+\infty}\mathbb{E}^{(1)}(Z_t^{(0)})\,dt$ will be shown to be the threshold quantity for system (1).

The following proposition can be proved with a similar technique (see [6])

Proposition 2. $G''(s) = 2d^2\pi^{(s)}(R(R(e))) = 2d^2\pi^{(s)}(h)$ *where*

$$h(m) = \left(1 - \frac{m}{N}\right)\int_0^\infty\left[\mathbb{E}^{(m+1)}Q(X_t^{(s)}) - \mathbb{E}^{(m)}Q(X_t^{(s)})\right]\,dt$$

$$Q(j) = \left(1 - \frac{j}{N}\right)\int_0^\infty(\mathbb{E}^{(j+1)}X_w^{(s)} - \mathbb{E}^{(j)}X_w^{(s)})\,dw.$$

5 Coupling Methods

In this Section, we prove by coupling methods (see, for instance, [14]) some results, needed to prove the properties of G, about rather general birth-and-death processes We consider a birth-and-death process $X := (X_t, t \ge 0)$ with birth and death rates $\lambda(i)$ and $\mu(i)$ respectively and state space $S = \{0, 1, 2, \ldots, N\}$. Assume that the function $\lambda(i)$ is concave in i and that the function $\mu(i)$ is convex and non-decreasing (and that $\mu(0) = 0$).

Proposition 3. *Let X be as above. Let $\mathbb{E}^{(m)}(X_t) = \mathbb{E}(X_t|X_0 = m)$. Then for all $m \geq 0$,*

$$\mathbb{E}^{(m+1)}X_t - \mathbb{E}^{(m)}X_t > 0$$

Proof. We consider a two-dimensional pure jump Markov process $(\underline{F}_t = (Y_t, W_t), t \geq 0)$; the processes $X^1 = Y$, $X^2 = Y + W$ will be Markov and have the same generator as X. Setting $Y(0) = m, W(0) = 1, \mathbb{E}^{(m+1)}X_t = \mathbb{E}X_t^1$ and $\mathbb{E}^{(m)}X_t = \mathbb{E}X_t^2$, so that $\mathbb{E}^{(m+1)}X_t - \mathbb{E}^{(m)}X_t = \mathbb{E}W_t$.

The transitions of the process $\underline{F}_t$ are the following, letting $\mathbf{n} = (i, j)$ and $\mathbf{e}^{(i)}$ the i-th coordinate vector. :

$$
\begin{aligned}
\mathbf{n} &\to \mathbf{n} - \mathbf{e}^{(1)} && \text{at rate } \mu(i) \\
\mathbf{n} &\to \mathbf{n} - \mathbf{e}^{(2)} && \text{at rate } \mu(i + j) - \mu(i) \\
\mathbf{n} &\to \mathbf{n} + \mathbf{e}^{(1)} && \text{at rate } \min(\lambda(i), \lambda(i + j)) \\
\mathbf{n} &\to \mathbf{n} + \mathbf{e}^{(2)} && \text{at rate } \lambda(i + j) - \min(\lambda(i), \lambda(i + j)) \\
\mathbf{n} &\to \mathbf{n} + \mathbf{e}^{(1)} - \mathbf{e}^{(2)} && \text{at rate } \lambda(i) - \min(\lambda(i), \lambda(i + j)).
\end{aligned}
$$

It is easy to see that X^1 and X^2 have the required properties, and that $V(t) \geq 0$.

Propositions 1 and 3 show that the function G, defined in the previous Section, is non-decreasing.

The assumptions on the concavity and convexity of birth and death rates play a key-role in the proof of the following proposition. This rather long construction represents the main paper of this contribution relatively to [6].

Proposition 4. *Let X as above. Then, for all $m \geq 0$,*

$$\mathbb{E}^{(m+1)}X_t - \mathbb{E}^{(m)}X_t > \mathbb{E}^{(m+2)}X_t - \mathbb{E}^{(m+1)}X_t.$$

Proof. We consider a four dimensional pure jump Markov process $(\underline{D}_t = (Y_t, W_t, U_t, V_t), t \geq 0)$; the aim of this construction is to have four processes $X^1 = Y$, $X^2 = Y + W$, $X^3 = Y + U$, $X^4 = Y + W + V$ which are Markov and have the same generator as the process X. Setting $Y(0) = m, W(0) = U(0) = V(0) = 1$, we will have $X^1(0) = m$, $X^2(0) = X^3(0) = m + 1$, $X^4(0) = m + 2$.

The state-space of the four dimensional process is

$$S = \{(i, j, k, l) : i \geq 0, j \geq 0, k \geq l \geq 0, \}$$

Letting $\mathbf{n} = (i, j, k, l)$, we describe the transitions of the process $\underline{D}_t$ together with the relative rates. First those representing deaths

- if $k \neq l$

$$
\begin{aligned}
\mathbf{n} &\to \mathbf{n} - \mathbf{e}^{(1)} \,\big|\, \mu(i) && \mathbf{n} \to \mathbf{n} - \mathbf{e}^{(2)} \,\big|\, \mu(i + j) - \mu(i) \\
\mathbf{n} &\to \mathbf{n} - \mathbf{e}^{(3)} \,\big|\, \mu(i + k) - \mu(i) && \mathbf{n} \to \mathbf{n} - \mathbf{e}^{(4)} \,\big|\, \mu(i + j + l) - \mu(i + j)
\end{aligned}
$$

- if $k = l$

$$
\begin{array}{ll}
\mathbf{n} \to \mathbf{n} - \mathbf{e}^{(1)} & \left| \mu(i) \right. \\
\mathbf{n} \to \mathbf{n} - \mathbf{e}^{(3)} - \mathbf{e}^{(4)} & \left| \mu(i+k) - \mu(i) \right. \\
\mathbf{n} \to \mathbf{n} - \mathbf{e}^{(4)} & \left| \mu(i+j+k) - \mu(i+j) - \mu(i+k) + \mu(i) \right.
\end{array}
\qquad
\mathbf{n} \to \mathbf{n} - \mathbf{e}^{(2)} \left| \mu(i+j) - \mu(i) \right.
$$

The transition rates representing births are as follows:

- if $k > l$
    - if $j, k, l > 0$

$$
\begin{array}{ll}
\mathbf{n} \to \mathbf{n} + \mathbf{e}^{(1)} - \mathbf{e}^{(2)} - \mathbf{e}^{(3)} & \left| \lambda(i) \right. \\
\mathbf{n} \to \mathbf{n} + \mathbf{e}^{(2)} - \mathbf{e}^{(4)} & \left| \lambda(i+j) \right.
\end{array}
\qquad
\begin{array}{ll}
\mathbf{n} \to \mathbf{n} + \mathbf{e}^{(3)} & \left| \lambda(i+k) \right. \\
\mathbf{n} \to \mathbf{n} + \mathbf{e}^{(4)} & \left| \lambda(i+j+l) \right.
\end{array}
$$

    - if $0 = j < l < k$

$$
\begin{array}{ll}
\mathbf{n} \to \mathbf{n} + \mathbf{e}^{(4)} \left| \lambda(i+l) \right. & \\
\end{array}
\qquad
\begin{array}{ll}
\mathbf{n} \to \mathbf{n} + \mathbf{e}^{(1)} - \mathbf{e}^{(3)} - \mathbf{e}^{(4)} & \left| \lambda(i) \right. \\
\mathbf{n} \to \mathbf{n} + \mathbf{e}^{(3)} & \left| \lambda(i+k) \right.
\end{array}
$$

    - if $0 = l < j, k$

$$
\begin{array}{ll}
\mathbf{n} \to \mathbf{n} + \mathbf{e}^{(2)} \left| \lambda(i+j) \right. & \\
\end{array}
\qquad
\begin{array}{ll}
\mathbf{n} \to \mathbf{n} + \mathbf{e}^{(1)} - \mathbf{e}^{(2)} - \mathbf{e}^{(3)} & \left| \lambda(i) \right. \\
\mathbf{n} \to \mathbf{n} + \mathbf{e}^{(3)} & \left| \lambda(i+k) \right.
\end{array}
$$

    - if $j = l = 0 < k$

$$
\mathbf{n} \to \mathbf{n} + \mathbf{e}^{(1)} - \mathbf{e}^{(3)} \left| \lambda(i) \right.
\qquad
\mathbf{n} \to \mathbf{n} + \mathbf{e}^{(3)} \left| \lambda(i+k) \right.
$$

- if $k = l$
    - if $j, k > 0$

$\mathbf{n} \to \mathbf{n} + \mathbf{e}^{(2)}$	$\lambda(i+j+k) - \min(\lambda(i+k), \lambda(i+j+k))$
$\mathbf{n} \to \mathbf{n} + \mathbf{e}^{(3)}$	$\lambda(i+k) - \min(\lambda(i) + \lambda(i+j+k), \lambda(i+k))$
$\mathbf{n} \to \mathbf{n} + \mathbf{e}^{(1)} - \mathbf{e}^{(3)} - \mathbf{e}^{(4)}$	$\lambda(i) + \min(\lambda(i+k), \lambda(i+j+k))$ $- \min(\lambda(i) + \lambda(i+j+k), \lambda(i+k))$
$\mathbf{n} \to \mathbf{n} + \mathbf{e}^{(3)} + \mathbf{e}^{(4)}$	$\min(\lambda(i+k), \lambda(i+j+k))$
$\mathbf{n} \to \mathbf{n} + \mathbf{e}^{(1)} - \mathbf{e}^{(2)}$	$\min(\lambda(i) + \lambda(i+j+k), \lambda(i+k))$ $- \min(\lambda(i+k), \lambda(i+j+k))$
$\mathbf{n} \to \mathbf{n} + \mathbf{e}^{(2)} - \mathbf{e}^{(4)}$	$\lambda(i+j) + \min(\lambda(i) + \lambda(i+j+k), \lambda(i+k))$ $-\lambda(i) - \lambda(i+j+k)$

    - if $0 = j < k$

$$
\mathbf{n} \to \mathbf{n} + \mathbf{e}^{(1)} - \mathbf{e}^{(3)} - \mathbf{e}^{(4)} \left| \lambda(i) \right.
\qquad
\mathbf{n} \to \mathbf{n} + \mathbf{e}^{(3)} + \mathbf{e}^{(4)} \left| \lambda(i+k) \right.
$$

    - if $0 = k < j$

$$
\mathbf{n} \to \mathbf{n} + \mathbf{e}^{(1)} - \mathbf{e}^{(2)} \left| \lambda(i) \right.
\qquad
\mathbf{n} \to \mathbf{n} + \mathbf{e}^{(2)} \left| \lambda(i+j) \right.
$$

    - if $j = k = 0$ $\qquad \mathbf{n} \to \mathbf{n} + \mathbf{e}^{(1)} \mid \lambda(i)$.

Note that all transitions are within the state space S, and that the assumptions on μ and λ guarantee that all rates are nonnegative.

We obtain $\mathbb{E}^{(m+1)} X_t - \mathbb{E}^{(m)} X_t = \mathbb{E} U_t$ and $\mathbb{E}^{(m+2)} X_t - \mathbb{E}^{(m+1)} X_t = \mathbb{E} V_t$. By construction, $U_t \geq V_t$, and we obtain the thesis. $\qquad \square$

These two propositions allow us to conclude that G is concave. In fact, we can compute $h(m)$, defined in Proposition 2, using the process (Y_t, W_t) used in the proof of Proposition 3. We obtain, in the notation of Proposition 2 and with $g(j, w) = \mathbb{E}^{(j)} X_w^{(s)}$:

$$\mathbb{E}^{(m+1)}Q(X_t^{(s)}) - \mathbb{E}^{(m)}Q(X_t^{(s)}) = \mathbb{E}(Q(Y_t + W_t) - Q(Y_t))$$

$$= \mathbb{E}\int_0^\infty \left[\left(1 - \frac{Y_t + W_t}{N}\right)(g(Y_t + W_t + 1, w) - g(Y_t + W_t, w))\right.$$

$$\left. - \left(1 - \frac{Y_t}{N}\right)(g(Y_t + 1, w) - g(Y_t, w))\right] dw$$

$$= \mathbb{E}\int_0^\infty \left[(g(Y_t + W_t + 1, w) - g(Y_t + W_t, w)) - (g(Y_t + 1, w) - g(Y_t, w))\right] dw$$

$$\times \left(1 - \frac{Y_t}{N}\right) - \mathbb{E}\int_0^\infty \frac{W_t}{N}(g(Y_t + W_t + 1, w) - g(Y_t + W_t, w))\, dw.$$

Proposition 4 yields $g(m+k+1, w) - g(m+k, w)) - (g(m+1, w) - g(m, w)) < 0$ for all $m, k \geq 0$ and $w \geq 0$; hence the first integral is negative. Similarly Proposition 3 shows that $g(m + 1, w) - g(m, w) > 0$. Hence $h(m) < 0$ for all $m \geq 0$ and $G''(s) < 0$.

6 Equilibria and Asymptotic Behavior

The results of Section 4 show that the function G is continuous and differentiable and satisfies $G(0) = 0$. Moreover, Propositions 1 and 2, together with Propositions 3 and 4 show that G is non-decreasing and concave.

It is then easy to obtain

Theorem 2. *If $G'(0) > 1$, then there exists a unique positive fixed point $s^\star$ of G; if $G'(0) \leq 1$, then $G(s) < s$ for all $s > 0$.*

Proof. The proof is straightforward. If $G'(0) \leq 1$, from the concavity of G it follows that $G(s) < s$. Otherwise, since it is clear that $G(s) < N$ for all s, there exists a unique $s \in (0, N)$ such that $G(s) = s$. $\square$

The quantity

$$G'_+(0) = d\int_0^\infty \mathbb{E}^{(1)} Z_t^{(0)}\, dt.$$

is then the threshold quantity for (1), and will be named R_0 (see [3] for a derivation of this quantity following the lines of [10]).

Remark 1. It is possible to obtain an explicit expression for $G'(0)$. In fact from

$$G'(s) = \sum_{j=1}^N j\frac{d}{ds}\left(\pi_j^{(s)}\right)$$ and using (5), we obtain, after lengthy computations,

$$R_0 = G'_+(0) = \sum_{j=1}^N j\pi'_j(0) = \frac{d}{c}\sum_{j=1}^N (\frac{c}{\gamma N})^j \binom{N}{j} j!.$$

In [6], stochastic comparison arguments, together with arguments from the theory of the dynamical systems are used to prove that all solutions converge to an equilibrium: the trivial equilibrium for $R_0 \leq 1$, the positive equilibrium for $R_0 > 1$. The same arguments would apply (more easily, because the system is finite-dimensional) to (1). It is, however, easier to use results from the theory of monotone dynamical systems either to (1) (relatively to $\overset{s}{\leq}$) or to (2) (relatively to the standard order).

Indeed, Theorem 2.3.1 from [15] shows that, for $R_0 \leq 1$, all solutions converge to the infection-free equilibrium. For $R_0 > 1$, one can use Theorem 2.3.2 from [15] to see that all solutions converge to an equilibrium; further, studying the linearization of (1) (restricted to the components 1 to N) at the infection-free equilibrium, it is easy to see that no solution starting with a non-zero fraction of infectives can converge to the infection-free equilibrium. This proves the main result of this paper:

Theorem 3. *If $R_0 \leq 1$, all solutions of (1) converge to the infection-free equilibrium; if $R_0 > 1$, all solutions of (1) with $\sum_{j=1}^{N} y_j > 0$ converge to the unique positive equilibrium.*

7 Different Household Sizes

The modelling assumption that all households are of the same size N seems rather unrealistic. More reasonably, we can let $n_i, i = 1, \ldots, N$ be the fraction of households with i individuals. Now N is the maximum number of individuals per household: this assumption allows us to deal with a finite-dimensional space, and is reasonable from the biological point of view.

We introduce the variables $\xi_l^i, i = 1, \ldots, N, l = 0, \ldots, i$: $\xi_l^i(t)$ is the fraction of households of size i that at time t have l infectives, so that $\sum_{l=0}^{i} \xi_l^i = 1$.

In this framework, the system of differential equations (1) becomes

$$
\begin{cases}
\dot{\xi}_j^i(t) = -\left[(i-j)\left(c\frac{j}{i} + ds(t) \right) + \gamma j \right] \xi_j^i \\
\qquad + \gamma j \xi_{j+1}^i + (i-j+1)\left(c\frac{j-1}{i} + ds(t) \right) \xi_{j-1}^i \\
\dot{\xi}_0^i(t) = \gamma \xi_1^i - \xi_0^i ds(t)
\end{cases}
\tag{7}
$$

with initial value $\xi_j^i(0) = y_j^i$ where $\sum_{j=0}^{i} y_j^i = 1$ and $y_j^i \geq 0$. The term

$$
s(t) = \frac{\left(\displaystyle\sum_{i=1}^{N} n_i \sum_{l=0}^{i} \xi_l^i(t) l \right)}{\displaystyle\sum_{i=1}^{N} i n_i}
$$

represents the average infective fraction in the population, and drives the infection transmission among different households. It is the only nonlinear term in the system, and indeed is the only term that 'mixes' the equations for households of different sizes.

If we assume that the quantity s is known, we deal with N different systems: each of them has the same structure as system (4) with $d_i = di$ instead of d:

$$\frac{d\underline{\xi}^i(t)}{dt} = A^i_s \underline{\xi}^i(t), \quad i = 1, \ldots, N. \tag{8}$$

The i-th system (8) has an equilibrium solution $\pi^{(s)i}$ and the function $G^i(s) = \sum_{l=0}^{i} l\pi_l^{(s)i}$ is increasing and concave.

It is easy to see that the function $G(s) = \dfrac{d\sum_{i=1}^{N} in_i G^i(s)}{\sum_{i=1}^{N} in_i}$ shares the same properties. Theorem 2 guarantees that, if $G'(0) > 1$, there exists a unique positive fixed point $s^\star$, and, thus, an endemic equilibrium for the system (7). On the other hand, when $G'(0) \le 1$, there is no positive equilibrium.

As in the previous Section, arguments from the theory of monotone dynamical systems (or the same arguments used in [6]) guarantee that all solutions of (7) converge to the infection-free equilibrium, below the threshold, and to the endmic equilibrium, above the threshold.

8 Discussion

We have shown here how the monotone structure of S–I–S epidemic models can be used, also in a metapopulation setting, to prove global convergence to the equilibria, thus yielding a sharp threshold result.

In order to obtain complete results, we had to establish the uniqueness of positive equilibria. This has been proved interpreting the solutions of the equations as the probabilities of a birth-and-death process; the required properties were obtained by studying the stationary distributions of the processes, extending the results of [6]. On the other hand, Ghoshal et al. [12] had proved uniqueness by direct computation.

We believe that our approach is more general, being easy to extend to the case of households of different size (Section 7), to nonlinear infection rules, and possibly to S–I–R models. The last extension would require us to consider the properties not of birth-and-death processes, but of two-dimensional stochastic epidemic models. Clearly, these have no monotonicity properties, but perhaps the fact that the function G is non-decreasing and concave might still hold.

A great limitation of this kind of metapopulation models is that the transmission of infection is the same among all patches. This is, however, an assumption inherent to the method, and cannot be relaxed. At the moment, metapopulation models with a real spatial (or network) structure can be studied only through simulations. The study of spatially implicit metapopulation models may shed some light on the relevance of the discrete nature of individuals and patches for the overall epidemic dynamics, and constitute a standard, against which to compare the result of spatially structured metapopulation simulation models.

References

1. Adke, S.R., Manjunath, S.M.: An introduction to finite Markov processes. Wiley, New York (1984)
2. Arino, J., van den Driessche, P.: A multi-city epidemic model. Math. Pop. Studies, **10**, 175–193 (2003)
3. Arrigoni, F., Pugliese, A.: Limits of a multi-patch SIS epidemic model, J. Math. Biol. **45**, 419–440 (2002)
4. Ball, F.: Stochastic and deterministic models for SIS epidemics among a population partitioned into households, Math. Biosci. **156**, 41–67 (1999)
5. Ball, F., Mollison. D., Scalia-Tomba, G.: Epidemics with two levels of mixing, Annals Appl. Prob. **7**, 46-89 (1997)
6. Barbour, A.D., Pugliese, A.: Asymptotic behavior of a metapopulation model, Annals Applied Probability **15**, 1306–1338 (2005)
7. Busenberg, S., Iannelli, M., Thieme, H.: Global behavior of an age–structured S-I-S epidemic model. SIAM J. Math. Anal. **22**, 1065–1080 (1991)
8. Capasso, V.: Mathematical structures of epidemic systems. Springer, Berlin (1993)
9. Ethier, S.N., Kurtz, T.G.: Markov processes. Wiley, New York (1986)
10. Diekmann, O., Heesterbeek, J.A.P.: Mathematical Epidemiology of Infectious Diseases. Wiley, New York (2000)
11. Ferguson, N.M., Cummings, D.A.T., Cauchemez, S., Fraser, C., Riley, S., Meeyai, A., Iamsirithaworn, S., Burke, D.S.: Strategies for containing an emerging influenza pandemic in Southeast Asia. Nature, **437**, 209–214 (2005)
12. Ghoshal, G., Sander, L.M., Sokolov, I.M.: SIS epidemics with household structure: the self-consistent field method , Math. Biosci. **190**, 71–85 (2004)
13. Hamza, K., and Klebaner, F.C.: Conditions for integrability of Markov chains., J. Appl. Prob. **32**, 541–547 (1995)
14. Lindvall, T.: Lectures on the coupling method. Wiley, New York, 1992
15. Smith, H.: Monotone dynamical systems. American mathematical society, Providence, USA (1995)

State Feedback Control of the Glucose-Insulin System

Pasquale Palumbo[1] and Andrea De Gaetano[2]

[1] Istituto di Analisi dei Sistemi "A. Ruberti", IASI-CNR, Viale Manzoni 30, 00185 Roma, Italy
`palumbo@iasi.cnr.it`
[2] Biomatlab of IASI-CNR, Università Cattolica del Sacro Cuore, Largo Gemelli 8, 00168 Roma, Italy
`andrea.degaetano@biomatematica.it`

Summary. The paper investigates the problem of tracking a desired level of plasma glucose concentration. The model for the glucose-insulin system considered here, and recently published, belongs to the class of single-distributed delay models. The control law is obtained according to the feedback linearization theory. Both the cases of hyperglycemic and hypoglycemic patients have been considered. Simulations support theoretical results and show the physical reliability of the approach proposed.

1 Introduction

The design of glucose/insulin infusion devices able to control plasma glucose concentration is of great importance when attempting to reduce the diabetic complications in selected clinical situations. From an applicative point of view, different therapeutic schemes can be considered, according to the accuracy of the glucose-insulin model adopted and to the technology available in actuating the scheme selected. Glucose control strategies are mainly actuated by subcutaneous or intravenous injections or infusions. The former consist of subcutaneous insulin injections, three or four times a day, with the dose adjusted on the basis of capillary plasma glucose concentration measurements: it has a wide field of application, especially in type 1 diabetes, because, thanks to its superior management and safety, the dose is administered by the patients themselves (see [1] and references therein). However, only open loop or semiclosed loop control strategies can be used, mainly due to the problem of modeling accurately the absorption from the subcutaneous depot in the plasma circulation (see [10] for a critical review of subcutaneous absorption models).

On the other hand, a closed loop control design, based on intravenous glucose/insulin administration, provides a wider range of possible strategies and ensures a rapid delivery with negligible delays (see [11] and references therein for a survey of the intravenous route to plasma glucose control). Naturally, the more accurate is the model of the glucose-insulin kinetics, the more appropriate and effective can the control law be. The modeling of the glucose-insulin system is an appealing and challenging topic in biomathematics: many different models have been presented in the last decades, mostly referring to the well-known experimental framework of the *Intra Venous Glucose Tolerance Test* (IVGTT), where a bolus of glucose is administered intra-venously and glucose and insulin concentrations are frequently sampled (see e.g. the ODEs of the Minimal Model [2], [12], or the more recent integro-differential equations models of [3], [9]). An interesting survey on a very wide class of most significative models available in literature and the software tools related to them can be found in [8]. The main role of these models is to evaluate glucose and insulin sensitivity in clinical patients [2], [12].

In this paper a closed loop approach is investigated in order to track a desired level of basal glycemia, by means of intravenous administration of either glucose or insulin. Taking into account the family of distributed-delay models recently developed in [9], a nonlinear ordinary differential system is achieved, whose components evolve on a suitably defined extended state space. The key-role is played by the *feedback linearization* of the system [7]. Differently from other control laws based on the linear *approximation* of the nonlinear model around the equilibrium point (e.g. [4, 5]), the proposed approach provides the *exact* linearization of the system (no approximations have been considered), by suitably designing the control law. Tracking is, then, achieved for the linearized system. Both the needs of increasing and decreasing the level of glycemia to the target have been considered.

Simulation results support the efficacy of the theoretical developments and show the physical reliability of the approach proposed.

2 The Glucose-Insulin Model

The glucose-insulin model here considered belongs to the family of single-distributed delay models [9], and is reported below; the names of the parameters have been maintained as in [9].

$$\frac{dG}{dt} = -b_1 G(t) - b_4 G(t)I(t) + b_7, \qquad \frac{dI}{dt} = -b_2 I(t) + b_6 \int_0^{+\infty} \omega(s)G(t-s)ds;$$

$$(1)$$

b_1 is the insulin-independent glucose disappearance rate, b_4 is the insulin dependent glucose disappearance rate per (μU/ml) of plasma insulin concentration, b_7 is the constant increase in plasma glucose concentration due to constant baseline liver glucose release, b_2 is the first-order insulin disappearance rate, b_6 is the second-phase insulin release rate per (mg/dl) of average plasma glucose concentration per unit time.

The kernel $\omega(s)$ in the insulin dynamics characterizes the choice of the model and is such that:

$$\int_0^{+\infty} \omega(s)ds = 1, \qquad \int_0^{+\infty} s\omega(s)ds = T < +\infty.$$

T represents the average time delay.

It has been proven in [9] that all the models provide unique, positive bounded solutions and admit a unique locally asymptotically stable equilibrium point, given by the basal glycemia and insulinemia, (G_b, I_b). We can then consider equilibrium concentrations and write:

$$b_1 G_b + b_4 G_b I_b = b_7, \qquad b_2 I_b = b_6 G_b. \tag{2}$$

Global asymptotical stability is ensured if the average time delay T is sufficiently small, [9].

According to standard identification procedures, mainly based on the IVGTT, basal values of glucose and insulin concentrations are acquired as measurements so that equations (2) are used to reduce the total amount of the parameters to be identified (e.g. b_7 and b_6 are computed from b_1, b_2, b_4, identified, and G_b, I_b, measured). The standard identification task is performed by injecting intravenously a glucose bolus and acquiring plasma glucose and insulin concentrations at frequent times for a period of about three hours. This means, by setting $t = t_0$ the injection time, that the initial conditions for the IVGTT are:

$$\begin{aligned} G(t) &\equiv G_b, \quad t \in (-\infty, t_0), & I(t) &\equiv I_b, \quad t \in (-\infty, t_0), \\ G(t_0) &= G_b + b_0, & I(t_0) &= I_b + b_3 b_0, \end{aligned} \tag{3}$$

where b_0 is the theoretical increase in plasma concentration over the basal glycemia after the bolus injection and b_3 is the first-phase insulin concentration increase per (mg/dl) increase in the glycemia, due to the injected bolus. b_0 and b_3 are further parameters to be identified.

As it has been done in [9], also in this paper $w(s)$ has been chosen as:

$$\omega(s) = \gamma^2 s e^{-\gamma s}, \qquad \gamma > 0,$$

so that, the integral in the insulin kinetics is written as:

$$\int_0^{+\infty} \omega(s)G(t-s)ds = \int_0^{+\infty} \gamma^2 s e^{-\gamma s}G(t-s)ds = \int_{-\infty}^{t} \gamma^2(t-\tau)e^{-\gamma(t-\tau)}G(\tau)d\tau.$$

By setting the following positions:

$$x_1(t) = G(t), \qquad x_3(t) = \int_{-\infty}^{t} \gamma^2(t-\tau)e^{-\gamma(t-\tau)}G(\tau)d\tau$$

$$x_2(t) = I(t), \qquad x_4(t) = \int_{-\infty}^{t} e^{-\gamma(t-\tau)}G(\tau)d\tau$$

due to the *linear chain trick* [6], the glucose-insulin system (1) evolves according to a 4-dimensional ordinary differential system:

$$\frac{dx_1}{dt} = -b_1 x_1(t) - b_4 x_1(t) x_2(t) + b_7, \qquad \frac{dx_2}{dt} = -b_2 x_2(t) + b_6 x_3(t),$$

$$\frac{dx_3}{dt} = -\gamma x_3(t) + \gamma^2 x_4(t), \qquad \frac{dx_4}{dt} = x_1(t) - \gamma x_4. \tag{4}$$

According to (3), the initial conditions for (4) in an IVGTT occurring at time $t = t_0$ become:

$$x_1(t_0) = G_b + b_0, \qquad x_2(t_0) = I_b + b_3 b_0, \qquad x_3(t_0) = G_b, \qquad x_4(t_0) = G_b/\gamma.$$

3 Glucose Control: the Case of Hyperglycemic Patients

The aim to decrease the level of plasma glucose concentration in a diabetic patient is of primary importance, in order to reduce or delay the long-term complications associated with sustained hyperglycemia. In such a framework, especially in type 1 diabetes, the control law needs to be a suitably defined insulin infusion, named $u_i(t)$, occurring in the insulin dynamics which is, then, modified as follows:

$$\frac{dx_2}{dt} = -b_2 x_2(t) + b_6 x_3(t) + u_i(t). \tag{5}$$

By taking into account (5), system (4) will be referred to as:

$$\frac{dx}{dt} = f\big(x(t)\big) + g_i\big(x(t)\big) u_i(t) \qquad \text{with} \qquad f(x) = \begin{pmatrix} -b_1 x_1 - b_4 x_1 x_2 + b_7 \\ -b_2 x_2 + b_6 x_3 \\ -\gamma x_3 + \gamma^2 x_4 \\ x_1 - \gamma x_4 \end{pmatrix} \tag{6}$$

and $g_i(x) = (0 \ 1 \ 0 \ 0)^T$. Consider the output function as the glucose measurements:

$$y(t) = h\big(x(t)\big) = x_1, \tag{7}$$

according to which, system (6) endowed with the output (7) has relative degree 2 [7]:

$$L_{g_i} h = \frac{dh}{dx} \cdot g_i = 0, \qquad L_{g_i} L_f h = \frac{dL_f h}{dx} \cdot g_i = -b_4 x_1 \neq 0, \qquad \forall x_1 > 0.$$

Note that the relative degree is global in the domain of x, whose components are strictly positive. Despite of a non-full relative degree, it is possible to design a state feedback control law, which linearizes the system equations w.r.t. the following change of coordinates:

$$z = T(x) = \begin{pmatrix} h(x) \\ L_f h(x) \\ x_3 \\ x_4 \end{pmatrix} = \begin{pmatrix} x_1 \\ -b_1 x_1 - b_4 x_1 x_2 + b_7 \\ x_3 \\ x_4 \end{pmatrix}, \tag{8}$$

with

$$T^{-1}(z) = \begin{pmatrix} z_1 \\ \dfrac{b_7 - b_1 z_1 - z_2}{b_4 z_1} \\ z_3 \\ z_4 \end{pmatrix}.$$

According to (8), system (4) becomes, in the new coordinates:

$$\frac{dz_1}{dt} = z_2(t), \qquad\qquad \frac{dz_2}{dt} = \varphi_i\big(T^{-1}(z)\big) - b_4 z_1(t) u_i(t),$$

$$\frac{dz_3}{dt} = -\gamma z_3(t) + \gamma^2 z_4(t), \qquad\qquad \frac{dz_4}{dt} = z_1(t) - \gamma z_4(t), \tag{9}$$

with:

$$\varphi_i(x) = L_f^2 h(x) = (b_1 + b_4 x_2)(b_1 x_1 + b_4 x_1 x_2 - b_7) + b_2 b_4 x_1 x_2 - b_4 b_6 x_1 x_3.$$

The linearizing feedback is, then, given by:

$$u_i(t) = u_i\big(x(t)\big) = \frac{1}{L_{g_i} L_f h\big(x(t)\big)}\Big(-\varphi_i\big(x(t)\big) + v_i(t)\Big) = \frac{\varphi_i\big(x(t)\big) - v_i(t)}{b_4 x_1(t)}, \tag{10}$$

with $v_i(t)$ an exogenous input to be assigned in order to achieve the desired tracking. According to (10) the equations (9) are linearized as:

$$\frac{dz}{dt} = A_i z(t) + B_i v_i(t), \qquad \text{with} \qquad A_i = \begin{bmatrix} 0 & 1 & 0 & 0 \\ 0 & 0 & 0 & 0 \\ 0 & 0 & -\gamma & \gamma^2 \\ 1 & 0 & 0 & -\gamma \end{bmatrix}, \quad B_i = \begin{bmatrix} 0 \\ 1 \\ 0 \\ 0 \end{bmatrix},$$

$$y(t) = C z(t),$$

$$C = \begin{bmatrix} 1 & 0 & 0 & 0 \end{bmatrix}. \tag{11}$$

The input v_i is chosen in order to stabilize the linearized closed loop and to assign the desired glucose level:

$$v_i(t) = F_i z(t) + K_i.$$

Notice that the pair (A_i, B_i) is controllable, which means that, for any chosen set of values $\Lambda = \{\lambda_1, \lambda_2, \lambda_3, \lambda_4\}$, there exists a suitably defined matrix $F_i = [f_{i,1} \ \ f_{i,2} \ \ f_{i,3} \ \ f_{i,4}]$ such that the spectrum of $A_i + B_i F_i$ is equal to Λ. The scalar gain K_i is designed in order to achieve the desired basal glucose level $G_d = \lim_{t \mapsto +\infty} y(t)$, so that, by naming $W_i(s)$ the input/output transfer function of (11):

$$G_d = \lim_{s \to 0} W_i(s) = \lim_{s \to 0} C(sI - A_i - B_i F_i)^{-1} B_i K_i = -\frac{\gamma K_i}{(f_{i,1} + f_{i,3})\gamma + f_{i,4}},$$

from which

$$K_i = -\frac{G_d\big((f_{i,1} + f_{i,3})\gamma + f_{i,4}\big)}{\gamma}.$$

The scheme of the control law is reported in Fig. 1.

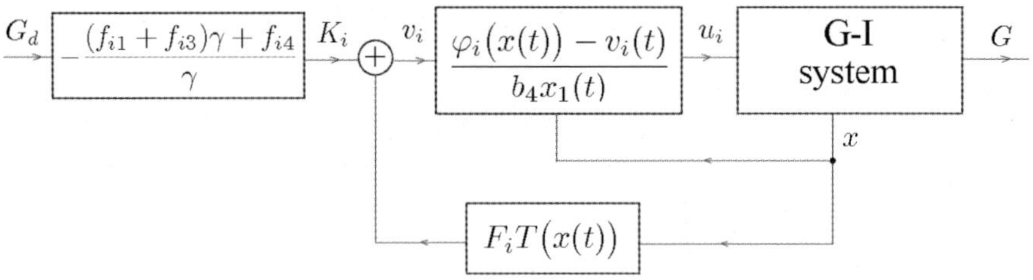

Fig. 1: Glucose control scheme: the hyperglycemic case.

Remark 1. By assigning the desired target glycemia, also the target insuline-mia changes. In this case:

$$\lim_{t \to +\infty} z_2(t) = 0 \quad \Rightarrow \quad \lim_{t \to +\infty} I(t) = \lim_{t \to +\infty} \frac{b_7 - b_1 z_1(t) - z_2(t)}{b_4 z_1(t)} = \frac{b_7 - b_1 G_d}{b_4 G_d}.$$

Remark 2. It has to be stressed that in a feasible framework the feedback law $u_i(t)$ can neither assume negative values, nor can produce negative sub-oscillations for the glucose/insulin evolutions. The first drawback is readily overcome by assuming to switch off the feedback when the input approaches the zero-level; nevertheless, even by adding such an input constrain, sub-oscillations can still appear. Moreover, as far as the plasma glucose concentration is concerned, sub-oscillations under 50mg/dl may produce permanent side effects, if occurring for too long a period. Preliminary simulations have, then, the task to determine the closed loop eigenvalues so as to prevent oscillations, besides converging to the desired glucose level.

4 Glucose Control: the Case of Hypoglycemic Patients

Consider the case of a basal level of plasma glucose concentration lower than the one desired to be tracked. A control law based on a glucose infusion is required in this case. By naming this control $u_g(t)$, the glucose dynamics is modified as follows:

$$\frac{dx_1}{dt} = -b_1 x_1(t) - b_4 x_1(t)x_2(t) + b_7 + u_g(t). \tag{12}$$

By taking into account (12), system (4) will be referred to as:

$$\frac{dx}{dt} = f\big(x(t)\big) + g_g\big(x(t)\big)u_g(t) \quad \text{with} \quad f(x) \quad \text{as in (6)} \quad \text{and} \quad g_g(x) = \begin{bmatrix} 1 \\ 0 \\ 0 \\ 0 \end{bmatrix}. \tag{13}$$

According to the output function (7), system (13) has relative degree 1:

$$L_{g_g} h = \frac{dh}{dx} \cdot g_g = 1 \neq 0.$$

Also in this case the relative degree is global in the domain of x. Nevertheless, the state feedback linearization can be obtained without a change of coordinates: the linearizing control law is readily given by

$$u_g(t) = -\varphi_g\big(x(t)\big) + v_g(t), \quad \text{with} \quad \varphi_g(x) = L_f h(x) = -b_1 x_1 - b_4 x_1 x_2 + b_7, \tag{14}$$

and $v_g(t)$ an exogenous input to be assigned in order to achieve the desired tracking. According to (14) the glucose-insulin system (4) is linearized as:

$$\frac{dx}{dt} = A_g x(t) + B_g v_g(t), \quad y(t) = Cx(t),$$

$$\text{with} \quad A_g = \begin{bmatrix} 0 & 0 & 0 & 0 \\ 0 & -b_2 & b_6 & 0 \\ 0 & 0 & -\gamma & \gamma^2 \\ 1 & 0 & 0 & -\gamma \end{bmatrix}, \quad B_g = \begin{bmatrix} 1 \\ 0 \\ 0 \\ 0 \end{bmatrix},$$

$$C = \begin{bmatrix} 1 & 0 & 0 & 0 \end{bmatrix}.$$

Also in this case, the input v_g is chosen in order to stabilize the linearized closed loop and to assign the desired glucose level:

$$v_g(t) = F_g x(t) + K_g;$$

the pair (A_g, B_g) is controllable which means that, for any chosen set of values $\Lambda = \{\lambda_1, \lambda_2, \lambda_3, \lambda_4\}$, there exists a suitably defined matrix $F_g = [f_{g,1} \;\; f_{g,2} \;\; f_{g,3} \;\; f_{g,4}]$ such that the spectrum of $A_g + B_g F_g$ is equal to Λ. The scalar gain K_g is designed in order to achieve the desired basal glucose level $G_d = \lim_{t \to +\infty} y(t)$, so that:

$$G_d = \lim_{s \to 0} C(sI - A_g - B_g F_g)^{-1} B_g K_g = -\frac{\gamma b_2 K_g}{(f_{g,1} b_2 + f_{g,2} b_6 + f_{g,3} b_2)\gamma + f_{g,4} b_2},$$

from which:

$$K_g = -\frac{G_d\big((f_{g,1} b_2 + f_{g,2} b_6 + f_{g,3} b_2)\gamma + f_{g,4} b_2\big)}{\gamma b_2}.$$

The scheme of the control law is reported in Fig. 2.

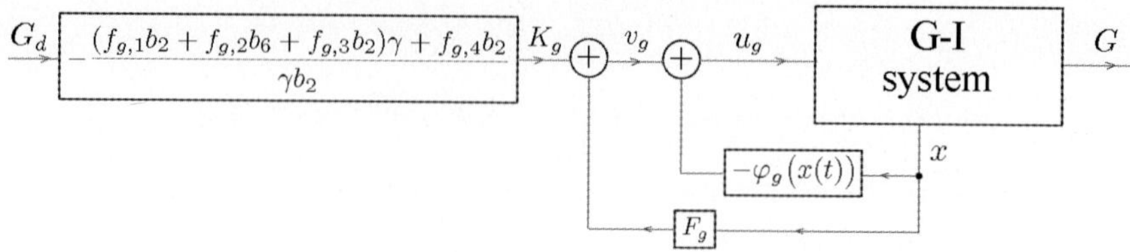

Fig. 2: Glucose control scheme: the hypoglycemic case.

Remark 3. By assigning the desired target glycemia, also the target insuline-
mia changes. In this case:

$$\lim_{t \mapsto +\infty} I(t) = \lim_{t \mapsto +\infty} x_2(t) = \frac{b_6 G_d}{b_2}.$$

Remark 4. Considerations written in Remark 2 can be repeated also for the
hypoglycemic case.

5 Numerical Simulations

In the following, simulations are proposed referring to a pair of hyperglycemic
patients and to a healthy subject. In all cases, the control law starts at the
initial time, set to zero, and the simulation goes on for 2 hours. The first case
is that of a type 2 diabetic patient, whose parameters are reported in Table 1.

Table 1: Type 2 diabetes parameters.

G_b	150	mg/dl
I_b	40	μU/ml
b_1	0.018063	$\min^{-1}$
b_2	0.041342	$\min^{-1}$
b_4	$1.484 \cdot 10^{-4}$	$(\mu$U/ml$)^{-1}\min^{-1}$
b_6	0.011	$(\mu$U/ml$)($mg/dl$)^{-1}\min^{-1}$
b_7	3.6	$($mg/dl$)\min^{-1}$
γ	0.1022	$\min^{-1}$

The desired target level of plasma glucose concentration is set to $G_d = 80$mg/dl. All eigenvalues of the closed loop dynamics are chosen equal to -0.1.
The evolution of glucose and insulin concentrations is reported in Fig. 3.

In this case the tracking of the desired target of glycemia is performed in
less than an hour.

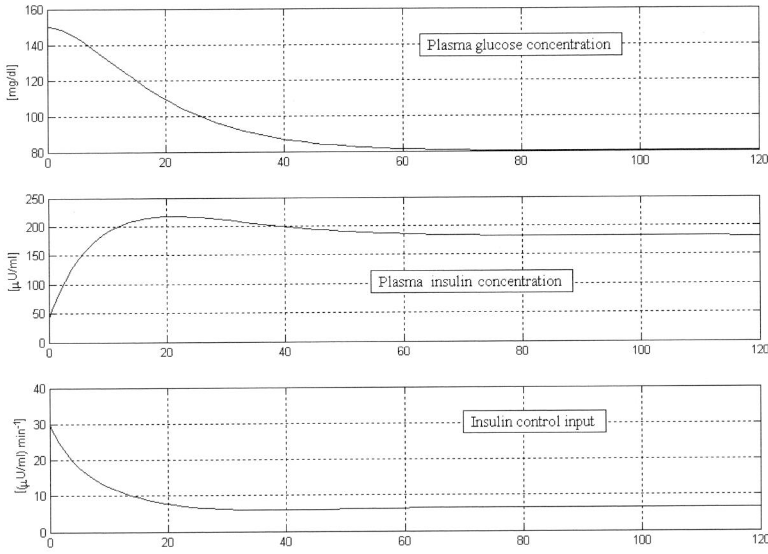

Fig. 3: Glucose/insulin evolution for a type 2 diabetic patient: $\lambda = -0.1$.

In Table 2, physical parameters are reported for a type 1 diabetic patient. Also in this case, the desired target level of plasma glucose concentration is set

Table 2: Type 1 diabetes parameters.

G_b	180	mg/dl
I_b	3	μU/ml
b_1	0.018063	min^{-1}
b_2	0.041342	min^{-1}
b_4	$6.457 \cdot 10^{-4}$	$(\mu\text{U/ml})\text{min}^{-1}$
b_6	$6.890 \cdot 10^{-4}$	$(\mu\text{U/ml})(\text{mg/dl})^{-1}\text{min}^{-1}$
b_7	3.6	$(\text{mg/dl})\text{min}^{-1}$
γ	0.1022	min^{-1}

to $G_d = 80\text{mg/dl}$ and the eigenvalues of the closed loop dynamics are chosen equal to -0.1. The evolution of the plasma glucose and insulin concentrations is reported in Fig. 4.

In order to test the effectiveness of the theoretical results when attempting to increase the desired glucose concentration, the following case has been considered (corresponding, for instance, to the establishment of a *clamped* hyperglycemic state in a normal subject). The parameters reported in table 3 refer to a healthy subject, whose basal glycemia has to be increased from

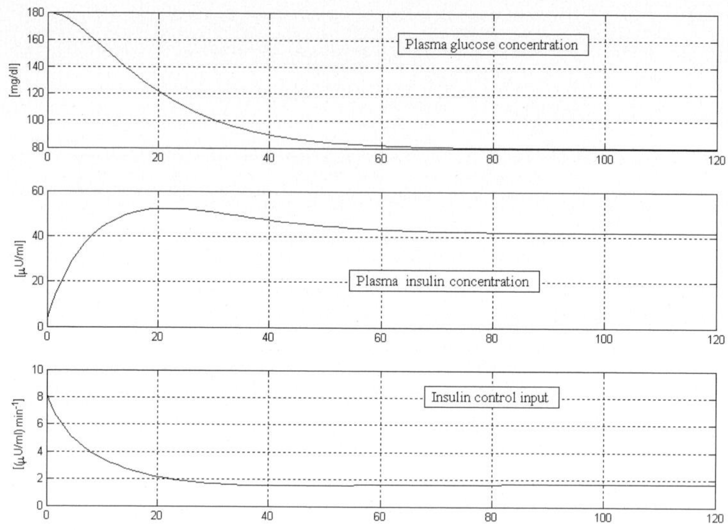

Fig. 4: Glucose/insulin evolution for a type 1 diabetic patient: $\lambda = -0.1$.

79mg/dl to 120mg/dl. In Fig. 5 simulations are reported, with the eigenvalues of the closed loop system chosen equal to -0.08.

Table 3: Healthy parameters.

G_b	79	mg/dl
I_b	62.5	μU/ml
b_1	0.018063	$\min^{-1}$
b_2	0.041342	$\min^{-1}$
b_4	$1 \cdot 10^{-5}$	$(\mu U/ml)^{-1}\min^{-1}$
b_6	0.032707	$(\mu U/ml)(mg/dl)^{-1}\min^{-1}$
b_7	1.4763	$(mg/dl)\min^{-1}$
γ	0.1022	$\min^{-1}$

Finally, taking into account the same healthy subject, a comparison between the natural response of the organism and the response under supplemental regulation (10) is reported in Fig. 6, when an intravenous glucose bolus is injected at time $t_0 = 10$min. According to (3), parameters b_0 and b_3 are set to $b_0 = 159.74$mg/dl and $b_3 = 2.827(\mu U/ml)(mg/dl)^{-1}$. Eigenvalues are chosen equal to -0.1. It is apparent that the proposed regulator provides a faster convergence to the target level without oscillations. It should be noted that the theoretical model chosen does not seem to reproduce well the secondary-phase insulin secretion *hump*, often seen in IVGTT's. This limitation leads naturally to the exploration of further models for the glucose-insulin system.

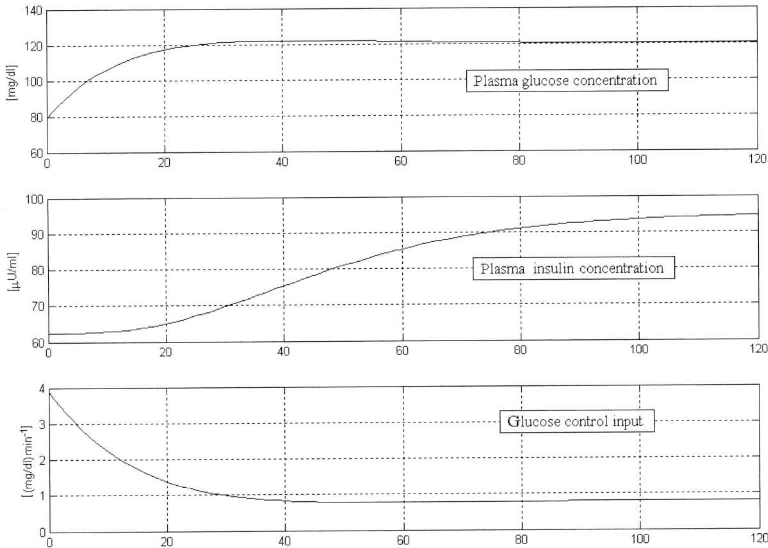

Fig. 5: Glucose/insulin evolution for a healthy subject: $\lambda = -0.08$.

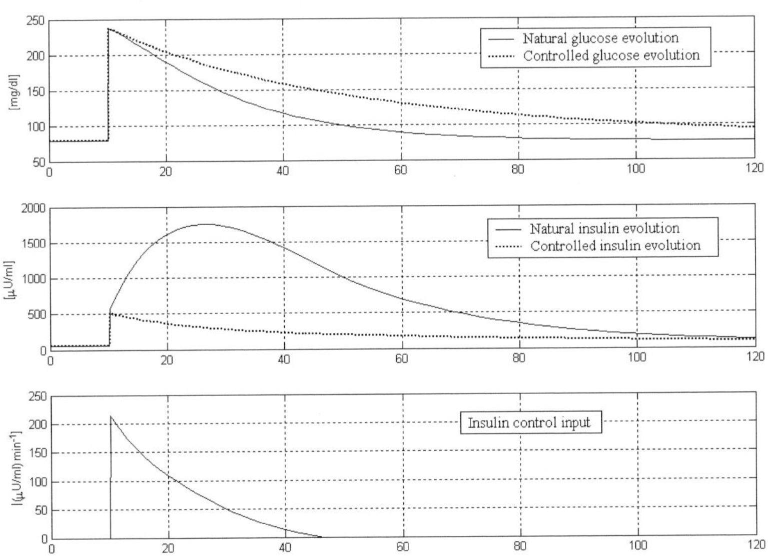

Fig. 6: Glucose/insulin evolution after an IVGTT for a healthy subject: $\lambda = -0.1$.

6 Conclusions

The tracking to a desired level of glycemia has been investigated according to intravenous therapy acting on a recently published single-distributed delay model of the glucose-insulin system. The control law design is based on the state feedback linearization theory and provides feasible glucose/insulin infusions, according to the simulations considered. The regulators proposed in the present work require the complete knowledge of the state of the system, which means complete glucose and insulin measurements. Nevertheless, according to the state-space methodology adopted, it may be possible to obtain essentially the same performance following an observer-based regulator approach, which only uses glucose measurements. This is work in progress by the same authors.

References

1. Bellazzi, R., Nucci, G., Cobelli, C.: The subcutaneous route to insulin-dependent diabetes therapy. IEEE Engineering in Medicine and Biology, **20**, 54–64 (2001).
2. Bergman, R.N., Ider, Y.Z., Bowden, C.R., Cobelli, C.: Quantitative estimation of Insulin sensitivity. Am. Journal on Physiology, **236**, 667–677 (1979).
3. De Gaetano, A., Arino, O.: Mathematical modelling of the intravenous glucose tolerance test. Journal of Mathematical Biology, **40**, 136–168 (2000).
4. Fisher, M.E., Teo, K.L.: Optimal insulin infusion resulting from a mathematical model of blood glucose dynamics. IEEE Engineering on Biomedical Engineering, **36**, 479–486 (1989).
5. Kovács, L., Paláncz, B., Benyó, Z.: Classical and modern control strategies in glucose-insulin stabilization. Proc. of 16-th IFAC World Congress on Autom. Contr. (IFAC05), Prague (2005).
6. Kuang, Y.: Delay Differential Equations with Applications in Population Dynamics. Vol 191 in the series of Mathematics in Science and Engineering, Academic Press, Boston (1993).
7. Isidori, A.: Nonlinear Control Systems. Third edition. Springer Verlag (1995).
8. Makroglou, A., Li, J., Kuang, Y.: Mathematical models and software tools for the glucose-insulin regulatory system and diabetes: an overview. to appear on Applied Numerical Mathematics.
9. Mukhopadhyay, A., De Gaetano, A., Arino, O.: Modeling the intra-venous glucose tolerance test: a global study for a single-distributed-delay model. Discrete and Cont. Dynam. Systems-Series B, **4**, 407–417 (2004).
10. Nucci, G., Cobelli, C.: Models of subcutaneous insulin kinetics. A critical review. Comp. Methods and Programs in Biomed., **62**, 249–257 (2000).
11. Parker, R.S., Doyle III, F.J., Peppas, N.A.: The intravenous route to blood glucose control. IEEE Engineering in Medicine and Biology, **20**, 65–73 (1996).
12. Toffolo, G., Bergman, R.N., Finegood, D.T., Bowden, C.R., Cobelli, C.: Quantitative estimation of beta cell sensitivity to glucose in the intact organism: a minimal model of insulin kinetics in the dog. Diabetes, **29**, 979–990 (1980).

An Algal Allelopathic Competition
with Internal and External Toxic Compounds

Paolo Fergola and Marianna Cerasuolo

Dipartimento di Matematica e Applicazioni "R. Caccioppoli", Università degli
Studi di Napoli Federico II, Via Cintia, 80126 Napoli (Italy)
paolo.fergola@dma.unina.it, marianna.cerasuolo@unina.it

A new mathematical model for an algal allelopathic competition is analyzed.
The competition takes place in a chemostat-like environment, in the presence
of a further concentration input of the same allelochemical compound produced by one of the two species. Steady-states and their asymptotic stability
properties are investigated in the two different cases: in the case of an instantaneous constant internal production of allelochemicals and in the case of
an instantaneous production linearly increasing with the concentration of the
producing species. Some numerical simulations, obtained by means of MATH-
EMATICA and performed by using recent experimental data are presented,
which confirm the allelopathic nature of the competition.

1 Introduction

In this paper we present some new results concerning the algal competition
between *Pseudokirkneriella subcapitata* and *Chlorella vulgaris*. Such a competition can be called allelopathic [4, 6, 7], because *C. vulgaris* produces an allelochemical compound called chlorellin which is noxious for the other species.

In [3] a mathematical model for such a competition has been studied by
assuming that it happens in a chemostat-like environment. This model has
been built on the basis of the experimental data obtained through several
new experiments, performed in our biochemical laboratories. These new data
specially concern the nutrient uptake rates of the two species, their yields, as
well as the nature of the effects of chlorellin on *P. subcapitata*.

In these laboratory experiments it has been easy to keep constant, during the competition, temperature, light, and the pH of the solution as well
as to consider it homogeneous. This has allowed to assume as mathematical
model a 4 ODE's system whose dynamics has resulted in a good agreement
with the outcomes of the laboratory experiments. However, because the concentration of chlorellin produced in those experiments has been very small,

further experiments are now in progress, in which the total chlorellin concentration present in the chemostat is due partially to the amount produced by *C.vulgaris*, partially to a further external concentration input of chlorellin previously collected from other experiments.

From a modelling point of view we have, in this case, a mixed toxicant problem, with two different sources for the same toxic compound, one internal the other one external. In this paper we start with the analysis of two different mathematical models representing such new scenario. In both models, according to experimental results, it has been assumed that the effect of chlorellin on *P. subcapitata* results to be of inhibitory type, i.e. able to reduce the potential growth of this species. In particular, such a reduction seems to be well represented by means of a decreasing exponential function. Furthermore, we assume that the production of chlorellin has a cost which is paid through the reduction of the growing potential of *C. vulgaris*. In other words, the overall energy coming to *C. vulgaris* from the assumption of nutrient is divided and devoted part to the growing process, part to the production of the allelochemicals. Hence, we consider two different mechanisms of production of chlorellin. Precisely, in Section 2, we assume that the production of chlorellin is instantaneous and constant; whereas in Section 3 we suppose that such a production is still instantaneous, but linearly increasing with *C. vulgaris'* concentration. The analysis of some biological meaningful steady-states and their local stability properties is performed for both cases, in the subsections 2.1 - 2.2 and 3.1 - 3.2 respectively. Finally, in Section 4, some numerical simulations, obtained by means of MATHEMATICA (Wolfram Research, 1988), are presented, which confirm the allelopathic nature of the competition, because they prove that the higher is the concentration of the chlorellin the faster *P. subcapitata* goes to the extinction.

2 The Mathematical Inhibitory Model

In this Section we study a 4 O.D.E.'s system describing the competition between two algal species which takes place in a chemostat-like environment. We suppose that one of the two species (*C. vulgaris*) produces a chemical compound noxious for the other one (*P. subcapitata*). We assume that the production of these allelochemicals is constant and has a cost. This cost is modelled by means of a reduction of the potential growth of this species, coming from the assumption of nutrient. We further assume that an additional concentration of the same allelochemicals (previously collected) is introduced in the continuous culture as an external input. Finally, we suppose that the nutrient uptake functions for both species are of Michaelis-Menten type.

Let us denote by $S(t)$ the nutrient concentration at time t in the culture vessel; $x(t)$, $y(t)$, the concentrations of the sensitive and producing algal species respectively, and $p(t)$ the concentration of allelochemicals.

The equations of the model take the form

$$\begin{cases} \dot{S} = (S^0 - S)D - f_1(S)e^{-\gamma p}\dfrac{x}{\eta_1} - f_2(S)\dfrac{y}{\eta_2} \\ \dot{x} = x[f_1(S)e^{-\gamma p} - D] \\ \dot{y} = y[(1-k)f_2(S) - D] \\ \dot{p} = (p^0 - p)D + kf_2(S)y \end{cases} \tag{1}$$

where all the parameters are supposed constant and positive. Moreover, S^0 is the constant input of the limiting nutrient; D is the constant washout rate and p^0 is the constant input of toxicant. S^0, p^0 and D are under the control of the experimenter; η_1, η_2 are the constant yields of populations x and y respectively; $f_i(S) = \frac{m_i S}{a_i + S}$ are the Michaelis-Menten functional responses, a_i the half saturation constants and m_i the maximal specific growth rates of the two populations $(i = 1, 2)$; γ is a measure of the inhibiting effect of chlorellin; k indicates the fraction of potential growth devoted to produce allelochemicals.

It is easy to check that when $p^0 = 0$ and $k = 0$ system (1) becomes asymptotic to the standard unpolluted chemostat model for the competition of two generic populations [8]. Moreover, when $p^0 \neq 0$ and $k = 0$ the system represents a polluted chemostat with an external toxicant input. Finally, if $k = 1$ (all efforts are devoted to producing toxicants) there is no growth of the producing population and thus its extinction follows. Therefore, we assume $0 < k < 1$.

In order to reduce the number of parameters the equations will be scaled, with the usual scaling for chemostat [8]. Specifically, let us set

$$S = \bar{S}S^0, \quad x = \bar{x}\eta_1 S^0, \quad y = \bar{y}\eta_2 S^0 \quad p = \bar{p}p^0, \quad m_1 = \bar{m}_1 D, \quad m_2 = \bar{m}_2 D,$$
$$t = \frac{\tau}{D}, \quad a_1 = \bar{a}_1 S^0, \quad a_2 = \bar{a}_2 S^0, \quad \gamma = \frac{\bar{\gamma}}{p^0}, \quad k_1 = k, \quad k_2 = \frac{S^0 \eta_2 k}{p^0}. \tag{2}$$

By substituing the new dimensionless variables and parameters and, dropping the bars, system (1) becomes

$$\begin{cases} \dot{S} = 1 - S - f_1(S)e^{-\gamma p}x - f_2(S)y \\ \dot{x} = x[f_1(S)e^{-\gamma p} - 1] \\ \dot{y} = y[(1-k_1)f_2(S) - 1] \\ \dot{p} = 1 - p + k_2 f_2(S)y. \end{cases} \tag{3}$$

Now, let us observe that (3) can be further simplified by introducing the following change of variables [5]

$$p = z + 1 + k_2 y/(1 - k_1). \tag{4}$$

In fact, from

$$z = p - 1 - k_2 y/(1 - k_1)$$

we have

$$\dot{z} = \dot{p} - \frac{k_2}{(1-k_1)}\dot{y} = 1 - p + k_2 f_2(S)y - \frac{k_2}{(1-k_1)}y[(1-k_1)f_2(S) - 1]$$
$$= 1 - p + k_2 f_2(S)y - k_2 f_2(S)y + \frac{k_2}{(1-k_1)}y = -\left(p - 1 - \frac{k_2}{(1-k_1)}y\right)$$

that is,

$$\dot{z} = -z.$$

Since $z(t) \to 0$ as $t \to \infty$, the obtained system admits a limiting system given by

$$
\begin{cases}
\dot{S} = 1 - S - f_1(S)e^{-\gamma\left(1 + \frac{k_2 y}{1 - k_1}\right)}x - f_2(S)y \\
\dot{x} = x[f_1(S)e^{-\gamma\left(1 + \frac{k_2 y}{1 - k_1}\right)} - 1] \\
\dot{y} = y[(1 - k_1)f_2(S) - 1].
\end{cases}
\tag{5}
$$

In the next Section we will limit ourselves to analyze the steady-state solutions of system (5).

2.1 Steady-State Solutions

Let us suppose $m_i > 1$, $i = 1, 2$ and denote with λ_i the root of the equation $f_i(S) = 1$, that is

$$\lambda_i = \frac{a_i}{m_i - 1}, \qquad i = 1, 2;$$

with $\hat{\lambda}_1$ the root of the equation $f_1(S) = e^{\gamma}$, that is

$$\hat{\lambda}_1 = \frac{a_1}{m_1 e^{-\gamma} - 1},$$

and $\hat{\lambda}_2$ the root of the equation $f_2(S) = \dfrac{1}{1 - k_1}$, that is

$$\hat{\lambda}_2 = \frac{a_2}{m_2(1 - k_1) - 1}.$$

With these assumptions it is easy to prove the following:

Theorem 1. *System (5) admits the following steady state solutions*

i $E_0 = (1, 0, 0)$ *always;*

ii $E_1 = \left(\hat{\lambda}_1, 1 - \hat{\lambda}_1, 0\right)$ *if* $\hat{\lambda}_1 < 1$;

iii $E_2 = \left(\hat{\lambda}_2, 0, (1 - k_1)(1 - \hat{\lambda}_2)\right)$ *if* $\hat{\lambda}_2 < 1$;

iv $E_3 = (S^*, x^*, y^*)$ *with*

$$S^* = \hat{\lambda}_2, \quad x^* = \left(1 - \hat{\lambda}_2 - \frac{y^*}{(1 - k_1)}\right), \quad y^* = -\frac{1 - k_1}{\gamma k_2}\left(\log \frac{1}{f_1(\hat{\lambda}_2)} + \gamma\right)$$

provided that

$$\hat{\lambda}_1 < \hat{\lambda}_2 \quad and \quad \gamma > -\frac{\log \frac{1}{f_1(\hat{\lambda}_2)}}{k_2(1 - \hat{\lambda}_2) + 1}.$$

2.2 Local Stability Properties

The stability analysis of the generic equilibrium $\bar{E} = (\bar{S}, \bar{x}, \bar{y})$ of system (5) can be performed by means of the characteristic equation associated to the linearized system of (5) with respect to $\bar{E}$. If we set

$$\alpha = e^{-\gamma\left(1 + \dfrac{k_2 \bar{y}}{1 - k_1}\right)}$$

and perform the change of variables

$$x_1 = S - \bar{S}, \quad x_2 = x - \bar{x}, \quad x_3 = y - \bar{y},$$

it is easy to show that this system can be written in the following form:

$$\begin{cases} \dot{x}_1 = \left(-1 - f_1'(\bar{S})\bar{x}\alpha - f_2'(\bar{S})\bar{y}\right) x_1 - f_1(\bar{S})\alpha x_2 \\ \qquad + \left(f_1(\bar{S})\dfrac{\gamma k_2}{1 - k_1}\alpha\bar{x} - f_2(\bar{S})\right) x_3 \\ \dot{x}_2 = f_1'(\bar{S})\bar{x}\alpha x_1 + [f_1(\bar{S})\alpha - 1]x_2 - \dfrac{\gamma k_2}{1 - k_1} f_1(\bar{S})\bar{x}\alpha x_3 \\ \dot{x}_3 = f_2'(\bar{S})\bar{y}(1 - k_1)x_1 + [(1 - k_1)f_2(\bar{S}) - 1]x_3. \end{cases}$$

Therefore, the Jacobian matrix in $\bar{E}$ is

$$J = \begin{bmatrix} -1 - f_1'(\bar{S})\bar{x}\alpha - f_2'(\bar{S})\bar{y} & -f_1(\bar{S})\alpha & f_1(\bar{S})\frac{\gamma k_2}{1-k_1}\alpha\bar{x} - f_2(\bar{S}) \\ f_1'(\bar{S})\bar{x}\alpha & f_1(\bar{S})\alpha - 1 & -\frac{\gamma k_2}{1-k_1}f_1(\bar{S})\bar{x}\alpha \\ f_2'(\bar{S})\bar{y}(1 - k_1) & 0 & (1 - k_1)f_2(\bar{S}) - 1 \end{bmatrix}. \tag{6}$$

To (6) corresponds the characteristic equation

$$\det |J - \rho I| = 0 \tag{7}$$

where I is the identity matrix in R^3. Equation (7) can be written as follows

$$\det \begin{bmatrix} -1 - f_1'(\bar{S})\bar{x}\alpha - f_2'(\bar{S})\bar{y} - \rho & -f_1(\bar{S})\alpha & f_1(\bar{S})\frac{\gamma k_2}{1-k_1}\alpha\bar{x} - f_2(\bar{S}) \\ f_1'(\bar{S})\bar{x}\alpha & f_1(\bar{S})\alpha - 1 - \rho & -\frac{\gamma k_2}{1-k_1}f_1(\bar{S})\bar{x}\alpha \\ f_2'(\bar{S})\bar{y}(1 - k_1) & 0 & (1 - k_1)f_2(\bar{S}) - 1 - \rho \end{bmatrix} = 0. \tag{8}$$

Hence, we can prove:

Theorem 2. *The following statements hold true*

i   If $\hat{\lambda}_1 > 1$ and $\hat{\lambda}_2 > 1$ then the equilibrium E_0 is asymptotically stable;

ii   If E_1 exists and $\hat{\lambda}_1 < \hat{\lambda}_2$ then E_1 is asymptotically stable;

iii   If E_2 exists and $\gamma > -\dfrac{\log \frac{1}{f_1(\hat{\lambda}_2)}}{k_2(1 - \hat{\lambda}_2) + 1}$ then E_2 is asymptotically stable;

iv   If E_3 exists then it is unstable.

Proof. i) In $E_0 = (1,0,0)$ equation (8) becomes

$$\det \begin{bmatrix} -1-\rho & -f_1(1)e^{-\gamma} & -f_2(1) \\ 0 & f_1(1)e^{-\gamma}-1-\rho & 0 \\ 0 & 0 & (1-k_1)f_2(1)-1-\rho \end{bmatrix} = 0.$$

By computing the roots of the characteristic equation we obtain

$$\rho_1 = -1, \quad \rho_2 = f_1(1)e^{-\gamma}-1, \quad \rho_3 = f_2(1)(1-k_1)-1.$$

Therefore the steady state E_0 turns out asymptotically stable if $\hat{\lambda}_1 > 1$ and $\hat{\lambda}_2 > 1$.

ii) In $E_1 = \left(\hat{\lambda}_1, (1-\hat{\lambda}_1), 0\right)$ the characteristic equation, obtained by (8), can be written as follows:

$$[(1-k_1)f_2(\hat{\lambda}_1)-1-\rho]\left[\rho^2 + \left(1+f_1'(\hat{\lambda}_1)\bar{x}e^{-\gamma}\right)\rho + f_1(\hat{\lambda}_1)f_1'(\hat{\lambda}_1)\bar{x}e^{-\gamma}\right] = 0. \tag{9}$$

By computing the roots of (9) we obtain

$$\rho_1 = (1-k_1)f_2(\hat{\lambda}_1)-1, \quad \rho_2 = -1, \quad \rho_3 = -f_1'(\hat{\lambda}_1)\bar{x}e^{-\gamma}.$$

Therefore, provided that E_1 exists, it is asymptotically stable if

$$f_2(\hat{\lambda}_1) < \frac{1}{1-k_1},$$

that is verified if $\hat{\lambda}_1 < \hat{\lambda}_2$.

iii) In $E_2 = \left(\hat{\lambda}_2, 0, (1-k_1)(1-\hat{\lambda}_2)\right)$ the characteristic equation, obtained by (8), can be written as follows:

$$[f_1(\hat{\lambda}_2)\alpha - 1 - \rho]\left[\rho^2 + \left(1+f_2'(\hat{\lambda}_2)\bar{y}\right)\rho + f_2(\hat{\lambda}_2)f_2'(\hat{\lambda}_2)\bar{y}(1-k_1)\right] = 0. \tag{10}$$

By computing the roots of (10) we obtain

$$\rho_1 = f_1(\hat{\lambda}_2)\alpha - 1, \quad \rho_2 = -1, \quad \rho_3 = -f_2'(\hat{\lambda}_2)\bar{y}.$$

Therefore, provided that E_2 exists, it is asymptotically stable if

$$e^{-\gamma(1+k_2(1-\hat{\lambda}_2))} < \frac{1}{f_1(\hat{\lambda}_2)}.$$

iv) Recalling that $E_3 = (S^*, x^*, y^*)$ with

$$S^* = \hat{\lambda}_2, \quad x^* = \left(1-\hat{\lambda}_2-\frac{y^*}{(1-k_1)}\right), \quad y^* = -\frac{1-k_1}{\gamma k_2}\left(\log\frac{1}{f_1(\hat{\lambda}_2)}+\gamma\right)$$

and by observing that

$$\alpha = \frac{1}{f_1(S^*)} \qquad \text{and} \qquad f_2(S^*) = \frac{1}{1-k_1},$$

we find, from (8), that the characteristic equation in E_3 can be written as follows:

$$\rho^3 + \left[1 + \frac{f_1'(S^*)}{f_1(S^*)}x^* + f_2'(S^*)y^*\right]\rho^2 - \left[\gamma k_2 f_2'(S^*)x^*y^* - f_2'(S^*)y^* + \frac{f_1'(S^*)}{f_1(S^*)}x^*\right]\rho - \gamma k_2 f_2'(S^*)x^*y^* = 0. \tag{11}$$

It is easy to check that E_3 is unstable whatever being the sign of the third coefficient in equation (11). In fact, the sequence of the coefficients of (11) has always only one change of signs. Therefore, due to the Descartes' rule of signs, we can conclude that (11) admits one positive root.

$\square$

In the following Table the previous sufficient conditions for the existence and the asymptotic stability of equilibria are resumed. We can observe that if $\hat{\lambda}_1 > \hat{\lambda}_2$ then $\gamma > -\dfrac{\log \frac{1}{f_1(\hat{\lambda}_2)}}{k_2(1-\hat{\lambda}_2)+1}$.

Table 1: Existence conditions and stability properties of equilibria E_0, E_1, E_2, E_3.

	Steady States	Conditions	Attractors
A	E_0	$\hat{\lambda}_1 > 1,\ \hat{\lambda}_2 > 1$	E_0
B	$E_0,\ E_1$	$\hat{\lambda}_1 < 1 < \hat{\lambda}_2$	E_1
C	$E_0,\ E_2$	$\hat{\lambda}_2 < 1 < \hat{\lambda}_1$	E_2
D	$E_0,\ E_1,\ E_2$	$\hat{\lambda}_1 < 1,\ \hat{\lambda}_2 < 1$ $\hat{\lambda}_1 < \hat{\lambda}_2$ $\hat{\lambda}_1 > \hat{\lambda}_2$	 E_1 E_2
E	$E_0,\ E_1,\ E_2,\ E_3$	$\hat{\lambda}_1 < \hat{\lambda}_2$ and $\gamma > -\dfrac{\log \frac{1}{f_1(\hat{\lambda}_2)}}{k_2(1-\hat{\lambda}_2)+1}$	$E_1,\ E_2$

3 A Concentration Dependent Toxicant Production

Some previous experiments [3] have shown that in the competition between *P. subcapitata* and *C. vulgaris* the production of chlorellin is proportional to *C. vulgaris* concentration. This suggests to sustitute the constant k in system (1) with a linear bounded function of the species concentration, that is:

$$k(y) = \theta y, \qquad \theta = const. > 0,\ \theta y < 1.$$

We observe that this type of function has been used in [2] and it can be viewed as a special case of the more general mathematical model introduced in [1] to

represent the biological mechanism called "quorum sensing".
Therefore, we consider the new system

$$\begin{cases} \dot{S} = (S^0 - S)D - f_1(S)e^{-\gamma p}\frac{x}{\eta_1} - f_2(S)\frac{y}{\eta_2} \\ \dot{x} = x[f_1(S)e^{-\gamma p} - D] \\ \dot{y} = y[(1 - \theta y)f_2(S) - D] \\ \dot{p} = (p^0 - p)D + \theta f_2(S)y^2. \end{cases} \tag{12}$$

By means of the same scaling procedure used in Section 2, we can write the
dimensionless version of (12) in the form

$$\begin{cases} \dot{S} = 1 - S - f_1(S)e^{-\gamma p}x - f_2(S)y \\ \dot{x} = x[f_1(S)e^{-\gamma p} - 1] \\ \dot{y} = y[(1 - \theta_1 y)f_2(S) - 1] \\ \dot{p} = 1 - p + \theta_2 f_2(S)y^2 \end{cases} \tag{13}$$

with $\theta_1 = \theta\eta_2 S^0$, $\theta_2 = \frac{\theta\eta_2^2 S^{02}}{p^0}$.

3.1 Steady-State Solutions

We observe that the change of variables (4) used in Section 2 is not helpful in
this case. However, it is easy to prove the following:

Theorem 3. *Suppose that $m_i > 1$, $i = 1, 2$, then system (13) admits the
following steady state solutions*

i $E_0 = (1, 0, 0, 1)$ *always;*

ii $E_1 = \left(\hat{\lambda}_1, 1 - \hat{\lambda}_1, 0, 1\right)$ *if $\hat{\lambda}_1 < 1$;*

iii $E_2 = \left(\lambda_S, 0, \frac{f_2(\lambda_S) - 1}{\theta_1 f_2(\lambda_S)}, 1 + \frac{\theta_2(f_2(\lambda_S) - 1)^2}{\theta_1^2 f_2(\lambda_S)}\right)$ *with*

$$\lambda_S = \frac{1 - m_2 + \theta_1 - \theta_1 a_2 + \sqrt{4\theta_1 a_2(1 + \theta_1) + (m_2 - 1 + \theta_1 - \theta_1 a_2)^2}}{2\theta_1}$$

if

$$\lambda_2 < 1.$$

3.2 Local Stability Properties

The stability analysis of the generic equilibrium $\bar{E} = (\bar{S}, \bar{x}, \bar{y}, \bar{p})$ can be performed by studying the characteristic equation associated to the linearized
system of (13) in $\bar{E}$. Precisely, by performing the change of variables

$$x_1 = S - \bar{S}, \quad x_2 = x - \bar{x}, \quad x_3 = y - \bar{y}, \quad x_4 = p - \bar{p},$$

we obtain

$$\begin{cases} \dot{x}_1 = \left(-1 - f_1'(\bar{S})\bar{x}\beta - f_2'(\bar{S})\bar{y}\right)x_1 - f_1(\bar{S})\beta x_2 - f_2(\bar{S})x_3 + \gamma f_1(S)\bar{x}\beta x_4 \\ \dot{x}_2 = f_1'(\bar{S})\bar{x}\beta x_1 + [f_1(\bar{S})\beta - 1]x_2 - \gamma\bar{x}f_1(S)\beta x_4 \\ \dot{x}_3 = f_2'(\bar{S})\bar{y}(1 - \theta_1\bar{y})x_1 + [(1 - 2\theta_1\bar{y})f_2(\bar{S}) - 1]x_3 \\ \dot{x}_4 = f_2'(\bar{S})\theta_2\bar{y}^2 x_1 + 2\theta_2\bar{y}f_2(\bar{S})x_3 - x_4 \end{cases}$$

where $\beta = e^{-\gamma\bar{p}}$. The Jacobian matrix in $\bar{E}$ is

$$J = \begin{bmatrix} \left(-1 - f_1'(\bar{S})\bar{x}\beta - f_2'(\bar{S})\bar{y}\right) & -f_1(\bar{S})\beta & -f_2(\bar{S}) & \gamma f_1(S)\bar{x}\beta \\ f_1'(\bar{S})\bar{x}\beta & [f_1(\bar{S})\beta - 1] & 0 & -\gamma\bar{x}f_1(S)\beta \\ f_2'(\bar{S})\bar{y}(1 - \theta_1\bar{y}) & 0 & [(1 - 2\theta_1\bar{y})f_2(\bar{S}) - 1] & 0 \\ f_2'(\bar{S})\theta_2\bar{y}^2 & 0 & 2\theta_2\bar{y}f_2(\bar{S}) & -1 \end{bmatrix}$$

to which corresponds the characteristic equation

$$\det |J - \rho I| = 0 \tag{14}$$

where I is the identity matrix in R^4. Equation (14) can be written as follows

$$\det \begin{bmatrix} \left(-1 - f_1'(\bar{S})\bar{x}\beta - f_2'(\bar{S})\bar{y}\right) - \rho & -f_1(\bar{S})\beta & -f_2(\bar{S}) & \gamma f_1(S)\bar{x}\beta \\ f_1'(\bar{S})\bar{x}\beta & [f_1(\bar{S})\beta - 1] - \rho & 0 & -\gamma\bar{x}f_1(S)\beta \\ f_2'(\bar{S})\bar{y}(1 - \theta_1\bar{y}) & 0 & [(1 - 2\theta_1\bar{y})f_2(\bar{S}) - 1] - \rho & 0 \\ f_2'(\bar{S})\theta_2\bar{y}^2 & 0 & 2\theta_2\bar{y}f_2(\bar{S}) & -1 - \rho \end{bmatrix} = 0.$$

We can prove the following:

Theorem 4. *These statements hold true*

i   If $\hat{\lambda}_1 > 1$ and $\lambda_2 > 1$ then the equilibrium E_0 is asymptotically stable;
ii   If E_1 exists and $\hat{\lambda}_1 < \lambda_2$ then E_1 is asymptotically stable;
iii If E_2 exists and $\hat{\lambda}_1 > \lambda_2$ then E_2 is asymptotically stable.

In Table 2 sufficient conditions for the existence and the asymptotic stability of equilibria are resumed.

Table 2: Existence conditions and stability properties of equilibria E_0, E_1, E_2.

	Steady States	Conditions	Attractors
A	E_0	$\hat{\lambda}_1 > 1,\ \lambda_2 > 1$	E_0
B	$E_0,\ E_1$	$\hat{\lambda}_1 < 1 < \lambda_2$	E_1
C	$E_0,\ E_2$	$\lambda_2 < 1 < \hat{\lambda}_1$	E_2
D	$E_0,\ E_1,\ E_2$	$\hat{\lambda}_1 < 1,\ \lambda_2 < 1$	
		$\hat{\lambda}_1 < \lambda_2$	E_1
		$\hat{\lambda}_1 > \lambda_2$	E_2

If we compare the sufficient conditions for the asymptotic stability of equilibrium E_2 in the Tables 1 and 2, we note that in the first case it is required $\lambda_2 < \hat{\lambda}_1$ and in the second case $\lambda_2 < \hat{\lambda}_1$. Therefore, by observing that $\lambda_2 < \hat{\lambda}_2$

and recalling that $f_2(\lambda_2) < f_2(\hat{\lambda}_2)$ being $f_2(S)$ a monotone increasing function, we can conclude that when the toxicant production is proportional to its own concentration, *C. vulgaris* is able to win the competition even with a growth rate which is lower than that one necessary when the toxicant production is constant. Moreover, it is easy to check that the stability properties of the equilibria are strictly dependent on the p^0 values. This can be immediately seen by using (2) and rewriting Table 2 in terms of the dimensional parameters of system (12) (Table 3).

Table 3: Existence conditions and stability properties with real parameters.

	Steady States	Conditions		Attractors
A	E_0	$S^0 < \frac{a_2 D}{m_2 - D}$	$p^0 > -\frac{1}{\gamma} log \frac{(a_1 + S^0)D}{m_1 S^0}$	E_0
B	$E_0,\ E_1$	$S^0 < \frac{a_2 D}{m_2 - D}$	$p^0 < -\frac{1}{\gamma} log \frac{(a_1 + S^0)D}{m_1 S^0}$	E_1
C	$E_0,\ E_2$	$S^0 > \frac{a_2 D}{m_2 - D}$	$p^0 > -\frac{1}{\gamma} log \frac{(a_1 + S^0)D}{m_1 S^0}$	E_2
D	$E_0,\ E_1,\ E_2$	$S^0 > \frac{a_2 D}{m_2 - D}$	$p^0 < -\frac{1}{\gamma} log \frac{(a_1 + S^0)D}{m_1 S^0}$	
			$p^0 < -\frac{1}{\gamma} log \frac{(a_1 m_2 - a_1 D + a_2 D)}{a_2 m_1}$	E_1
			$p^0 > -\frac{1}{\gamma} log \frac{(a_1 m_2 - a_1 D + a_2 D)}{a_2 m_1}$	E_2

4 Discussion

In this Section we compare the simulations performed with MATHEMATICA related to system (6) of [3], which is

$$\begin{cases} \dot{S} = 1 - S - f_1(S)N_1 e^{-\gamma p} - f_2(S)N_2 \\ \dot{N}_1 = N_1 \left[f_1(S)e^{-\gamma p} - 1 \right] \\ \dot{N}_2 = N_2 \left[f_2(S)(1 - k_1 N_2) - 1 \right] \\ \dot{p} = k_2 f_2(S)N_2^2 - p \end{cases}$$

and system (13) of this paper. Provided that we identify the letter k with the letter θ, N_1 with x and N_2 with y, we observe that the differences between these systems are only two. The first one consists in the presence in $(13)_4$ of a term corresponding to the external toxicant concentration input which is absent in $(6)_4$. The other difference is due to the fact that in (6) $f_1(S)$ is an Andrews function $\left(\frac{m_1 S}{a_1 + S + h_1 S^2} \right)$ whereas in (13) $f_1(S)$ is a Michaelis-Menten function. As it is easy to check on the expressions of these functions, actually this difference can be neglected in all the cases in which the numerical value of the coefficient h_1 is small enough. This exactly happens in the experiments presented and discussed in [3] where the external input of toxicants is absent ($p^0 = 0$) and the numerical values of the parameters, drawn from those experiments, are

$$D = 1, \ S^0 = 2.47, \ m_1 = 1.19295, \ m_2 = 1.25535, \ a_1 = 0.0157469,$$
$$a_2 = 0.00158039, \ \gamma = 19.3, \ \theta_1 = 0.8151, \ \theta_2 = 1.6302. \tag{15}$$

Therefore, with respect to simulations performed by using the numerical values given in (15), we can assume that the only difference between the two systems is due to the presence in (13) of a further toxicant external input.

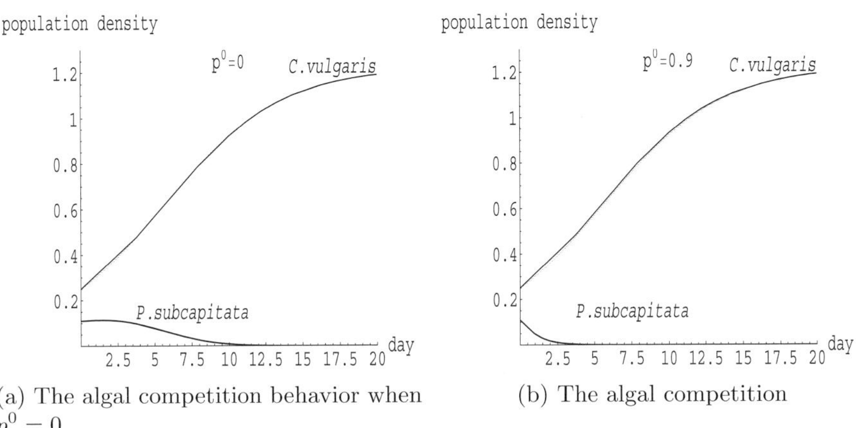

(a) The algal competition behavior when $p^0 = 0$

(b) The algal competition

Fig. 1: Algal competition.

In Figure 1 we reproduce the behaviors of the competition obtained with MATHEMATICA according to [3, system (6)] (Fig. 1a) and to system (13) (Fig. 1b) respectively.

By the comparison of the two figures clearly it comes out the remarkable inhibithory effect of the chlorellin on the growth of *P. subcapitata*. In fact, we observe that even a small concentration of a further external chlorellin input is sufficient to push this algal population to the extinction (about 3 days) much more quickly than when it is absent (about 10.5 days). These behaviours, further supported by new experiments now in progress, reinforce the idea that we are in presence of an allelopathic competition.

References

1. J.P. Braselton, P. Waltman, *A Competition model with dynamically allocated inhibitor production*. Mathematical Biosciences, 173, 55–84, 2001.
2. P. Fergola, F. Aurelio, M. Cerasuolo, A. Noviello, *Influence of mathematical modelling of nutrient uptake and quorum sensing on the allelopathic competitions*. Proocedings "WASCOM 2003" 12th Conference on Waves and Stability in Continuous Media, 191–203, 2004.

3. P. Fergola, M. Cerasuolo, A. Pollio, G. Pinto and M. Della Greca, *Allelopathy and Competition between* Chlorella vulgaris *and* Pseudokirchneriella subcapitata*: Experiments and mathematical model*, to appear.

4. E.M. Gross, *Allelopathy of aquatic autotrophs (invited review)*. Critical Reviews in Plant Science 22, 313–339, 2003.

5. S.B. Hsu, P. Waltman, *Competition in the Chemostat when One Competitor Produces a Toxin*. Jpn. J. Ind. Appl. Math., 15, 471–490, 1998.

6. R. Pratt, *Studies on Chlorella vulgaris. V. Some properties of the growth-inhibitor formed by chlorella cells*, Amer. Jour. Bot. 29, 142–148, 1942.

7. R. Pratt, *Studies on Chlorella vulgaris. XI. Relation between surface tension and accumulation of Chlorellin*, Amer. Jour. Bot. 35, 634–637, 1948.

8. H.L. Smith, P. Waltman, The Theory of the Chemostat – Dynamics of Microbial Competition. Cambridge Studies in Mathematical Biology, 1995.

Subsoil Decontamination with Biological Techniques: a Bio-Fluid Dynamics Problem

Filippo Notarnicola

Istituto per le Applicazioni del Calcolo, IAC-CNR, Via Amendola 122-D, 70126 Bari, Italy
f.notarnicola@ba.iac.cnr.it

Summary. A subsoil cleanup technology is called *bioventing*: bacteria are used to biodegrade pollutants and air is injected to enhance their activity. In this paper a general mathematical model describing the physical phenomenon is presented. The model is based on the theory of fluid dynamics in porous media. A multi-component and multi-phase fluid is considered and the system of partial differential equations is coupled with a population bacteria equation.

1 Introduction

Some kinds of contaminants can be removed from polluted subsoil by bacteria populations which transform the contaminants into less hazardous components in an aerobic situation. It is an *in situ* method since no soil removal is required. The bacteria biodegradation activity requires oxygen, so fresh air is supplied by means of forced air injection and/or extraction. This technique is called *bioventing* and it is often used in the unsaturated part of the soil: air and water - and contaminants too - are present in the void space of the porous media. The mathematical model of the physical phenomenon comprises a biological part - that is the description of the bacteria population dynamics and the pollutant biodegradation kinetic - and a fluid dynamics one, describing the subsoil fluid movements.

Since we refer to the unsaturated zone, gases and liquids are present in the soil and, therefore, we shall use a *multiphase model*. The oxygen concentration plays a significant rule in the biodegradation reaction and then the air is divided into two components: oxygen and non–oxygen parts. Moreover, other chemical components are present: water and a pollutant; therefore the model describes transport and concentrations of the components in the different phases. Part of the pollutant is assumed to be adsorbed by the solid matrix. Bacteria are described by a spatial concentration. They do not migrate in the space but they spread by a diffusion like–phenomenon.

The paper is organized as follows: Sect. 2 describes the transport of fluids. Sect. 3 is devoted to the biological phenomena and Sect. 4 to the adsorption process. In Sect. 5 the reactive and external source terms of the equations are specified. Finally Sect. 6 reports the complete model and some conclusions.

2 The Multiphase and Multicomponent Transport Equations

The fluid transport mathematical model is based on the theory of dynamics of multiphase and multicomponent fluids in porous media [1], [5], [2].

We suppose that three different phases are present: the *gas* phase, the liquid *wetting* phase (whose main component is water) and the liquid *non–wetting* phase (whose main component is the pollutant). The wetting and the non–wetting phases are unmiscible and therefore, although both are liquid, we treat them as different phases. The following components are present in the system: oxygen, non–oxygen part of the air, water and pollutant (a hydrocarbon). Moreover we suppose that the wettability phase order is wetting, non–wetting and gas, as shown in Fig. 1.

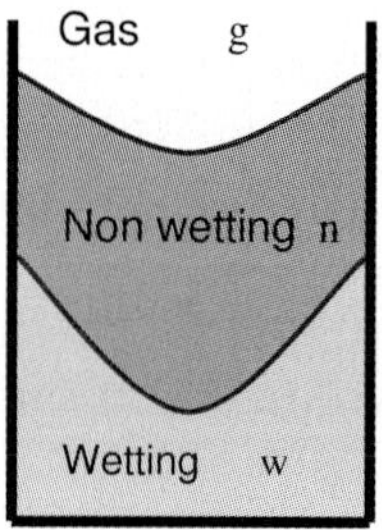

Fig. 1: Phases wettability.

Small amounts of all the components can be dissolved in the three phases. To describe the different variables of the model it is useful to introduce the following notations.

2.1 Introductory Notations

Component Notations

h water
C organic pollutant component

O oxygen part of air

N non oxygen part of air.

Phase Notations

w wetting

n non wetting phase

g gas phase

Porous Media Notations

Φ the volume of the pore space.

Φ_α volume of the phase α in the pore space, for $\alpha \in \{w, n, g\}$.
The following equality holds:

$$\Phi = \Phi_w + \Phi_n + \Phi_g$$

Saturation Definitions

$$S_\alpha = \frac{\text{volume of the phase } \alpha}{\text{pore space volume}} = \frac{\Phi_\alpha}{\Phi} \qquad \text{for} \qquad \alpha = w, n, g$$

Therefore S_w, S_n, S_g indicate the saturations of the wetting, non wetting and gas phases, respectively. The following relation holds:

$$S_w + S_n + S_g = 1 \tag{1}$$

Mass Fraction Definition of the Components

We assume that in each phase all the components can be present. Then we have the following definition. The mass fraction X_α^γ denotes the relative concentration of the component $\gamma \in \{h, C, O, N\}$ in the phase $\alpha \in \{w, n, g\}$, referred to the total mass of the phase α. That is:

$$X_\alpha^\gamma = \frac{\text{mass of component } \gamma \text{ in phase } \alpha}{\text{total mass of phase } \alpha}$$

Therefore the following relation holds for each phase:

$$X_\alpha^h + X_\alpha^C + X_\alpha^O + X_\alpha^N = 1 \qquad \text{for} \qquad \alpha \in \{w, n, g\} \tag{2}$$

2.2 Fluid Dynamics Equations

Component Equations

Mass conservation allows the following continuity equation to be written for the component $\gamma \in \{h, C, O, N\}$ in the phase $\alpha \in \{w, n, g\}$:

$$\frac{\partial}{\partial t}\left(\Phi S_\alpha X_\alpha^\gamma \rho_\alpha^\gamma\right) = -\,\mathbf{div}\,\left(X_\alpha^\gamma \rho_\alpha^\gamma \boldsymbol{v}_\alpha\right) +$$

$$\mathbf{div}\,\left(\Phi S_\alpha \boldsymbol{D}_\alpha^\gamma\,\mathbf{grad}\,X_\alpha^\gamma \rho_\alpha^\gamma\right) + F_\alpha^\gamma + q_\alpha^\gamma + a_\alpha^\gamma + r_\alpha^\gamma \quad (3)$$

where for each component γ in each phase α:

$\rho_\alpha^\gamma\,$ is the density;
$\boldsymbol{D}_\alpha^\gamma$ is the dispersion tensor;
$F_\alpha^\gamma\,$ is the inter phase mass transfer rate for a unit of volume;
$q_\alpha^\gamma\,$ is the reactive source term rate for a unit of volume;
$a_\alpha^\gamma\,$ is the adsorption source term rate for a unit of volume;
$r_\alpha^\gamma\,$ is the external source term rate for a unit of volume, that is the component injection or extraction due to an action outside the system.

The Darcy velocity of the phase α is denoted by $\boldsymbol{v}_\alpha$ and can be described by the generalized Darcy law:

$$\boldsymbol{v}_\alpha = -\frac{k_\alpha}{\mu_\alpha}\boldsymbol{K}\left(\mathbf{grad}\,p_\alpha - \rho_\alpha \boldsymbol{g}\right) \quad \text{for} \quad \alpha \in \{w, n, g\} \quad (4)$$

where:

$\boldsymbol{K}\,$ is the intrinsic permeability tensor;
$k_\alpha\,$ is the relative permeability of the phase α;
$p_\alpha\,$ is the pressure of the phase α;
$\boldsymbol{g} = (0, 0, -g)^T\,$ is the gravitational acceleration vector;
$\mu_\alpha\,$ and ρ_α are the dynamic viscosity and the density of the phase α, respectively.

It should be pointed out that, since the phase α can have several components, then in (4):

$$\rho_\alpha = \sum_\gamma \rho_\alpha^\gamma X_\alpha^\gamma \quad (5)$$

and also:

$$\mu_\alpha = \sum_\gamma \mu_\alpha^\gamma X_\alpha^\gamma \quad (6)$$

where μ_α^γ is the dynamic viscosity of the component γ in the phase α.
If we substitute (4) into (3) we have:

$$\frac{\partial}{\partial t}\left(\Phi S_\alpha X_\alpha^\gamma \rho_\alpha^\gamma\right) = \mathbf{div}\,\left(X_\alpha^\gamma \rho_\alpha^\gamma \frac{k_\alpha}{\mu_\alpha}\boldsymbol{K}\left(\mathbf{grad}\,p_\alpha - \rho_\alpha \boldsymbol{g}\right)\right) +$$

$$\mathbf{div}\,\left(\Phi S_\alpha \boldsymbol{D}_\alpha^\gamma\,\mathbf{grad}\,X_\alpha^\gamma \rho_\alpha^\gamma\right) + F_\alpha^\gamma + q_\alpha^\gamma + a_\alpha^\gamma + r_\alpha^\gamma \quad (7)$$

and then the phase velocity disappears from the continuity equation.

2.3 Capillary Pressure Relationships

In a multi phase system, at the interface between different phases, surface tension forces appear (see [1, p. 441-449], [5, p. 50-60]) and this leads to pressure discontinuity. The inter facial difference of pressure is called capillary pressure and is defined as follows. If we assume that phase w (*wetting phase*) wets phase n (*non wetting phase*) we have:

$$pc_{nw} = p_n - p_w$$

where p_n is the pressure of the *non wetting phase* and p_w is the pressure of the *wetting phase*. Moreover we suppose that phase n wets phase g and therefore we have:

$$pc_{gn} = p_g - p_n$$

As described in [1, p.441-449] and [5, p.50-60] the inter facial capillary pressure depends on the pore space geometry (and therefore on the soil characteristics) and on the phase saturations. That means the following relations hold:

$$p_n - p_w = pc_{nw}(S_w, S_n, S_g) = f_1(S_w, S_n, S_g)$$

$$p_g - p_n = pc_{gn}(S_w, S_n, S_g) = f_2(S_w, S_n, S_g)$$

(8)

The functions $f_1(S_w, S_n, S_g)$ and $f_2(S_w, S_n, S_g)$ are considered to be known and they represent the relationships between capillary pressures and saturations; several expressions of them have been proposed and a summary can be found in [5] p. 54-60.

3 Bacteria Population and Biodegradation Kinetic

In this section, the bacteria equation, the pollutant and oxygen consumptions will be treated. For simplicity, as first step, in Subsect. 3.1 we shall consider a spatially homogeneous distribution of microorganism, pollutant and oxygen. Therefore the population dynamics will be described with a system of ordinary differential equations. As second step, in Subsect. 3.3 a reaction diffusion equation for non uniformly spatial distributed bacteria will be given.

3.1 The Homogeneous Model

Let us denote the spatial homogeneous microorganism, pollutant and oxygen concentrations variables with $\widetilde{B}(t)$, $\widetilde{C}(t)$ and $\widetilde{O}(t)$, respectively. The contaminant is the primary substrate for microorganism and all variables are time dependent.

A common description of the bacteria population dynamics is based on *Monod*-type growth terms [3, p. 364] and in order to build the model, two assumptions will be adopted.

First Assumption

We assume that bacteria rise only where both oxygen and pollutant are available and so the microbial growth will be described with a double Monod term; moreover we assume that bacteria death decay is a linear function of the bacteria concentration itself. Thus, for the microorganism, $\widetilde{B}(t)$, the equation is:

$$\frac{d}{dt}\widetilde{B}(t) \;=\; g(\widetilde{C}(t),\widetilde{O}(t))\ \widetilde{B}(t) - \delta\ \widetilde{B}(t). \tag{9}$$

where $g(\widetilde{C}(t),\widetilde{O}(t))$ is the microorganism growth rate:

$$g(\widetilde{C}(t),\widetilde{O}(t)) = \frac{\beta_C \widetilde{C}(t)}{K_C + \widetilde{C}(t)}\ \frac{\beta_O \widetilde{O}(t)}{K_O + \widetilde{O}(t)} \tag{10}$$

where:

$$\frac{\beta_C \widetilde{C}(t)}{K_C + \widetilde{C}(t)} \tag{11}$$

is the Monod term corresponding to the *pollutant specific growth rate*, and:

$$\frac{\beta_O \widetilde{O}(t)}{K_O + \widetilde{O}(t)} \tag{12}$$

is the Monod term corresponding to the *oxygen specific growth rate*. Moreover, in (11) and (12) β_C and β_O are the *asymptotic maximum specific growth rates*; K_C and K_O are the *half specific velocity constants* (that is, when $\widetilde{C}(t) = K_C$ then the *pollutant specific growth rate* has value $\beta_C/2$ and, also, when $\widetilde{O}(t) = K_O$ then the *oxygen specific growth rate* has value $\beta_O/2$); δ is a constant and represents the specific microorganism decay rate.

Second Assumption

Pollutant plays the role of nutrient for bacteria and then we assume that pollutant and oxygen are converted into microbial cell mass and they are also used for the endogenous metabolism.

At the end of the cycle life, bacteria release some of the oxygen consumed in the cell mass growth process but they do not release pollutant since we suppose that biodegradation is an irreversible reaction.

The transformation from pollutant to cell mass term expresses that, in a time unit, the decrement of $\widetilde{C}(t)$ is proportional to the growth of $\widetilde{B}(t)$, that is to $g(\widetilde{C}(t),\widetilde{O}(t))$; the consumption rate term of $\widetilde{C}(t)$ due to the metabolic process is based on a kind of mass action law. In terms of equations:

$$\frac{d}{dt}\widetilde{C}(t) = -\frac{1}{Y_C}g(\widetilde{C}(t),\widetilde{O}(t))\widetilde{B}(t) - M_C\widetilde{C}(t)\widetilde{O}(t)\widetilde{B}(t) \tag{13}$$

where Y_C and M_C are the pollutant *yield coefficient* and the *metabolic consumption constant*, respectively.

The equation of the oxygen dynamics is:

$$\frac{d}{dt}\widetilde{O}(t) = -\frac{1}{Y_O}\frac{d}{dt}\widetilde{B}(t) - M_O\widetilde{C}(t)\widetilde{O}(t)\widetilde{B}(t) \tag{14}$$

where Y_O and M_O are the oxygen *yield coefficient* and the *metabolic consumption constant*, respectively.

In equation (14) the metabolic consumption term is similar to the corresponding one in the pollutant equation (13); moreover, the rate of the oxygen change due to biomass growth is proportional to the change in time of the bacteria population that is to $d/dt\,\widetilde{B}(t)$.

Substituting (9) into (14) we obtain:

$$\frac{d}{dt}\widetilde{O}(t) = -\frac{1}{Y_O}g(\widetilde{C}(t),\widetilde{O}(t))\widetilde{B}(t) + \frac{1}{Y_O}\delta\widetilde{B}(t) - M_O\widetilde{C}(t)\widetilde{O}(t)\widetilde{B}(t) \tag{15}$$

We explicitely observe that in the above equation the term $\frac{1}{Y_O}\delta\widetilde{B}(t)$ describes the oxygen released in the bacteria death decay process.

The mathematical model for the microbial dynamic is formed by equations (9), (13) and (15). It is useful to stress that, in the present subsection, the unknowns of the homogeneous model depend only on time.

In Subsect. 3.3 equation (9) will be used to obtain the evolution equation for a non uniform spatial bacteria distribution. Equations (13) and (15) will be used in Subsect. 5.1 to define the reactive terms in equations (7).

3.2 A Simpler Model

Some simplification can be introduced in the microorganism, pollutant and oxygen mathematical model. For example, a simpler version of the growth rate defined in (10) and based on the mass action law is the following:

$$g(\widetilde{C}(t),\widetilde{O}(t)) = \lambda\widetilde{O}(t)\widetilde{C}(t) \tag{16}$$

where λ is the reproduction constant coefficient. Then the bacteria equation is:

$$\frac{d}{dt}\widetilde{B}(t) \;= \lambda\widetilde{O}(t)\widetilde{C}(t)\widetilde{B}(t) - \delta\,\widetilde{B}(t). \tag{17}$$

Moreover, in (13) and (14) we can only consider the metabolic consumption terms, obtaining:

$$\frac{d}{dt}\widetilde{C}(t) = -M_C\widetilde{O}(t)\widetilde{C}(t)\widetilde{B}(t) \tag{18}$$

and:

$$\frac{d}{dt}\widetilde{O}(t) = -M_O\widetilde{O}(t)\widetilde{C}(t)\widetilde{B}(t) \tag{19}$$

Therefore, in place of equations (9) (13) and (15), an alternative simpler model is formed by equations (17), (18) and (19).

3.3 The Equation of a Spatial non Homogeneously Distributed Bacteria Population

Let us consider the subsoil model. In this subsection equation (9) will be adapted to a non uniform spatial distribution; bacteria are fixed in space and spread by diffusion.

Let us denote with denote B the punctual microorganism density, depending on space and time. Then we have:

$$\frac{\partial}{\partial t}B = D\boldsymbol{\Delta}B + g(C_T, O_T)B - \delta B \tag{20}$$

where $\boldsymbol{\Delta}$ is the Laplace operator; D is the bacteria diffusion coefficient and $g(C_T, O_T)$, δ, represent the microorganism growth and decay rate, respectively; δ is a positive constant. According to equations (10) and (16), it is:

$$g(C_T, O_T) = \frac{\beta_C C_T}{K_C + C_T}\frac{\beta_O O_T}{K_O + O_T} \tag{21}$$

or

$$g(C_T, O_T) = \lambda O_T C_T \tag{22}$$

where C_T is the total punctual contaminant concentration:

$$C_T = \Phi\left(\rho_w^C X_w^C S_w + \rho_n^C X_n^C S_n + \rho_g^C X_g^C S_g\right) \tag{23}$$

and O_T is the total punctual oxygen concentration:

$$O_T = \Phi\left(\rho_w^O X_w^O S_w + \rho_n^O X_n^O S_n + \rho_g^O X_g^O S_g\right) \tag{24}$$

4 Adsorbed Contaminant Equation

The pollutant can be adsorbed or released by the solid matrix. Adsorption [4, p. 22] is the contaminant transfer from the non–solid phase to the surface of the solid matrix; it depends on rocks and pollutant characteristics and on pollutant concentrations in non–solid phase and solid surface.

In bioremediation, adsorption plays an important role: as the contaminant is removed from the three non-solid phases, the deadsorption process reintegrates it in the same phases, and the time scale of the deadsorption process could be much longer than that of the bioremediation process. It is, thus, necessary to describe this physical phenomena in the mathematical model.

If we denote the concentration of the adsorbed pollutant (per unit of volume of the solid phase) with A, and the weighted pollutant mass per unit of volume of the non–solid phase with $\widehat{C}_T$, the following isothermal nonequilibrium continuity equation holds [1, p. 618]:

$$\frac{\partial}{\partial t}\rho_A A = -\tau_A\{A\rho_A - \widehat{C}_T\} \tag{25}$$

where ρ_A is the adsorbed contaminant density; τ_A is the time contaminant transmission coefficient between the solid matrix and the non-solid phases. Moreover $\widehat{C}_T$ is defined as:

$$\widehat{C}_T = \epsilon_w \rho_w^C X_w^C S_w + \epsilon_n \rho_n^C X_n^C S_n + \epsilon_g \rho_g^C X_g^C S_g$$

where ϵ_w, ϵ_n and ϵ_g are dimensionless coefficients related with the adsorptive properties between the solid phase and the pollutant contained in each of the fluid phases. We assume that ρ_A, τ_A and ϵ_w, ϵ_n, ϵ_g are constants.

5 Source Term Specifications

5.1 Reactive Terms

The reactive source terms represent the change of mass due to contaminant biotransformation and their expressions are based on the homogeneous model described in Subsect. 3.1.

Since the non–oxygen part of the air is not involved in biodegradation, in (7) we have:

$$q_w^N = q_n^N = q_g^N = 0$$

From (13), the reactive terms of the pollutant in (7) are:

$$q_\alpha^C = -\left\{ \frac{1}{Y_C} g(C_T, O_T) B + M_C O_T C_T B \right\} \frac{\Phi S_\alpha X_\alpha^C \rho_\alpha^C}{C_T}$$

$$\text{for} \quad \alpha \in \{w, n, g\}$$

where the function g is defined by expression (21) or (22); Y_C, M_C are defined in Sect. 3.1 and C_T, O_T are defined in (23), (24), respectively. We assume that the total consumed pollutant is subdivided among the different phases proportionally to its mass in each phase.

Biodegradation is an oxygen consuming phenomena. Then, from (15) the oxygen reactive source terms in (7) are:

$$q_\alpha^O = -\left\{ \frac{1}{Y_O} \left(g(C_T, O_T) - \delta \right) B + M_O O_T C_T B \right\} \frac{\Phi S_\alpha X_\alpha^O \rho_\alpha^O}{O_T}$$

$$\text{for} \quad \alpha \in \{w, n, g\}$$

where Y_O and M_O are defined in Sect. 3.1. Also, consumed oxygen is subdivided among the different phases proportionally to its mass in each phase.

During the biodegradation process a quantity of water is produced in the three phases, proportionally to X_w^h, X_n^h and X_g^h. Then the water source term for each component in each phase is:

$$q_\alpha^h = \frac{1}{Y_h} O_T C_T B \left\{ \frac{\Phi S_\alpha X_\alpha^h \rho_\alpha^h}{h_T} \right\} \quad \text{for} \quad \alpha \in \{w, n, g\} \tag{26}$$

where the parameter Y_h is constant and represents the water *yield* coefficient and:

$$h_T = \Phi \left(\rho_w^h X_w^h S_w + \rho_n^h X_n^h S_n + \rho_g^h X_g^h S_g \right)$$

In (26) it is assumed that water is produced only in the metabolic bacteria activity.

5.2 Adsorption Terms

We only consider contaminant adsorption and thus, for water and air, it is: $a_\alpha^h = a_\alpha^O = a_\alpha^N = 0$ for $\alpha \in \{w, n, g\}$. From (25) the adsorption/deadsorption source terms for pollutant are:

$$a_\alpha^C = \Phi \, X_\alpha^C \, \frac{\epsilon_\alpha}{\epsilon_w + \epsilon_n + \epsilon_g} \, \tau_A \{ A \rho_A - \widehat{C}_T \} \quad \text{for} \quad \alpha \in \{w, n, g\}$$

The hypothesis is that the total adsorbed/deadsorbed contaminant is subdivided among the three phases, proportionally to $\epsilon_\alpha / (\epsilon_w + \epsilon_n + \epsilon_g)$.

5.3 External Source Terms

We suppose that only air will be injected or extracted in the subsoil in the gas phase. Therefore all the external sources terms r_α^γ are null except: $r_g^O = p$ and $r_g^N = (1 - p)\Sigma$.

The function Σ, defined in the spatial domain, is the punctual air injection or extraction flow rate and p is the oxygen fraction of the air. If the air souces are punctual then Σ is a summation of Dirac delta functions.

5.4 Component Phase Migrations

In a multiphase and multicomponent environment, components can cross interphase boundaries for physical/chemical equilibrium reasons. Examples are water and pollutant evaporation or condensation, air dissolution in liquid phases, pollutant dissolution in water and so on. The phase changes of the components give rise to source terms in continuity equations and this section deals with them.

The terms F_α^γ in equations (7), describe the component exchanges among the fluid phases; that is, for a unit of volume, F_α^γ is the total interphase mass transfer rate of the component γ in the phase α.

Moreover if, for $\gamma \in \{h, C, O, N\}$, and for $\alpha, \beta \in \{w, n, g\}$, $\alpha \neq \beta$, we denote with $F_{\beta \to \alpha}^\gamma$ the transfer rate of component γ from the phase β in the contiguous phase α, then we have:

$$\begin{aligned}
F_w^\gamma &= F_{n \to w}^\gamma + F_{g \to w}^\gamma \\
F_n^\gamma &= F_{w \to n}^\gamma + F_{g \to n}^\gamma \\
F_g^\gamma &= F_{w \to g}^\gamma + F_{n \to g}^\gamma
\end{aligned} \qquad (27)$$

Each of the terms $F^\gamma_{\beta \to \alpha}$ is defined as follows:

$$F^\gamma_{\beta \to \alpha} = \Phi S_\alpha \rho^\gamma_\alpha \mathcal{T}^\gamma_{\beta \to \alpha} (\bar{X}^\gamma_{\beta \leftrightarrow \alpha} - X^\gamma_\alpha)$$

where $\bar{X}^\gamma_{\beta \leftrightarrow \alpha}$ is the mass fraction of the component γ in the phase α in equilibrium with the component γ in the phase β; $\mathcal{T}^\gamma_{\beta \to \alpha}$ is the mass transfer rate coefficient from phase β to phase α. The equilibrium terms $\bar{X}^\gamma_{\beta \to \alpha}$ are obtained, for isothermal ideal fluids, by Raoult's and Henry's laws.

6 The complete Model and Conclusions

At the end of the presentation it is useful to summarize the model; it is formed by the following twenty equations:

- twelve *continuity equations* (7),
- three *relations between components in each phase* (2),
- one *phase saturation relation* (1),
- two *relations between the phase pressures*, established by the capillary pressures (8),
- one *population dynamic equation* (20)
- one *adsorbed pollutant equation* (25)

containing the following twenty unknowns, which depend on space and time:

- X^γ_α for $\gamma \in \{h, c, O, N\}$ and $\alpha \in \{w, n, g\}$, the *phase relative concentrations of the components*,
- S_α for $\alpha \in \{w, n, g\}$, the *phase saturations*,
- p_α for $\alpha \in \{w, n, g\}$, the *phase pressures*,
- B, the *bacteria concentration*
- A, the *adsorbed pollutant concentration*.

We can observe that the derived model is general and includes a large number of equations. From a practical point of view, like in numerical simulations, it is difficult to use. The aim of this paper is to offer a sufficiently large framework describing the main processes involved in the bioventing phenomenon so that it can be specialised according to the different contexts by identifying, case by case, the essential physical phenomena and obtaining, as a consequence, a more treatable model.

Different levels of simplification are possible. A first possibility consists of neglecting the presence of all the components in each phase, that is: water is the only component in the wetting phase; pollutant is the only component in the non–wetting phase; water and pollutant are not present in the gas phase and, therefore, only air is in the gas phase. Since oxygen is essential to the biodegradation phenomenon, air is considered as a two component phase: the oxygen part and the non–oxygen part. In this way only the following phase–relative component concentrations and phase saturation remain unknown: X_g^O, X_g^N, S_w, S_n, S_g, instead of the initial fifteen. Moreover the component inter–phase migration terms defined in (27) are not present in the equations of the model.

Another simplification consists of considering the wetting and non–wetting phases immobile, for example, in the form of residual saturation. The only mobile phase is air, made up of the two components oxygen and non–oxygen. In this case X_g^O, X_g^N, S_n, S_g remain unknown but a simpler model is obtained: S_n is not involved in transport but only in a simpler punctual decay equation; S_w does not change in time and, therefore, it is not unknown and can be considered part of the solid matrix.

From a conceptual point of view we can imagine that biodegradation is formed of two distinct phenomena: the first acts on the pollutant in the non–wetting phase and the second acts on the adsorbed pollutant; the time scale of the two phenomena is very different. The adsorbing phenomenon can ever be neglected, however in this case the long time scale biodegradation is not considered and the model can become inaccurate.

References

1. Bear J.: Dynamics of fluids in porous media. Elsevier, New York (1972)
2. Bear J., Bachmat Y.: Introduction to modeling of transport phenomena in porous media. Kluwer, Dordrecht (1991)
3. Cookson J.T.: Bioremediation engineering: design and application. Mc GrawHill, New York (1995)
4. de Marsily G.: Quantitative hydrogeology. Academic Press, San Diego (1986)
5. Helmig R.: Multi phase Flow and Transport Processes in the Subsurface. Springer, Berlin (1997)

Part III

Mathematical Problems in Industry and Economics

Modelling and Optimizing Batch Processes in the Chemical Industry

Rainer E. Burkard[1] and Johannes Hatzl[2]

[1] Graz University of Technology `burkard@tugraz.at`
[2] Graz University of Technology `hatzl@opt.math.tu-graz.ac.at`

Dedicated to Professor Capasso on the occasion of his 60th birthday

Summary. In this paper we investigate two different models for minimizing the makespan of batch processes by mixed-integer linear programming models. Special emphasis is laid on a small number of binary variables and on valid constraints. After a reformulation of the objective function, it is for the first time possible to find optimal solutions for medium-sized benchmark problems. Furthermore, a powerful iterative construction heuristic for larger-sized problems is developed.

1 Introduction

In the chemical and pharmaceutical industry, production planning based on batch processes play an important role. This means that there is no continuous stream of resources, but well defined steps in the production process at which the input or output of a task is consumed (respectively, received). The task is to determine the order in which different batches are carried out on different equipment and to find a detailed timing of the execution of all processes and the corresponding batch sizes in order to minimize the makespan. Problems of this kind were considered by several authors. For surveys of this field see, for example, Kallrath [8], Reklaitis et al. [12] and Schilling [15].

In order to give a detailed description of the production process and its components (processing units, batches and resources) Kondili, Pantelides and Sargent [9] introduced the widely used State-Task-Network (STN), that is able to describe the major characteristics of real batch production processes involving variable batch sizes, shared intermediates, flexible proportions of output products, cyclic material flows and non-storable resources.

In this paper two different mixed-integer linear programs are stated for this kind of problem. The first one is called UDM and is based on a uniform discretization of time, which involves restrictions on the times at which a batch could start. The large number of binary variables needed to state MILPs of this type and the enormous computational time to solve even small problems encouraged to think about different formulations of the model and LP-based heuristics to obtain near-optimal solutions.

The second class of models discussed in this paper avoids a uniform discretization of time. This idea was suggested by Sahinidis and Grossman [13] for the first time and has been revived again in different forms by Mockus and Reklaitis [10] and by Schilling and Pantelides [14]. Another step forward was made in the papers by Ierapetritou and Floudas [6, 7]. They proposed an approach that leads to a smaller MILP that has fewer binary variables. Instead of using a binary variable for every time unit, the time horizon is divided into a number of periods such that each point on the time grid corresponds to an event representing the start and end of a batch.

In the following, we analyze these approaches. We discuss how the integrality gap between the optimal solution of the relaxed linear programming representation and its mixed-integer counterpart can be reduced.

Due to the large size of the mixed-integer programming formulations, large instances are still intractable. Thus, heuristical approaches are of special interest. In Burkard et al. [3], a greedy algorithm for makespan minimization for chemical batch processes is proposed. The running times of their approach are moderate even for large instances. Loosely speaking, the running time of the greedy algorithm depends linearly on the makespan of the whole process. In this paper, we revive the idea of this greedy algorithm, but modify some concepts suggested in [3] substantially. Computational experiments show that the new heuristic approach works fast and is satisfactory from the quality point of view.

2 A Problem Formulation Using State-Task-Networks

One of the first attempts to standardize the representation of batch processes was given by Reklaitis [11] in terms of recipe networks. These are similar to the flowsheet representation of continuous plants and are intended to describe the process itself rather than a specific plant. Each node on a recipe network corresponds to a task and directed arcs between nodes represent the task precedences. Due to the fact that resources are omitted, some ambiguities may occur when applied to more complex processing structures. This drawback arises because a recipe network does not distinguish the process operations from the resources that may be used to execute them. State-Task-Networks (STN) are an alternative representation that repair this disadvantage by including both the individual batch operations as well as raw materials, intermediate and final products explicitly as network nodes.

An STN is a description of the process recipe in terms of the set of transformations of material taking place. It is a directed graph which consists of three elements:

1. *state* nodes represent the feeds, intermediate and final products.

2. *task* nodes represent the process operations which transform material from one or more input states into one or more output states. The tasks are processed by facilities and are performed in batch mode.
3. *arcs* indicate the flow of material.

An instance of the problem is characterized by a set S of *states* (raw materials, intermediates and final products), a set T of *tasks* or *batch types* and a set M of *machines* or *production units*. For each state $i \in S$, we are given an *initial stock size* S_i^{init}, a *minimal* and *maximal stock size* $0 \leq S_i^{\text{min}} \leq S_i^{\text{max}}$ describing the storage conditions due to technological reasons, and an *external demand* $d_i \geq 0$. Note that using this notation we are able to model non-storable intermediate products which have to undergo further processing steps immediately by setting $S_i^{\text{min}} = S_i^{\text{max}} = 0$. Without loss of generality, we can assume that $S_i^{\text{min}} = 0$, otherwise we reduce the initial amount S_i^{init} and the maximum stock size S_i^{max} suitably and solve the modified problem.

The *batch processing time* $\tau_b \in \mathbb{N}$ as well as the *minimum* and *maximum batch size* $0 \leq z_b^{\text{min}} \leq z_b^{\text{max}}$ are associated with each task $b \in T$. Thereby, we assume that the processing times are constant per batch, i.e., they do not depend on the particular batch size.

Finally, we need to know the *consumption intensities* $\gamma_{b,i}$ and lower and upper bounds $0 \leq \pi_{b,i}^{\text{min}} \leq \pi_{b,i}^{\text{max}} \leq 1$ on the *production intensities*. A production plan is called *feasible* if the following conditions are satisfied:

1. At any given time, only one batch can run on each machine $m \in M$.
2. The size of each batch $b \in T$ has to be within the limits given by z_b^{min} and z_b^{max}.
3. The proportion of the produced resources of batches that allow variable output has to be within the given limits.
4. The storage capacity constraints for the resources and the mass conservation have to be satisfied at any time.

Using the model described above, a solution is fully specified by the starting times for each batch, the production intensities and the corresponding batch sizes. Concluding we give the key parameters used in the STN representation:

$S = \{s_1, \ldots, s_r\}$ representing the states
$T = \{b_1, \ldots, b_s\}$ representing the tasks or batch types
$T = T^{\text{fix}} \uplus T^{\text{flex}}$ representing the tasks with fixed and variable output
$M = \{M_1, \ldots, M_t\}$ representing the machines
$T(m) \subset T$ representing the tasks
                       that can be processed on machine m.

$S_i^{\text{init}} \geq 0$ initial stock size, $\forall i \in S$
$S_i^{\text{min}} \geq 0$ minimal stock size, $\forall i \in S$
$S_i^{\text{max}} \geq S_i^{\text{min}}$ maximal stock size, $\forall i \in S$
$d_i \geq 0$ external demand, $\forall i \in S$
$\tau_b > 0$ processing time, $\forall b \in T$

$$z_b^{\min} \geq 0 \qquad\qquad \text{minimal batch size, } \forall b \in T$$
$$z_b^{\max} \geq z_b^{\min} \qquad\quad \text{maximal batch size, } \forall b \in T$$
$$0 \leq \gamma_{b,i} \leq 1 \qquad\quad \text{consumption intensity, } \forall b \in T, \forall i \in S$$
$$0 \leq \pi_{b,i}^{\min} \leq 1 \qquad\quad \text{minimum proportion of product } i$$
$$\text{produced in batch } b, \forall b \in T, \forall i \in S$$
$$\pi_{b,i}^{\min} \leq \pi_{b,i}^{\max} \leq 1 \quad \text{maximum proportion of product } i$$
$$\text{produced in batch } b, \forall b \in T, \forall i \in S$$

3 Models Using a Uniform Discretization of Time (UDM)

In this model, we divide the entire time horizon $[0, t_{\max}]$ into a number of smaller periods, i.e., $0 = t_1 < \ldots < t_K = t_{\max}$, of equal length. As a consequence, each batch starts and ends at a time t_k and we only have to calculate the starting points of batch $b \in T$. Thus, we introduce the variable $\lambda_{b,k}$, which is equal to 1 if and only if a batch of type b starts at time t_k. Additionally, we have to find its batch size $z_{b,k}$ in order to describe a feasible solution. ¿From now on we will assume without loss of generality that the length of one time interval is 1, i.e., $t_{k+1} - t_k = 1$ for $k = 1, \ldots, K - 1$.

We may formulate the problem as a mixed integer linear program (MILP) with the following variables:

MS	makespan of the process
$x_{i,k}$	stock size of state i at time t_k
$q_{b,i,k}$	quantity of state $i \in S$ consumed by batch b starting at t_k
$z_{b,k}$	size of batch $b \in B$ starting at t_k
$\lambda_{b,k}$	binary variable equal to 1 if and only if task of type $b \in B$ starts at t_k.

Using the terms introduced in the STN and the variables defined above, we can formulate this model in the following way:

The objective function - minimizing the makespan - is given by

$$\min \ \mathrm{MS} \tag{1}$$

where we have to claim that

$$\mathrm{MS} \geq k \cdot \lambda_{b,k} + \tau_b - 1 \qquad \forall b \in T, \ k = 1, \ldots, K.$$

The stock balance constraints

$$x_{i,1} = S_i^{\mathrm{init}} - \sum_{b \in T} \gamma_{b,i} \cdot z_{b,1} \qquad \forall i \in S,$$

and

$$x_{i,k} = x_{i,k-1} + \sum_{\{b \in T : k-\tau_b \geq 1\}} q_{b,i,k-\tau_b} - \sum_{b \in T} \gamma_{b,i} \cdot z_{b,k} \quad \forall i \in S, \ k = 2, \ldots, K.$$

describe the mass conservation.

In order to model the variable output proportion, we need that

$$\pi_{b,i}^{\min} \cdot z_{b,k} \leq q_{b,i,k} \leq \pi_{b,i}^{\max} \cdot z_{b,k} \qquad \forall b \in T, \ i \in S, \ k = 1, \ldots, K$$

and

$$\sum_{i \in S} q_{b,i,k} = z_{b,k} \qquad b \in T, \ k = 1, \ldots, K$$

hold.

The bounds on the batch sizes are given by

$$z_b^{\min} \cdot \lambda_{b,k} \leq z_{b,k} \leq z_b^{\max} \cdot \lambda_{b,k} \qquad \forall b \in T, \ k = 1, \ldots, K,$$

whereas the storage capacities are described by

$$S_i^{\min} \leq x_{i,k} \leq S_i^{\max} \qquad \forall i \in S, \ k = 1, \ldots, K.$$

To ensure that at the end of the process the external demand is satisfied and that no batch is active any more, we state that

$$d_i \leq x_{i,K} \qquad \forall i \in S,$$

and

$$\lambda_{b,K} = 0 \qquad \forall b \in T.$$

Finally, we have to ensure that at each time only one batch can run on each machine using

$$\sum_{b \in T(m)} \sum_{j=\max(1,k-\tau_b)}^{k-1} \lambda_{b,j} \leq 1 \qquad \forall m \in M, \ k = 1, \ldots, K. \tag{2}$$

Finally, we require that

$$\lambda_{b,k} \in \{0,1\} \qquad \forall b \in T, \ k = 1, \ldots, K$$

and

$$z_{b,k} \geq 0 \qquad \forall b \in T, \ k = 1, \ldots, K.$$

4 A Continuous Time Model (CTM)

The number of binary variables needed in UDM is highly effected by the number K of intervals. This number depends on the processing times of the tasks and the time horizon t_{max}. As an alternative we state another model, whose number of binary variables is not significantly influenced by a different choice of the processing times. Here we just deal with the real variables t_n for $n = 1, \ldots, N$ representing the starting or ending times of batches. Therefore, we need an upper bound on the number N of batch starting or ending times. Binary variables $\lambda_{b,n,j}$ are introduced for describing whether a task of type $b \in T$ starts at time t_n and is still active during the interval $[t_j, t_{j+1})$. In the MILP below, we use the following variables:

t_n n-th time at which some batch can start or end ($n = 1, \ldots, N$)

$x_{i,n}$ stock size of state i at time t_n

$z_{b,n,j}$ size of batch b starting at time t_n
           and still being active during the interval $[t_j, t_{j+1})$

$\lambda_{b,n,j}$ binary variable equal to 1 if and only if a task of type b starts at
           time t_n and is still being active during the interval $[t_j, t_{j+1})$.

$q_{b,n,i}$ quantity of state $i \in S$ obtained from batch b ending at t_n.

Now we can state the MILP. The objective function is given by

$$\min t_N$$

subject to the following constraints. In this model, the mass conservation can be expressed by

$$x_{i,1} = S_i^{init} - \sum_{b \in T} \gamma_{b,i} \cdot z_{b,1,1} \qquad \forall i \in S$$

and

$$x_{i,n} = x_{i,n-1} - \sum_{b \in T} \gamma_{b,i} \cdot z_{b,n,n} + \sum_{b \in T} q_{b,n,i} \quad \forall i \in S, \ n = 2, \ldots, N.$$

To model the variable output of the batches, we state

$$\pi_{b,i}^{min} \sum_{j=1}^{n-1} (z_{b,j,n-1} - z_{b,j,n}) \leq q_{b,n,i},$$

$$q_{b,n,i} \leq \pi_{b,i}^{max} \sum_{j=1}^{n-1} (z_{b,j,n-1} - z_{b,j,n}) \qquad \forall i \in S, \forall b \in T, \ n = 1, \ldots, N,$$

and

$$\sum_{i \in S} q_{b,n,i} = \sum_{j=1}^{n-1} (z_{b,j,n-1} - z_{b,j,n}) \qquad \forall b \in T, \ n = 1, \ldots, N, \ j = n, \ldots, N.$$

Keeping in mind that $\sum_{j=1}^{n-1}(z_{b,j,n-1} - z_{b,j,n})$ is the output of batch b at time t_n, these are exactly the same constraints as in the previous model.

The following inequalities (3) and (4) guarantee that during the time intervals in which a batch is running its size remains constant:

$$z_{b,n,j+1} \leq z_{b,n,j} \qquad \forall b \in T, \ n = 1, \ldots, N, \ j = n, \ldots, N-1, \qquad (3)$$

$$z_{b,n,n} - z_{b,n,j} \leq z_b^{\max}(1 - \lambda_{b,n,j}) \quad b \in T, \ n = 1, \ldots, N, \ j = n, \ldots, N. \qquad (4)$$

By claiming

$$x_{i,N} \geq d_i \qquad \forall i \in S,$$

we ensure the production of the demand d_i for each state i.

In order to fulfill the bounds on the batch sizes when a batch is running, we need to satisfy

$$z_b^{\min} \cdot \lambda_{b,n,j} \leq z_{b,n,j} \leq z_b^{\max} \cdot \lambda_{b,n,j} \qquad \forall b \in T, \ n = 1, \ldots, N, \ j = n, \ldots, N.$$

To force the binary variables to be non-zero for one consecutive range of intervals, we need

$$\lambda_{b,n,j+1} \leq \lambda_{b,n,j} \qquad \forall b \in T, \ n = 1, \ldots, N, \ j = n, \ldots, N-1.$$

By setting

$$\lambda_{b,n,N} = 0 \qquad \forall b \in T,$$

we guarantee that all batches are stopped at the end of the production process.

To avoid that one machine has to execute two processes at the same time we require that

$$\sum_{n \leq j}\sum_{b \in T(m)} \lambda_{b,n,j} \leq 1 \qquad \forall m \in M, j = 1, \ldots, N.$$

In the next constraints, we model that $t_n \leq t_{n+1}$ and the fact that there exist some indices i and j such that every batch starts at t_i and finishes at t_j. To include the ending times, let M be a sufficiently large integer in (6). Note that $\lambda_{b,n,j} - \lambda_{b,n,j+1}$ equals to 1 if and only if batch b ends at t_{j+1} and 0 otherwise. Thus (6) is redundant in the first case, but is satisfied with equality otherwise because of (5).

$$t_{j+1} - t_n \geq \tau_b(\lambda_{b,n,j} - \lambda_{b,n,j+1}) \qquad \forall b \in T, \ n = 1, \ldots, N, \ j = n, \ldots, N-1, \qquad (5)$$

$$t_{j+1} - t_n \leq \tau_b(\lambda_{b,n,j} - \lambda_{b,n,j+1}) + M(1 - (\lambda_{b,n,j} - \lambda_{b,n,j+1})) \qquad (6)$$
$$\forall b \in T, \ n = 1, \ldots, N, \ j = n, \ldots, N-1.$$

Finally, we have the obvious constraints

$$S_i^{\min} \le x_{i,n} \le S_i^{\max}, \qquad \forall i \in S, \ n = 1, \ldots, N,$$

and

$$\lambda_{b,n,j} \in \{0,1\} \qquad b \in T, \ n = 1, \ldots, N, \ j = n, \ldots, N.$$

5 Modifications of the Mixed-integer Linear Programs

Basically, there are two essential features for solving MILPs within a reasonable amount of time. Because of the fact that most optimizers exploit a branch-and-bound algorithm, the number of binary variables plays a key role. Thus, we should try to keep it as small as possible. On the other hand, a small integrality gap also enhances the performance of the solution procedure due to tighter bounds. This gap can be reduced by a reformulation of the objective function and by introducing strong valid inequalities. These inequalities are commonly referred to as cuts and produce a better approximation of the convex hull of integer points by removing several fractional solutions. As a consequence, the branch-and-bound algorithm becomes more effective.

In the following, we give some examples for possible reformulations of the stated mixed integer linear programs. For a more detailed discussion we refer to [4]. Let us assume that we know a lower bound D_i for the amount of state i that has to be produced to guarantee that the external demand is fulfilled at the end. Then, we can state the new constraint

$$\sum_{\{b \in T : \pi_{b,i}^{\max} > 0\}} \sum_{k=1}^{K} \lambda_{b,k} \ge \left\lceil \frac{D_i}{\max_{b : \pi_{b,i}^{\max} > 0} \left(\pi_{b,i}^{\max} z_b^{\max} \right)} \right\rceil \qquad \forall i \in S$$

for UDM which forces batches to start that produce resource i sufficiently often. A corresponding constraint for CTM can be obtained in a similar way. The value D_i can be determined by an appropriate linear program which just takes the mass conservation and the external demand into account.

The objective function (1) in UDM interacts only in a weak way with the constraints of the model. Thus, it is useful to introduce further binary variables f_k, $k = 1, \ldots, K$, which are equal to 1 if and only if the the process is still going on during the interval $[t_{k-1}, t_k)$ and 0 otherwise, satisfying $f_{k+1} \le f_k$ for $k = 1, \ldots, K - 1$. If we change constraint (2) to

$$\sum_{b \in T(m)} \sum_{j=\max(1, k-\tau_b)}^{k-1} \lambda_{b,j} \le f_k$$

the objective function (1) can be equivalently reformulated as

$$\min \sum_{k=1}^{K} k^2 f_k.$$

6 An Iterative Construction Algorithm

It is easy to show that the batch processing problem under discussion is $\mathcal{NP}$-hard in the strong sense since it contains the standard job shop scheduling problem as special case. Thus, we tried to use local search methods that have proved to be very efficient for many scheduling problems in real world applications. However, for the problem discussed in the previous sections, classical metaheuristics based on neighborhood search do not work satisfactorily. The problem is that starting from a feasible solution neighborhood search leads almost immediately to infeasible solutions. It turns out to be rather hard to restore feasibility again. A theoretical result by Burkard et al. [3] confirms this. In this paper it is shown that it is $\mathcal{NP}$-complete to decide whether there exists a feasible solution. The corresponding $\mathcal{NP}$-completeness proof does not even involve many features of the process scheduling problem such as minimum and maximum batch sizes, storage capacities and variable production intensities.

In this section, we propose a construction heuristic that tries to find feasible production plans. The performance of this algorithm has been extensively tested in [5] using different State-Task-Networks from the literature and there was no instance for which no feasible production plan was obtained.

The main contribution of this approach is the fact that it is not based on large MLIPs. Thus the algorithm solves large instances within moderate running times. We give here the key ideas of the algorithm. The idea of the algorithm is to start with the first time period as current one. As long as there are free processing units, we start batches that can be processed on free machines. If all units are occupied, the current time period is increased by one. This loop is repeated until the external demand is satisfied.

The core of the proposed construction algorithm is shown in Algorithm 4. We have three different subroutines:

- PossibleBatchSize
- Wait
- StartBatch

Algorithm 4 Construction Algorithm

1: **while** demand is not fulfilled **do**
2:     Start PossibleBatchSize to get p_b for all $b \in T$
3:     **if** $p_b = 0$ for all $b \in T$ **then**
4:         Start Wait
5:     **else**
6:         Start StartBatch
7:     **end if**
8: **end while**

The aim of the subroutine PossibleBatchSize is to calculate the current maximum allowable batch size p_b for each batch type $b \in T$.

If $p_b = 0$ for all $b \in T$, no batch can be started due to lack of ingredients, storage capacities or free processing units. As a consequence, the start of the subroutine Wait is necessary, which decides when a first batch should be started due to further free units or increased material resources.

If there is a $b \in T$ for which $p_b \neq 0$, it is allowed to start a batch of type b. Now it has to be decided which batch type is started or if we abstain from starting any process. This may be the case, or example, if the external demand of a certain state has already been fulfilled and it is not advantageous to overfill that request. In the subroutine StartBatch, the usefulness of starting a batch of type b is measured. Based on this evaluation it is decided whether b is started or not. Note that the production process always stays feasible during the algorithm in the sense that mass conservation, machine scheduling and storage capacities are always fulfilled.

One drawback of the algorithm is the fact that decisions are based on the production plan so far. The next starting batch type is chosen without considering any future aspects. A made decision, which later may turn out to be unfavorable, cannot be revised. To overcome this difficulty, we divide the entire time horizon into a number of smaller periods. By adding some randomness in the Startbatch subroutine we are able to compute more than just one feasible solution for the first period. Based on certain decision rules we keep good solutions and discard the others. Starting from good solutions we will use the same idea for the next period. These strategies are called diversification and intensification strategies and are widely used in local search algorithms. Here intensification means to restart from high quality solutions of the previous time period, whereas diversification accomplished by the randomness drives the search to examine new solutions.

7 Numerical Results

We used the MILPs described above and the iterative construction heuristic to solve instances of a benchmark problem proposed by Kallrath [8]. An STN representation of this problem can, for example, be found in Burkard and Hatzl [4]. It consists of 24 different tasks, 19 resources and 9 machines, shared intermediates, non-storable products and batches with flexible output. Furthermore there are five endproducts that have to be produced. Thus, this problem is a challenging one and it is sometimes hard to even find feasible solution by trial and error. The MILPs were implemented using the modeling language AMPL, and were solved by the optimization software CPLEX 7.1. During the tests, it turned out that UDM works better due to a smaller relative integrality gap relative to that of CTM. However, CTM typically has fewer binary variables. Thus, a topic for further research is to take advantage of this fact and to develop special branching and node selection strategies that are adjusted for this type of problem. More detailed computational results about other benchmark problems are discussed in Blömer and Günther [1, 2] and Burkard and Hatzl [4, 5].

In the table below, the results of 15 different instances are shown. The external demand of the endproducts is given in the first five columns. In the column denoted by C_{max}, we list the values for the obtained duration of the production process using UDM as discussed above. Finally, we also give the results obtained by the iterative construction heuristic. Optimal solutions are shown in bold letters. Best known solutions are written in italic. Instances 12-15 have not been considered in other papers, because they could not deal such big instances. We also tried exact methods discussed in this paper to judge the quality of the construction method for larger instances, but could not find a feasible solution for instances 12, and 14 within 3 hours. The best makespan obtained for instance 13 was 99; for instance 15, we get a production process that lasts 101 units of time.

Table 1: Objective function values for the instances proposed by Kallrath [8].

	d_{15}	d_{16}	d_{17}	d_{18}	d_{19}	C_{max}	heuristic
1	10	10	20	20	30	**42**	45
2	10	20	30	20	10	**38**	39
3	18	18	18	18	18	**38**	39
4	15	15	30	30	45	*60*	63
5	45	30	30	15	15	*54*	52
6	15	30	45	30	15	*54*	59
7	27	27	27	27	27	*54*	58
8	20	20	40	40	60	*72*	81
9	60	40	40	20	20	66	*64*
10	20	40	60	40	20	*66*	72
11	36	36	36	36	36	*66*	71
12	30	30	60	60	90		114
13	90	60	60	30	30		97
14	30	60	90	60	30		107
15	54	54	54	54	54		99

Concluding it can be said that batch processes for a STN of moderate size can be solved exactly with MILPs. UDM is a powerful approach to find the minimum makespan especially if the batch processing times are similar. We also described a competitive heuristic, which enables to give suboptimal solutions for instances with a large external demand and a long production duration. The heuristic works fast and the results are satisfactory from a quality point of view for all the instances we considered. Feasible production plans can be completed within seconds, which was not possible thus far. Thus, it may be concluded that the iterative construction heuristic is well-suited for practical purposes.

References

1. Blömer, F., Günther, H.: Numerical Evaluation for Scheduling Chemical Batch Processes. Discussion Paper 1999/05, TU Berlin (1999).
2. Blömer, F., Günther, H.: LP-based Heuristics for Scheduling Chemical Batch Processes. International Journal of Production Research, **38**, 1029–1051 (2000).
3. Burkard, R.E., Hujter, M., Klinz, B., Rudolf, R., Wennink, M.: A Process Scheduling Problem Arising from Chemical Production Planning. Optimization Methods and Software, **10**, 175–196 (1998).
4. Burkard, R.E., Hatzl, J.: Review, Extenisons and Computational Comparison of MILP Formulations for Scheduling of Batch Processes. Computers and Chemical Engineering, **29**, 1752–1769 (2005).
5. Burkard, R.E., Hatzl, J.: A Complex Time Based Construction Algorithm for Batch Scheduling Problems in the Chemical Industry. European Journal of Operational Research, 174, 1162–1183 (2006).
6. Ierapetritou, M., Floudas, C.: Effective Continuous-Time Formulation for Short-Term Scheduling. 1. Multipurpose Batch Processes. Industrial and Engineering Chemistry Research, **37**, 4341–4359 (1998).
7. Ierapetritou, M., Floudas, C.: Effective Continuous-Time Formulation for Short-Term Scheduling. 2. Continuous and semicontinuous processes. Industrial and Engineering Chemistry Research, **37**, 4360–4374 (1998).
8. Kallrath, J.: Planning and scheduling in the process industry. OR Spectrum, **24**, 219–250 (2002).
9. Kondili, E., Pantelides, C., Sargent R.: A General Algorithm for Short-Term Scheduling of Batch Operations - I. MILP Formulation. Computers and Chemical Engineering, **17**, 211–227 (1993).
10. Mockus, L., Reklaitis, G.: Mathematical Programming Formulation for Scheduling of Batch Operations Based on Nonuniform Time Discretization. Computers and Chemical Engineering, **21**, 1147–1156 (1997).
11. Reklaitis, G.: Perspective of scheduling and planning of process operations. Proc. PSE'91 Conf., (1991).
12. Reklaitis, G., Sunol, A., Rippin, D., Hortascu. Ö. (eds.): Batch Processing Systems Engineering, Springer Verlag, NATO ASI Series (1996).
13. Sahinidis, N., Grossmann, I.: Reformulation of Multiperiod MILP Models for Planning and Scheduling of Chemical Processes. Computers and Chemical Engineering, **15**, 255–272 (1991).
14. Schilling, G., Pantelides, C.: A Simple Continuous-Time Process Scheduling Formulation and a Novel Solution Algorithm. Computers and Chemical Engineering, **20**, 1221–1226 (1996).
15. Schilling, G.: Algorithms for Short-Term and Periodic Process Scheduling and Rescheduling. Ph.D. Thesis, Department of Chemical Engineering and Chemical Technology, Imperial College of Science, Technology and Medicine, University of London (1997).

Kinetics of Nucleation and Growth: Classical Nucleation and Helium Bubbles in Nuclear Materials

Luis Bonilla[1], Ana Carpio[2], and John C. Neu[3]

[1] Grupo de Modelización, Simulación Numérica y Matemática Industrial, Universidad Carlos III de Madrid, Avenida de la Universidad 30, 28911 Leganés, Spain
`bonilla@ing.uc3m.es`
[2] Departamento de Matemática Aplicada, Universidad Complutense de Madrid, 28040 Madrid, Spain
`ana_carpio@mat.ucm.es`
[3] Department of Mathematics, Universidad de California at Berkeley, Berkeley, CA 94720, USA
`neu@math.berkeley.edu`

Dedicated to Vincenzo Capasso on the occasion of his 60th birthday

Summary. Discrete kinetic equations describe homogeneous nucleation and many other processes such as the formation and growth of helium bubbles due to self-irradiation in plutonium. A key ingredient in the analysis of these equations is a wave front expansion which is the equivalent of boundary layer theory for discrete equations. This expansion solves approximately the nucleation problem, but it needs to be patched to an outer solution describing sizes not too close to the maximum size for the helium bubble problem. The composite theory yields an integrodifferential equation for the monomer concentration of single helium atoms which compares well with numerical solution of the full discrete model.

1 Introduction

Vincenzo Capasso coordinated and led very successfully the ECMI Special Interest Group on Polymers in the late 1990s. In this SIG, there participated groups from the universities of Milan, Barcelona, Florence, Genoa, Eindhoven and my own University, Carlos III de Madrid, the Polish Academy of Sciences and industries from Austria (PCD), Italy (Montell), and the Netherlands (Dow Chemicals, Geleen and Axxicon Moulds, DSM). The book [1] gives a good idea of the work produced by the SIG members. Part of this work dealt with polymer crystallization according to the Ziegler-Natta industrial process.

In this process, tiny spherulites are sown in an undercooled monomer solution and act as nucleation sites to grow polymer crystals to macroscopic sizes. Capasso and his collaborators M. Burger, A. Micheletti and C. Salani modeled this process by assuming that crystal creation is a random process in space and time with a given rate $\alpha(x, t)$ and that the growth of crystals at a given rate $G(x, t)$ is described by level sets. They then derived a homogenized description of the process at macroscopic scales in terms of partial differential equations for the crystallinity, the temperature and the average surface and oriented surface densities; see Chapters 5 and 6 in [1].

In this work, we consider discrete kinetic models of nucleation and growth which are simpler than the polymer models and discuss how to approximate their solutions by singular perturbation methods. Firstly, we present the Becker-Döring equations of classical homogeneous nucleation, and approximate the transient stage until a steady nucleation rate of supercritical clusters by using a wave front expansion [2]. Related work can be found in Chapter 2 of [1]. Secondly, we consider a model for the formation and pure growth of helium bubbles in nuclear materials due to Schaldach and Wolfer [3]. We describe the continuum approximation of this discrete model, which is a first order hyperbolic PDE for the size distribution function having a similarity solution. This solution has a singularity for large cluster sizes which should be fixed by adding a boundary layer. However, boundary layers are typical of PDE problems, and the single minded device of finding the boundary layer for a diffusively regularized PDE fails: the boundary layer solution does not match the similarity solution and neither solution approximates correctly that of the discrete equations. We do two things: (i) correct the first order hyperbolic PDE to include effects due to discreteness, which gives us an outer approximation to the discrete equations, and (ii) we use a wave front expansion to produce a boundary layer solution of the discrete equations which matches the outer solution.

2 Transient Homogeneous Nucleation

2.1 Discrete Kinetic Model

We consider nucleation in a lattice in which there are many more binding sites, M, than particles, N, [2]. We shall consider the thermodynamic limit, $N \to \infty$ with fixed particle density per site, $\rho \equiv N/M$. Let p_k be the number of clusters with k particles (monomers) or, in short, k clusters, and let $\rho_k \equiv p_k/M$ be the density of k clusters. Note that the number densities per site, ρ and ρ_k, are both dimensionless. Number densities per unit volume are obtained dividing ρ and ρ_k by the molecular volume, $v = V/M$. The Becker-Döring equations (BDE) describing homogeneous nucleation are

$$\dot{\rho}_k = j_{k-1} - j_k \equiv -D_- j_k, \quad k \geq 2, \tag{1}$$

$$j_k = d_k \left\{ e^{\frac{D_+ \varepsilon_k}{k_B T}} \rho_1 \rho_k - \rho_{k+1} \right\}. \tag{2}$$

Here $D_{\pm} j_k = \pm(j_{k\pm1} - j_k)$ are the usual finite differences, k_B is the Boltzmann constant and T is the temperature. The rate at which k clusters become $(k+1)$ clusters is the flux j_k in size space, given by the mass action law. We see that clusters grow or decay by adding or shedding one monomer at a time. Notice that d_k is the coefficient for decay of a $(k+1)$ cluster, and we have selected the kinetic coefficient for monomer aggregation so that

$$\tilde{\rho}_k = \rho_1^k \exp\left(\frac{\varepsilon_k}{k_B T} \right) \equiv \rho_1 e^{-g_k}, \tag{3}$$

is the equilibrium size distribution solving $j_k = 0$ (detailed balance assumption). In (2), ε_k is the binding energy of a k cluster, required to separate it into its monomer components and g_k is the free energy per monomer measured in units of $k_B T$. For spherical aggregates,

$$\varepsilon_k = \left((k-1)\alpha - \frac{3}{2}\sigma(k^{\frac{2}{3}} - 1) \right) k_B T.$$

$\alpha k_B T$ is the monomer-monomer bonding energy and

$$\sigma = 2\gamma_s (4\pi v^2/3)^{\frac{1}{3}} / (k_B T),$$

in which γ_s is the surface tension. Note that α and σ are both dimensionless. The monomer density ρ_1 can be obtained from the conservation identity

$$\sum_{k=1}^{\infty} k\rho_k = \rho, \tag{4}$$

in which the total particle density ρ is constant. In (1), $\dot{\rho}_k = d\rho_k/dt$. The time t, the discrete diffusivity d_k and the flux j_k are nondimensional. t and d_k are related to the dimensional time $\tilde{t}$ and decay coefficient $\tilde{d}_k$ as follows [2]

$$t = \Omega \tilde{t}, \quad d_k = \tilde{d}_k / \Omega.$$

Here the factor Ω has units of frequency. Assuming that a monomer has to overcome an activation energy barrier for its transfer across the interface of a cluster, we obtain the Turnbull-Fisher (TF) model for d_k [2]:

$$d_k = k^{2/3} e^{D + g_k/2}, \quad \Omega = 12 D_0 v^{-2/3} e^{-Q/(RT)}.$$

Here $D = D_0 e^{-Q/(RT)}$ is the diffusion coefficient in the liquid, Q is the activation energy for diffusion and $R = k_B N_A$ is the gas constant. In the classical theory, d_k is proportional to the surface area of a k cluster. In other models, d_k is selected so as to yield the known expression for the adiabatic growth of a nucleus of critical size by diffusion, and it is proportional to the cluster radius, thereby to $k^{1/3}$.

2.2 Approximate Description of Transient Nucleation

Inserting the equilibrium solution (3) in (4), we find

$$e^{\alpha}\rho = \sum_{k=1}^{\infty} k \left(e^{\alpha}\rho_1\right)^k e^{-\sigma_k} = \sum_{k=1}^{\infty} k \, e^{k\varphi-\sigma_k}, \tag{5}$$

$$\sigma_k = \frac{3}{2}\sigma\left(k^{\frac{2}{3}}-1\right),$$

$$\varphi = \ln\left(e^{\alpha}\rho_1\right).$$

The series (5) converges for $e^{\alpha}\rho_1 = e^{\varphi} \leq 1$ ($\varphi \leq 0$), and diverges for $e^{\alpha}\rho_1 > 1$ ($\varphi > 0$). At the critical micelle concentration, $\rho_1 = e^{-\alpha}$ ($\varphi = 0$), we obtain the critical density above which equilibrium is no longer possible,

$$e^{\alpha}\rho_c = 1 + \sum_{k=2}^{\infty} k \, e^{-\sigma_k}.$$

For $\rho > \rho_c$, the BDE predict phase segregation, i.e., indefinite growth of ever larger clusters, and there remains a residual monomer concentration whose density $\rho_1 e^{\alpha} \to 1$ as $t \to \infty$. Numerical solutions of the BDE with initial condition $\rho_k = 0$ for $k \geq 2$ and $\rho_1 = \rho$ show that, after a short transient during which φ tends to a constant $\tilde{\varphi}$ and ρ_k becomes a continuous function of k, ρ_k approximates a moving wave front in size space k, as indicated in Fig. 1. Behind the wave front, $\rho_k \approx \tilde{\rho}_k$ (equilibrium distribution), whereas $\rho_k = 0$ ahead of the wave front. The leading edge of the wave front advances until it arrives at the critical size, at which the free energy per monomer, g_k, has a maximum: $k_c \approx (\sigma/\varphi)^3$. Then nucleation of clusters over the critical size begins and, after a certain time, the flux of supercritical clusters reaches a stationary value (the Zeldovich nucleation rate) and transient nucleation ends.

How do we describe approximately these processes until nucleation of supercritical clusters becomes stationary?

It is convenient to redefine the size distribution function to factor out equilibrium,

$$\rho_k = \rho_1 e^{-g_k} s_k = e^{-\alpha} e^{k\varphi-\sigma_k} s_k,$$

so that the BDE (1) and the constraint (4) become ($k \geq 2$):

$$\dot{s}_k + u_k(s_{k+1} - s_k) = -k\dot{\varphi}s_k + d_{k-1}\left(s_{k-1} - 2s_k + s_{k+1}\right), \tag{6}$$

$$u_k = d_{k-1} - d_k e^{\varphi-D+\sigma_k}, \tag{7}$$

$$s_1 \equiv 1 \quad (\forall t > 0), \tag{8}$$

$$e^{\varphi(0)} = e^{\varphi} + \sum_{k=2}^{\infty} k \, e^{k\varphi-\sigma_k} s_k. \tag{9}$$

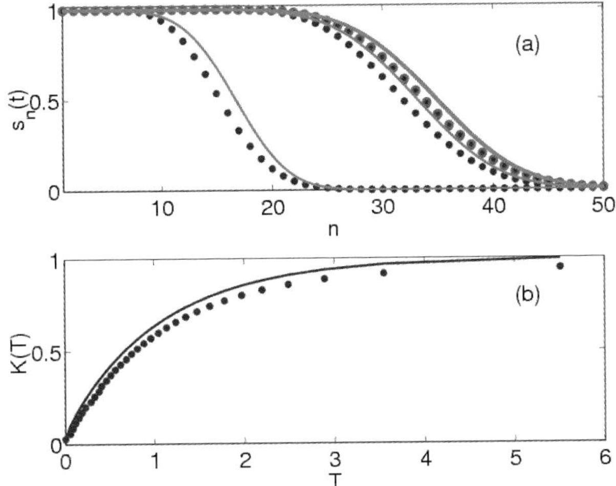

Fig. 1: (a) Comparison of $s_k(t)$ evaluated (at different times) from the numerical solution of the discrete equations (6) - (9) to the asymptotic result (16) (solid line). (b) $K(\tau)$ calculated from Eq. (10) with $K(0) = \epsilon^3$ (solid line) is compared to the numerically obtained position of the wave front. Data correspond to disilicate glass at 820 K with $k_c = 34$. All variables are written in dimensionless units.

In the s_k representation, the wave front described above connects 1 to 0, as k moves across it. For nucleation processes in many materials, the critical size is large. This occurs in particular for devitrification of disilicate glass which provided the parameters used in the numerical simulations depicted in Fig. 1. Then we can use $\epsilon = \tilde{\varphi}/\sigma = k_c^{-1/3}$ as a small parameter and seek an asymptotic description of transient nucleation in the limit as $\epsilon \to 0+$. We shall consider the situation after φ has relaxed to $\tilde{\varphi}$, so that $\dot{\varphi} = 0$ in (6), and we can ignore (9) because it holds identically for all times.

In the numerical solutions shown in Fig. 1(a), the graphs of s_k vs. k at fixed time have clear inflection points at some k, where $s_k \approx 1/2$. The inflection point is taken as the *position* of the wave front. In the continuum model, the front position $k = k_f(t)$ is a smooth function which obeys $\dot{k}_f = u(k_f)$, with $u(k) = u_k$. If we scale $k_f = K/\epsilon^3$, this equation becomes

$$\frac{dK}{d\tau} = U(K), \quad \tau = \epsilon t, \tag{10}$$

$$U(K) \equiv \lim_{\epsilon \to 0}[\epsilon^2 u(\epsilon^{-3} K)] = 2K^{2/3} \sinh\left(\frac{\tilde{\varphi}}{2}(K^{-1/3} - 1)\right), \tag{11}$$

in the limit as $\epsilon \to 0$. Fig. 1(b) compares the wave front position calculated by solving (10) with $K(0) = \epsilon^3$ to the numerical solution of (6) - (9). Note that the solution of (10) presents a time shift with respect to the numerical solution of the discrete model. This time shift reflects the breakdown of the continuum limit as $K \to 0$, due to discreteness, and also the transient in $\varphi(t)$ before it settles to $\tilde{\varphi}$. If the solution of Eq. (10) - (11) is forced to agree with the numerical $K(\tau)$ when the latter is, say, 0.1, the comparison fares much better.

To find the shape of the wave front, we have to describe a layer centered at $K(T)$ in which s_k decreases from 1 to 0 as k increases through it. The continuum representation of s_k in this layer is

$$s_k = S(X, \tau; \epsilon), \quad X = \epsilon^{3/2}\left(k - \frac{K}{\epsilon^3}\right). \tag{12}$$

Inserting (12) into (6), and then using (10), we obtain

$$\frac{\partial S}{\partial \tau} + U'(K)X\frac{\partial S}{\partial X} = D(K)\frac{\partial^2 S}{\partial X^2}, \tag{13}$$

$$D(K) \equiv \lim_{\epsilon \to 0}\left[d\left(\frac{K}{\epsilon^3}\right) - \frac{1}{2}u\left(\frac{K}{\epsilon^3}\right)\right]\epsilon^2 = K^{2/3}\cosh\left(\frac{\tilde{\varphi}}{2}(K^{-1/3} - 1)\right) \tag{14}$$

in the limit as $\epsilon \to 0$. The definition of X has been chosen so that the dominant balance between time derivative of S, diffusion and convection (once (10) has been used) yields (13); see [2]. It is convenient to seek a similarity solution of (13), considering S as a function of a similarity variable:

$$\xi = \frac{X}{2\sqrt{A(\tau)}} = \epsilon^{3/2}\frac{k - \frac{K(\tau)}{\epsilon^3}}{2\sqrt{A(\tau)}}.$$

The equation for $S(\xi)$ is

$$-\left[\frac{1}{2A}\frac{dA}{d\tau} - U'(K)\right]\xi\frac{dS}{d\xi} = \frac{D(K)}{4A}\frac{d^2 S}{d\xi^2},$$

which is

$$\frac{d^2 S}{d\xi^2} + 2\xi\frac{dS}{d\xi} = 0, \tag{15}$$

provided A satisfies

$$\frac{dA}{d\tau} - 2U'(K)\,A = D(K).$$

The solution of (15) satisfying $S(-\infty) = 1$ and $S(\infty) = 0$ is

$$S = \frac{1}{2}\operatorname{erfc}\xi = \frac{1}{2}\operatorname{erfc}\left[\frac{X}{2\sqrt{A(T)}}\right]. \tag{16}$$

This approximate wave front solution can be used to calculate the transient flux of supercritical clusters in excellent agreement with numerical solution of the kinetic BDE [2].

3 Formation of Helium Bubbles in Nuclear Materials

3.1 Discrete Kinetic Model

There are simple kinetic models of irreversible aggregation, in which a cluster with k monomers grows by absorbing one monomer but it cannot decrease in size by shedding part of its mass. An interesting example is the formation and growth of helium bubbles in plutonium alloys as a consequence of alpha decay due to self-irradiation [3, 4]. As an alloy ages, there is an initial transient stage during which self-irradiation produces dislocation loops that tend to saturate within approximately two years. The alpha particles created during irradiation become helium atoms. These atoms come to rest at unfilled vacancies generated during their slowing-down process, before they are captured at existing helium bubbles. A helium atom diffuses through the lattice until it finds another helium atom and form a stable dimer or until it finds a helium bubble (a stable cluster with k atoms or, in short, a k-cluster), which absorbes it. Helium bubbles are attached to lattice defects, do not move and do not shed helium atoms. The following kinetic model based on these observations has been proposed by Schaldach and Wolfer [3]:

$$\dot{\rho}_k = 4\pi D\,\tilde{c}\,a_{k-1}\rho_{k-1} - 4\pi D\,\tilde{c}\,a_k\rho_k, \quad k \geq 3, \tag{17}$$

$$\dot{\rho}_2 = 8\pi D\,\tilde{c}^2\,a_1 - 4\pi D\,\tilde{c}\,a_2\rho_2, \tag{18}$$

$$\tilde{c} + \sum_{k=2}^{\infty} k\rho_k = \int_0^{\tilde{t}} g(t')\,dt'. \tag{19}$$

Here $\dot{\rho}_k = d\rho_k/d\tilde{t}$, ρ_k is the number density of k clusters having effective radii $a_k = a_1 k^{1/3}$ (when the center of a monomer comes within distance a_k of the cluster center, it is absorbed), c is the number of monomers per unit volume, D is the diffusion coefficient and $g(\tilde{t})$ is the number of monomers created per unit volume and per unit time. Eq. (19) means that the helium number density should equal the time integral of $g(\tilde{t})$. In Eqs. (17) and (18), $(k-1)$ clusters can grow to be k clusters by capturing one monomer at a rate $4\pi D\tilde{c}a_{k-1}$ (for $k > 2$), but they do not decay. The rate of creation of an immobile dimer by the collision of two mobile monomers is twice this quantity, $8\pi D\tilde{c}a_1$ [3].

It is interesting to observe that a related kinetic system was proposed and solved in 1914 by McKendrick as a model of leucocyte phagocytosis [5]. In McKendrick's model, ρ_k is the density of leucocytes which have ingested k bacteria, and its rate equation is (17) for $k \geq 0$, with a known function of time $\tilde{c}(\tilde{t}) > 0$ and $\rho_{-1} \equiv 0$. McKendrick's solution method involved solving the equation for ρ_0 in terms of $\int \tilde{c}\,d\tilde{t}$ and solving recursively all other equations for ρ_k as functions of ρ_0. His method cannot be used to solve the system (17) - (19), but an useful closure of this infinite system to only three differential equations was introduced in [3], and compared to experiments, [3, 4].

We shall study the solution of the system (17) - (19) with an initial condition corresponding to the absence of helium bubbles, i.e., $\tilde{c}(0) = 0$ and

298   Luis Bonilla, Ana Carpio, and John C. Neu

$\rho_k(0) = 0$ for $k \geq 2$. We assume a constant production rate, $g(\tilde{t}) = g\tilde{t}$. It is convenient to write the equations (17) - (19) in dimensionless form by using:

$$t = \tilde{t}\sqrt{4\pi Da_1 g}, \quad c = \tilde{c}\sqrt{\frac{4\pi Da_1}{g}}, \quad r_k = \rho_k\sqrt{\frac{4\pi Da_1}{g}},$$

with the result:

$$\frac{dr_k}{dt} = c\left[(k-1)^{1/3}r_{k-1} - k^{1/3}r_k\right], \quad k \geq 3, \tag{20}$$

$$\frac{dr_2}{dt} = 2c^2 - 2^{1/3}c\,r_2, \tag{21}$$

$$c + \sum_{k=2}^{\infty} kr_k = t. \tag{22}$$

These nondimensional kinetic equations should be solved with initial conditions $r_k(0) = 0$, $c(0) = 0$. Defining an adaptive time

$$\frac{ds}{dt} = c, \quad s(0) = 0, \tag{23}$$

we can rewrite (20) and (21) in the more convenient form:

$$\frac{dr_k}{ds} = (k-1)^{1/3}r_{k-1} - k^{1/3}r_k, \quad k \geq 3, \tag{24}$$

$$\frac{dr_2}{ds} = 2c - 2^{1/3}r_2. \tag{25}$$

Time differentiating (22), we obtain

$$c\frac{dc}{ds} + 4c^2 + cM_{1/3} = 1, \tag{26}$$

in which we have defined the moments of the size distribution function $r_k(s)$:

$$M_\mu(s) = \sum_{k=2}^{\infty} k^\mu r_k.$$

M_0 and M_1 are the number densities of bubbles and of helium, respectively. They satisfy $M_\mu(0) = 0$ and:

$$\frac{dM_0}{ds} = 2c, \quad \frac{dM_1}{ds} = 4c + M_{1/3}. \tag{27}$$

3.2 Outer Solution and Relation to the Continuum Limit Equations

A first attempt at approximating the model equations consists of taking the continuum limit of (24) and (22). Assuming that $r_k(s) = r(k, s)$, and Taylor expanding r in (24) up to first order terms, we obtain

$$\frac{\partial r}{\partial s} + \frac{\partial}{\partial k}(k^{1/3}r) = 0, \tag{28}$$

$$\int_0^\infty k\, r\, dk = t. \tag{29}$$

Integrating (28) over $k > 0$, we obtain $(d/ds)\int_0^\infty r\, dk = \lim_{k\to 0}(k^{1/3}r)$, and (27) implies the following signaling condition:

$$\lim_{k\to 0}(k^{1/3}r) = 2c. \tag{30}$$

The method of characteristics provides the following solution to (28) and (30) with initial condition $c(0) = 0$:

$$r(k, s) = 2k^{-1/3}\, c\,(s - a(k))\, \theta\,(s - a(k)), \tag{31}$$

$$a(k) = \frac{3}{2}\, k^{2/3}, \tag{32}$$

in which $\theta(x) = 1$, $x > 0$, and $\theta(x) = 0$, $x < 0$, is the unit step function.

The problem (28) - (30) has the following similarity solution [6]

$$r(\chi, s) = \frac{R_0 s^{-5/4}\chi^{-1/3}}{\left(1 - \frac{3}{2}\chi^{2/3}\right)_+^{3/4}}, \quad \chi = \frac{k}{s^{3/2}}, \tag{33}$$

$$c(s) = \frac{1}{2}R_0\, s^{-3/4}, \quad s = \left(\frac{7}{8}R_0\, t\right)^{4/7}, \quad R_0 = \frac{(27\pi)^{1/4}}{\Gamma(1/4)} \approx 0.837042.$$

Here $f(x)_+ = f(x)\,\theta(x)$. (33) has integrable singularities at $\chi = 0$ and at $\chi = \chi_0 \equiv (2/3)^{3/2}$ (corresponding to the maximum cluster size $k_f(s)$). Related similarity solutions have been recently found by Wattis for a system of equations comprising (17) for $k \geq 2$, $a_k \equiv a_1$ and a closed system of equations for c and M_0 containing source terms proportional to t^w. These equations modelled irreversible aggregation with monomer input [7]. It is not known how well Wattis's similarity solutions approximate $r_k(t)$ because they are not compared to the numerical solution of the full model in [7].

Figure 2 shows that (33) is a relatively poor approximation to the numerical solution of the full model. We need to correct it by including the effects of discreteness and by approximating better $c(s)$. To find the effects of discreteness, we solve the linear equations (24) using the Laplace transform:

$$\hat{r}_k(\sigma) = \frac{(k - 1)^{1/3}\hat{r}_{k-1}}{\sigma + k^{1/3}},$$

for $k > 2$, from which it follows $k^{1/3}\,\hat{r}_k(\sigma) = 2\,\hat{c}(\sigma)\,\hat{R}_k(\sigma)$, thereby

$$r_k(s) = 2k^{-1/3}\int_0^s R_k(s - s')\, c(s')\, ds', \tag{34}$$

$$\hat{R}_k(\sigma) \equiv \prod_{j=2}^{k}\frac{1}{1 + \sigma\, j^{-1/3}}. \tag{35}$$

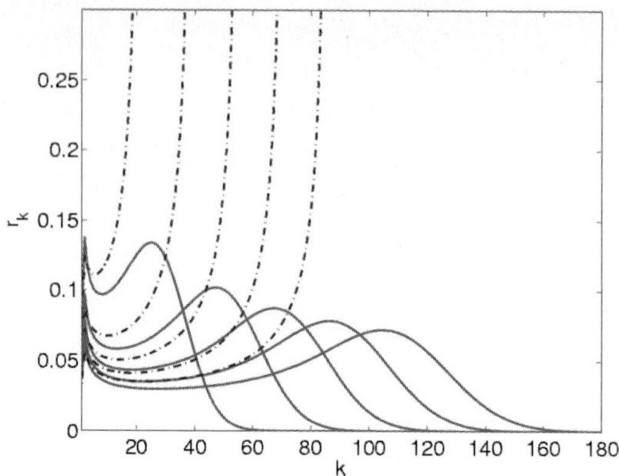

Fig. 2: Nondimensional size distribution function $r_k(t)$ evaluated by solving the full model system of discrete equations (solid line) and the similarity solution (dashed line) at the nondimensional times 100, 200, 300, 400 and 500.

Inserting (34) in (26) yields the integrodifferential equation

$$c\frac{dc}{ds} + 4c^2 + 2c \int_0^s \left[\sum_{k=2}^{\infty} R_k(s-s')\right] c(s')\, ds' = 1, \tag{36}$$

to be solved with $c(0) = 0$. Unfortunately, (36) contains an infinite series of inverse Laplace transforms of (35), which makes impractical using it. An approximate form of (34) follows from assuming that $R_k(s)$ has a narrow peak about its mean value:

$$a(k) \equiv \frac{\int_0^{\infty} s\, R_k(s)\, ds}{\int_0^{\infty} R_k(s)\, ds} = -\frac{\hat{R}_k'(0)}{\hat{R}_k(0)} = \sum_{j=2}^{k} j^{-1/3} \sim \frac{3}{2} k^{2/3} - 3 + \frac{1}{2\,k^{1/3}}, \tag{37}$$

as $k \to \infty$. Provided $c(s)$ is a smooth function (which is not always the case), we may approximate $R_k(s) \sim \delta(s - a(k))$, so that the distribution is given by (31) with $a(k)$ replaced by (37). Eq. (36) becomes

$$c\frac{dc}{ds} + 4c^2 + 2c \sum_{k=2,\, a(k)<s} c(s - a(k)) = 1. \tag{38}$$

For large s, the maximum cluster size is such that $a(k_f) \sim 3k_f^{2/3}/2 - 3 = s$. Then we can approximate the sum in (38) by an integral over k from $k = 0$ to $k = k_f(s)$. Changing variables in the integral, (38) becomes

$$c\frac{dc}{ds} + 4c^2 + 2\sqrt{\frac{2}{3}}\, c \int_0^s (s - s' + 3)^{1/2}\, c(s')\, ds' = 1. \tag{39}$$

In terms of the time t, (23), (31) and (39) become the following local theory

$$r_k(t) = 2k^{-1/3}\, c(s(t) - a(k))\, \theta(s(t) - a(k)),$$

$$\frac{dc}{dt} + 4c^2 + 2\sqrt{\frac{2}{3}}\, c \int_0^t [s(t) - s(t') + 3]^{1/2}\, [c(s(t'))]^2\, dt' = 1, \qquad (40)$$

$$\frac{ds}{dt} = c, \quad \text{with} \quad c(0) = s(0) = 0.$$

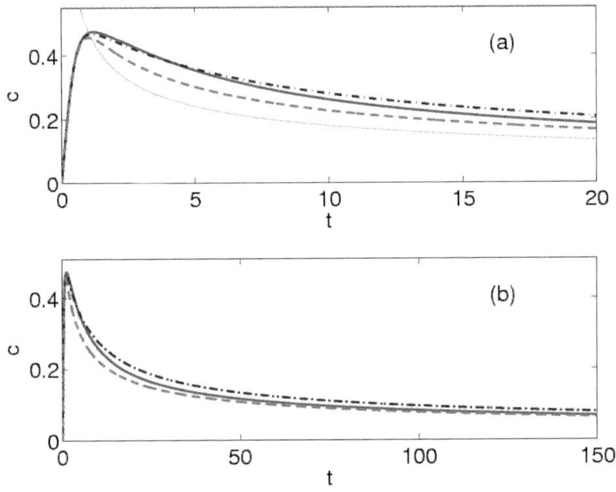

Fig. 3: (a) Monomer concentration $c(t)$ evaluated using: (i) the numerical solution of the discrete equations of the model (solid line), (ii) the local theory (40) (dashed line), (iii) the SW moment equations (dot-dashed line), and (iv) the similarity solution (33) (thin solid line). (b) Same as in (a) for a larger range of times.

Figure 3 shows a comparison between the monomer concentration evaluated by solving the full discrete model equations, the local theory (40), the similarity solution and the three moment equations used by Schaldach and Wolfer (SW) [3]. In Fig. 3(a), we observe that the SW approximation is better for short times, but that the local theory given by (40) provides the best approximation as time goes to infinity, cf. Fig. 3(b). Figure 4 shows the size distribution function calculated at different times by using the local theory (40) (dashed lines) and the numerical solution of the full discrete model. The local theory yields higher cluster densities than the exact solution, a much higher maximum density but it predicts a maximum size which is very close to the local maximum of the real distribution function at large sizes.

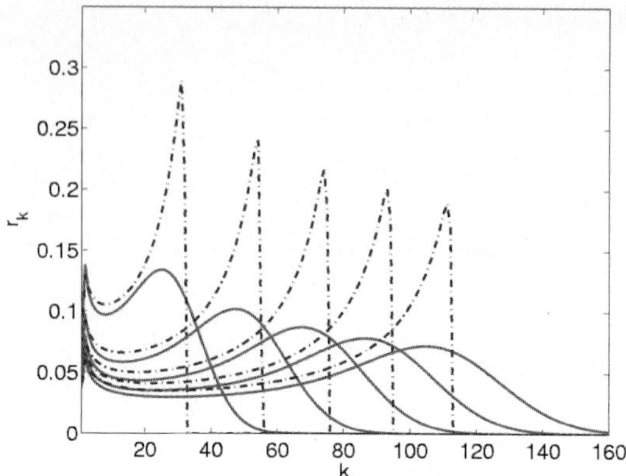

Fig. 4: Bubble distribution $r_k(t)$ calculated from the numerical solution of the full discrete model (solid line) and from the local theory (40) (dashed line).

3.3 Leading Edge of the Size Distribution Function (Inner Solution)

The previous local description of the size distribution function differs substantially from the numerical solution of the model equations for large sizes. However, the maximum of the numerical r_k coincides with the peak of the approximate r_k at $k = k_f(s)$. To improve our asymptotic theory, we should insert a moving boundary layer there. A naive way to do that is to keep an additional diffusive term in the continuum approximation (28), $(1/2)\partial^2(k^{1/3}r)/\partial k^2$, and calculate the corresponding boundary layer correction. In terms of the similarity variable χ of (33), the boundary layer equation is:

$$s\frac{\partial r}{\partial s} + \frac{\partial}{\partial \chi}(\chi^{1/3}r) - \frac{3}{2}\chi\frac{\partial r}{\partial \chi} = \frac{1}{2\,s^{3/2}}\frac{\partial^2}{\partial \chi^2}(\chi^{1/3}r). \tag{41}$$

We now define $X = \chi - \chi_0$, about the approximate location of the maximum size for the outer solution, $\chi_0 = (2/3)^{3/2}$, expand $\chi^{1/3} \sim \chi_0^{1/3} + \chi_0^{-2/3}X/3 = \sqrt{2/3} + X/2$, and substitute in (41). After some algebra and using $\chi = \chi_0$ in the diffusion coefficient, we find

$$s\frac{\partial r}{\partial s} - X\frac{\partial r}{\partial X} + \frac{r}{2} = \frac{\chi_0^{1/3}}{2\,s^{3/2}}\frac{\partial^2 r}{\partial X^2}.$$

We now Fourier transform this equation with respect to X, solve the resulting hyperbolic equation by characteristics and invert the Fourier transform. Then

$$r(X,s) = \sqrt{\frac{ss_0}{4\pi\chi_0^{1/3}(\sqrt{s}-\sqrt{s_0})}}\int_{-\infty}^{\infty} r\left(\frac{X_0 s}{s_0},s_0\right)e^{-\frac{s^2(X-X_0)^2}{4\chi_0^{1/3}(\sqrt{s}-\sqrt{s_0})}}dX_0.$$

We can include the effects of discreteness by using (31), (37) and replacing $X = \chi - \tilde{\chi}_0$, $\tilde{\chi}_0(s) \equiv \chi_0 (1 + 3/s)^{3/2}$, instead of X. The result is

$$r(X,s) = \sqrt{\frac{ss_0 X^2}{\pi \tilde{\chi}_0(\sqrt{s} - \sqrt{s_0})}} \int_0^\infty c\left(\frac{|X|\, s}{s_0 \tilde{\chi}_0^{1/3}}\,\eta\right) e^{-\frac{s^2 X^2 (\eta + \mathrm{sign}\, x)^2}{4\tilde{\chi}_0^{1/3}(\sqrt{s} - \sqrt{s_0})}}\, d\eta. \quad (42)$$

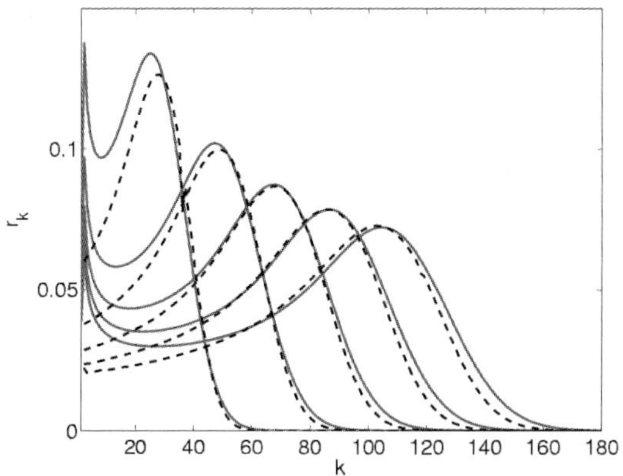

Fig. 5: Bubble distribution $r_k(t)$ from (42) with c given by (40) (dashed line) and the numerical solution of the full discrete model (solid line).

Figure 5 shows that the boundary layer formula approximates the maximum of the bubble distribution at large sizes much better than the other approximations so far discussed. However, this boundary layer approximation cannot match the outer solution which is systematically above the numerical solution of the full model.

An obvious reason for the previous failure of boundary layer theory is that we did not correct the integral kernel in (40) despite the large area underneath the leading edge of the size distribution. Not to mention the cavalier and ad hoc way in which we included the effects of discreteness. Fortunately, we have seen in Section 2 a better way to do boundary layer theory for discrete equations, namely the wave front expansion (12). To use it, we shall rewrite (24) and (26) as

$$\frac{d\sigma_k}{ds} = k^{1/3}\left(\sigma_{k-1} - \sigma_k\right), \quad k \geq 3, \quad (43)$$

$$c\frac{dc}{ds} + 4c^2 + c\sum_{k=2}^\infty \sigma_k = 1, \quad (44)$$

for $\sigma_k = k^{1/3} r_k$, and assume

$$\sigma_k \equiv k^{1/3} r_k = S(X, s), \quad X = k - K(s), \quad 1 \ll X \ll K. \tag{45}$$

$K(s)$ is the position of the inflection point in the leading edge of the wave front. Substitution of (45) in (43) yields

$$\frac{\partial S}{\partial s} - \frac{\partial S}{\partial X}\frac{dK}{ds} = \left(K^{1/3} + \frac{1}{3}K^{-2/3}X + \cdots\right)\left(-\frac{\partial S}{\partial X} + \frac{1}{2}\frac{\partial^2 S}{\partial X^2} + \cdots\right).$$

Provided

$$\frac{dK}{ds} = K^{1/3}, \tag{46}$$

the distinguished limit of the previous equation for S gives

$$\frac{\partial S}{\partial s} + \frac{1}{3}K^{-2/3}X\frac{\partial S}{\partial X} = \frac{1}{2}K^{1/3}\frac{\partial^2 S}{\partial X^2}. \tag{47}$$

If we change variables from s and X to the front location K and the similarity variable $\xi = X/\sqrt{K}$, respectively, (47) becomes

$$K\frac{\partial S}{\partial K} - \frac{\xi}{6}\frac{\partial S}{\partial \xi} = \frac{1}{2}\frac{\partial^2 S}{\partial \xi^2}, \quad \xi = \frac{k - K(s)}{\sqrt{K(s)}}, \tag{48}$$

to be solved with $S(\infty, K) = 0$ and an appropriate matching condition as $\xi \to -\infty$. The solution of (46) is

$$K(s) = \left(\frac{2s}{3} + K_0^{2/3}\right)^{3/2},$$

in which K_0 is an arbitrary positive constant to be selected later. The solution (31) with $a(k) \sim -3 + 3k^{2/3}/2$ yields the matching condition

$$\sigma_k = 2c\left(s + 3 - \frac{3}{2}k^{2/3}\right)_+ \sim 2c\left(3 - \frac{3}{2}K_0^{2/3} - \xi K^{1/6}\right)_+,$$

in the overlap region: $\sqrt{K} \ll (K - k) \ll K$, as $\xi \to -\infty$. The solution of (48) satisfying boundary and matching condition is [6]

$$S(\xi, K) = \frac{2}{\sqrt{6\pi(K^{1/3} - K_0^{1/3})}} \int_0^t [c(t')]^2\, e^{-\frac{\left[\xi K^{1/6} + s(t') - 3 + \frac{3}{2}K_0^{2/3}\right]^2}{6(K^{1/3} - K_0^{1/3})}}\, dt'. \tag{49}$$

Clearly, the front solution (49) contributes to the moment $M_{1/3}$ in (26) for small times corresponding to k in the overlap region. Since S is matched to a variable outer solution, it is convenient to pick a time $t_p(t)$ corresponding to k in the overlap region to split the time interval $(0, t)$ in (40) into two subintervals. For $0 < t' < t_p(t)$, we use the front approximation (45) and (49) whereas we use the outer approximation (31) with (37) for times in $(t_p(t), t)$. The patching time solves

$$s(t_p) = \xi_p \, [K(s(t))]^{1/6} + 3 - \frac{3}{2} K_0^{2/3},$$

for ξ_p in the overlap region. Since the width of the gaussian in (49) is $\sqrt{6}$, we may choose $\xi_p \geq \sqrt{6}$. Up to the patching time, the contribution of the leading edge (49) to the moment $M_{1/3}$ in (26) is $\int_{-\infty}^{\infty} S(\xi, K) \, K^{1/2} d\xi = 2 \, K^{1/3} \int_0^{t_p} [c(t')]^2 \, dt'$. Taking into account the approximation (31), we obtain

$$\frac{dc}{dt} + 4 c^2 + 2\sqrt{\frac{2}{3}} \, c \int_{t_p(t)}^{t} [s(t) - s(t') + 3]^{1/2} [c(t')]^2 dt'$$

$$+2 \, [K(s(t))]^{1/3} \, c \int_0^{t_p(t)} [c(t')]^2 dt' = 1. \tag{50}$$

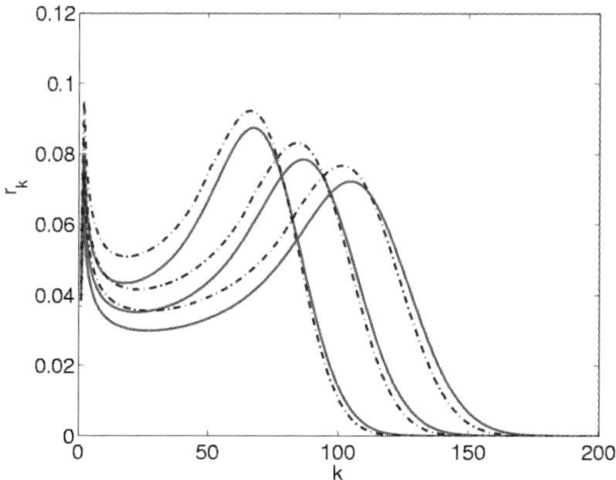

Fig. 6: Nondimensional size distribution function $r_k(t)$ evaluated using the composite solution (50) - (51) (dashed line) and the numerical solution of the full model discrete equations (solid line) at the nondimensional times 300, 400 and 500.

Figure 6 compares the numerical solution of the full discrete model equations to the composite solution:

$$r_k = 2k^{-1/3} c(s(t) - a(k))_+ \theta(K - \xi_p\sqrt{K} - k)$$

$$+\frac{2\,\theta(k - K + \xi_p\sqrt{K})}{\sqrt{6\pi(K^{1/3} - K_0^{1/3})}} \int_0^t [c(t')]^2 \, e^{-\frac{\left[\xi K^{1/6} + s(t') - 3 + \frac{3}{2} K_0^{2/3}\right]^2}{6\,(K^{1/3} - K_0^{1/3})}} \, dt', \tag{51}$$

plus (50) for c. We have used the convenient numerical values $K_0 = 0.5$ and $\xi_p = \sqrt{6}$ without looking for an optimal fit to the numerical solution of the full model equations by varying K_0 and ξ_p. Our final theory agrees much better than (40) with the numerical solution of the full model, but the great differences between the outer solution and the numerical solution at large sizes precludes better agreement between (51) and the numerical solution.

4 Conclusions

We have presented asymptotic descriptions of two problems modeled by discrete kinetic equations coupled to a mass constraint. Transient homogeneous nucleation described by the Becker-Döring equations reduces to the motion of a wave front in size space connecting 1 to zero as the size increases. The leading edge of the wave front is successfully described by an expansion about its inflection point, which is the equivalent of boundary layer theory for spatially discrete equations. The formation of helium bubbles in nuclear materials is modeled by seemingly simpler kinetic equations but with a time dependent mass constraint. As a result, the bubble size distribution is approximated by a composite theory of an outer solution which solves a hyperbolic partial differential equation (corrected by discreteness effects) and an inner solution similar to the wave front expansion of nucleation. Both solutions are functionals of the monomer concentration and both contribute terms to the integrodifferential equation whose solution yields the monomer concentration.

Acknowledgements

This work has been supported by the Spanish MEC grants MAT2005-05730-C02-01 and MAT2005-05730-C02-02, and by the US NSF grant 0515616.

References

1. Capasso, V., editor, 2003. *Mathematical Modelling for Polymer Processing*. Mathematics in Industry **2**. Springer, Berlin.
2. Neu, J.C., Bonilla, L.L., Carpio, A., 2005. Igniting homogeneous nucleation. Phys. Rev. E **71**, 021601 (14 pages).
3. Schaldach, C.M., Wolfer, W.G., 2004. Kinetics of Helium bubble formation in nuclear and structural materials, in *Effects of Radiation on Materials: 21st Symposium*. M.L. Grossbeck; T.R. Allen; R.G. Lott; A.S. Kumar, eds. ASTM STP 1447, ASTM International, West Conshohocken.
4. Schwartz, A.J., Wall, M.A., Zocco, T.G., Wolfer, W.G., 2005. Characterization and modelling of helium bubbles in self-irradiated plutonium alloys. Phil. Mag. **85**, 479–488.

5. McKendrick, A.G., 1914. Studies on the theory of continuous probabilities, with special reference to its bearing on natural phenomena of a progressive nature. Proc. London Math. Soc. **13**, 401–416.
6. Bonilla, L.L., Carpio, A., Neu, J.C., Wolfer, W.G., 2005. Kinetics of helium bubble formation in nuclear materials. Preprint.
7. Wattis, J.A.D., 2004. Similarity solutions of a BeckerDring system with time-dependent monomer input. J. Phys. A **37**, 7823–7841.

Polymer Crystallization Processes

Giacomo Aletti[1] and Diane Saada[2]

[1] ADAMSS and Dipartimento di Matematica, Università di Milano, 20133 Milan, Italy
giacomo.aletti@unimi.it
[2] Department of Statistics, Hebrew University, Jerusalem, Israel
dianes@mscc.huji.ac.il

> *May your heart always be joyful,*
> *May your song always be sung,*
> *May you stay forever young!*
>> Dedicated to Professor Vincenzo Capasso
>> in the occasion of his sixtieth birthday.

Summary. This paper deals with the process of crystallization. We first present two major models that describe this phenomenon either as a birth-and-growth process or in terms of a Johnson-Mehl random tessellation. Then, we estimate the parameters of these models and we establish the asymptotic law of the estimators for the geometrical aspect of this phenomenon. Simulations of these laws are also provided in some cases.

1 The Problem

Due to the influence of temperature, crystals appear randomly in space and time and start to grow. The starting point of any crystal is called a nucleus. According to the assumptions made on this process, the way of covering the space and the models adopted to study this covering will be different. The problem is that, even if the nuclei are generated independently and also grow independently, they are very strongly connected for the two following reasons:

- A new nucleus cannot be born inside an already grown crystal.
- The crystals stop growing at the contact points, when they meet. This phenomenon is called impingement.

The shape of the interface depends on the conditions imposed on the growth and the underlying processes. Moreover, the number of crystals that meet at the same time is controlled and limited by the choice of the model. Some models do not take into account the impingement and deal only with the occupied space and its complement, the free space. The question is, on one hand, to know at any given time whether a point has been covered or not, and on the other, how much of the space has been covered and by how many crystals. Obviously, since nucleation is a random process, the answer is a random variable and we intend to estimate its expected value. The first model we will explain is developed by Capasso et al. [5, 6]. It mainly deals with the free space and with tools and characteristics related to random closed sets as developed in Stoyan et al. [11]. The second one, that deals more with the geometric aspect of these crystals, is developed by Møller [9]. As most of the parameters of these models are non-observable and therefore unknown, we use [2] to estimate them. Finally, we compute or simulate the asymptotic law of some estimators that has been obtained. We start with a review of some well known results on stationary Poisson processes and of the Boolean model as a source for reference.

2 The Boolean Model

Definition 1. *A stationary Poisson process is a point process $\Phi = \{x_i, i \in \mathbb{N}\}$ regarded as a random sequence. It satisfies:*

1. *The number of points of Φ in a bounded Borel set B has a Poisson distribution with mean $\lambda \nu_d(B)$, for some constant λ;*
2. *The numbers of points of Φ in k disjoint Borel sets form k independent random variables.*

Here, ν_d stands for the Lebesgue measure on $\mathbb{R}^d$, it will also be denoted by $|\cdot|$. The intensity measure Λ of the process is defined by $\Lambda(B) = \mathbb{E}[\Phi(B)]$, for any Borel set B, where $\Phi(B)$ is the number of points that fall in the set B.

Define $\Phi_x = \{x_n + x\}$ for any point $x \in \mathbb{R}^d$. Then Φ is stationary if $\mathbb{P}(\Phi \in Y) = \mathbb{P}(\Phi_x \in Y)$, for any measurable set of configurations Y, and for any x. If the distribution of the process is rotation-invariant, it is said to be isotropic.

When the Poisson process is stationary, $\Lambda(B) = \lambda \nu_d(B)$. Thus Λ may be interpreted as the mean number of points of of Φ per unit volume.

Suppose now that $\Phi = \{x_n\}$ is a stationary Poisson process in $\mathbb{R}^d$ of intensity λ. Let $\Sigma_1, \Sigma_2, \cdots$ be a sequence of independent and identically distributed random closed sets in $\mathbb{R}^d$, that are independent from the Poisson process Φ. Σ_n are called grains. The Boolean model is defined as $\Sigma = \cup_{n=1}^{\infty}(\Sigma_n + x_n)$. Due to the stationarity of Φ and the identical distribution of Σ_i's, the process Σ itself is stationary. Furthermore, if the grains are convex, the process is ergodic.

Let Σ_0 denote a random compact set that is distributed like the Σ_n's and independent of them and of Φ. It is called the primary grain of Σ. The distribution of a Boolean model is uniquely determined by its hitting distribution T_Σ (capacity functional), defined by $T_\Sigma(K) = \mathbb{P}(\Sigma \cap K \neq \emptyset)$, for any K compact. It can be shown that $T_\Sigma(K) = 1 - \exp(-\lambda \mathbb{E}[\nu_d(\check{\Sigma}_0 \oplus$

$K)]) = 1 - \exp(-\lambda\mathbb{E}[\nu_d(\Sigma_0 \oplus \check{K})])$, where $\check{A} = -A$ and $\oplus$ is the Minkowski sum.

3 Stochastic Model for the Crystallization Process

The nucleation process is modeled as a stochastic spatial space-time and marked point process N whose random measure is $N = \sum_{n=1}^{\infty} \delta_{(T_n, X_n)}$, where

- T_n represents the random time of birth of the n-th nucleus;
- X_n represents the random spatial location of the nucleus born at time T_n.

The *crystalline phase* at time t corresponds to the function of the space that has been occupied by time t. It involves the definition of the occupied space, $\Theta^t = \cup_{T_j \leq t} \Theta_j^t$ which is the union of all the crystals born up to time t and freely grown up to t. Θ_j^t is the crystal born at time T_j and grown until time t. Then the *degree of crystallinity* at location x and time t is

$$\xi(x,t) = \mathbb{P}(x \in \Theta^t) = \mathbb{E}[\mathbb{1}_{\Theta^t}(x)].$$

Since $\xi(x,t)$ is an important component of the model and is usually unknown, *it has to be estimated*. We denote the compensator of N by ν, and we assume it is given by $\nu(dt \times dx) = \alpha(x,t)(1 - \mathbb{1}_{\Theta^{t-}}(x))dtdx$, where α is called the nucleation rate. We call $\nu_0(dt \times dx) = \alpha(x,t)dtdx$ the free space intensity. Note that if we define the process $N(t) = \sum_{j=1}^{\infty} \mathbb{1}_{\{T_j \leq t\}}$ then its intensity, which is the process λ such that $N - \int \lambda$ is a martingale, is the probability rate of nucleation. It is defined by $\lambda_t dt = \mathbb{P}(N(t + dt) - N(t-) = 1)|\mathcal{F}_{t-})$. The same definition is not given in our case because we do not want to define here a bi-parameter filtration (with respect to space and time).

The corresponding deterministic measure is $\Lambda([0,t] \times B) = \mathbb{E}[N([0,t] \times B)] = \mathbb{E}[\nu([0,t] \times B)] = \alpha(x,t)(1 - \xi(x,t))dtdx$.

Remark 1. Such processes may be viewed as set-indexed processes. If we denote by $Y_n = (X_n, T_n)$ the random variable that characterizes the n-th nucleus, the set-indexed process $N_A = \sum_n \mathbb{1}_{\{Y_n \in A\}}$, where if $T = \mathbb{R}^d \times \mathbb{R}_+$, then A is a compact subset of T of the form $A = B \times [0,t]$, is a marked Poisson process, where the marks correspond to the locations of the crystals.

As before, the occupied space is completely characterized by its hitting functional $T_{\Theta^t}(K) = \mathbb{P}(\Theta^t \cap K \neq \emptyset)$. Note the dynamical aspect of this function. In particular, $T_{\Theta^t}(\{x\}) = \xi(x,t)$. There are several manners to compute ξ, introduced by Capasso et al., see [5] and [4]. A crystal can be born in x, at time t, if the point x was not covered by an already existing crystal by time t. Therefore,

$$\xi(x,t) = 1 - \mathbb{P}(x \notin \Theta^t) = 1 - \mathbb{P}(\text{no nucleation occurs in } A(x,t)),$$

where $A(x,t)$ is the causal cone of a point x at time t, that is the set of possible nuclei that could cover x. The previous quantity is shown to be equal to

$$\xi(x,t) = 1 - \mathbb{P}(N(A(x,t)) = 0) = 1 - e^{-\nu_0(A(x,t))},$$

see [4] in the current book for more details on this topic. Also, if $T(x)$ defines the time of survival of point x with respect to its occupation, then $\mathbb{P}(x \notin \Theta^t) = \mathbb{P}(T(x) > t)$ and this is equal to $1 - \xi(x,t)$. This quantity is denoted by $S(x,t)$ and is called the survival function of $T(x)$. It follows that ξ can also be computed by means of the hazard function associated with $T(x)$. The computation is made in [4].

The next step is to recall some results stated in the paper by Møller [9], which will be useful in the following.

4 Random Johnson-Mehl Tessellations

Definition 2. *A* tessellation *of* $\mathbb{R}^d$ *or a mosaic is a subdivision* $\mathbb{R}^d = \cup_i C_i$ *into d-dimensional non-overlapping sets* C_i*. These sets are called cells or crystals.*

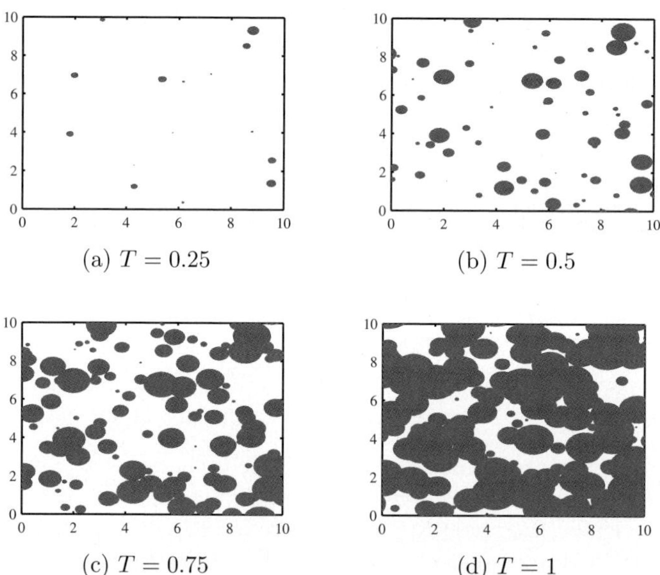

(a) $T = 0.25$ \qquad (b) $T = 0.5$

(c) $T = 0.75$ \qquad (d) $T = 1$

Fig. 1: Johnson-Mehl tessellation with free-rate nucleation $\Lambda(t) = 2.5\sqrt{t}$ and growth speed $v = 1$ at different values of T.

Suppose $\Phi = \{a_1, a_2, \cdots\}$ is a time non-homogeneous Poisson process, where $a_i = (x_i, t_i) \in \mathbb{R}^d \times [0, \infty)$. We denote its intensity measure by $dx\Lambda(dt)$. These points correspond to the nuclei that can potentially be born and grow. Now imagine a point x_i starts to grow with a constant speed $v > 0$ in all directions. It will cover a given area that will increase with time but may also stop increasing in some directions, whenever an impingement occurs. A point y in the space is reached by a_i at time $T_i(y) = t_i + \|x_i - y\|/v$. We can define

$$C_i = C(a_i|\Phi) = \{y \in \mathbb{R}^d | \forall j \neq i; T_i(y) \leq T_j(y)\}$$

which is the set of points in $\mathbb{R}^d$ first reached by a_i. The cells C_i form a *Johnson-Mehl tessellation*. In the case of a *Voronoi tessellation*, i.e. when all nuclei are assumed to be born at the same time t_0 ($\Lambda(dt) = \alpha\delta_{t_0}$), there is no reason to specify the birth time and therefore, $C(x_i|\Phi) = \{y \in \mathbb{R}^d; \|x_i - y\| \leq \|x_j - y\|$, for all $x_j \in \mathbb{R}^d\}$. It consists of all points that have x_i as nearest nucleus. In an equivalent manner, one has $C(x_i|\Phi) = \cap_{j;j \neq i} H(x_i, x_j)$ where $H(x_i, x_j)$ is the closed half-space $H(x_i, x_j) = \{y \in \mathbb{R}^d; (y - z_{ij}) \cdot (x_i - x_j) \geq 0\}$ that contains x_i and bounded by the bisecting hyperplane $G(x_i, x_j)$ of x_i and x_j, with $z_{ij} = \frac{1}{2}(x_i + x_j)$. Such characterization does not hold for general Johnson-Mehl tessellations, but still the notion of interfaces deserves a definition, since it will be of interest for us.

The paper assumes the following consistency assumptions.

1. For any $(x, t) \in \Phi$ and any unit vector $u \in \mathbb{R}^d$, there exists (y, s) with $(y - x) \cdot u > v(s - t)$.
2. No nucleus is born at the point y at the time at which another growing nucleus reaches y.
3. No $m + 1$ nuclei lie on an $(m - 1)$-dimensional affine subspace of $\mathbb{R}^d$, $m = 1, \cdots, d$.
4. No $d + 2$ arrivals reach any point at the same time.

The first condition implies that any crystal is bounded and has only a finite number of neighboring crystals. The second condition ensures that the crystals constitute a tessellation and that each of them is a domain ($C_i = \overline{C_i^\circ}$). The third and fourth ones are concerned with the *n-facets* to be defined as follows.

Define $F_n = \cap_{i=0}^m C_i$ with $m = d - n \geq 0$. For $n = d$ a d-facet is a crystal. When $d = 3$, the 0-facet is a vertex obtained as the intersection of 4 crystals, the 1-facet is an edge, the 2-facet is a face. The third condition is equivalent to assuming that any n-facet has dimension n. For $0 \leq n \leq d$, we define a virtual object,

$$G_n = G(a_0, \cdots, a_m) = \{y \in \mathbb{R}^d; T(y, a_0) = \cdots = T(y, a_m)\}.$$

This would have been the interface of the crystals $a_0, \cdots, a_m$, if there had been no other crystals in this neighborhood. In particular, this set may be empty in the real tessellation, and non-empty if we deal only with these crystals. This set is called a mathematical n-facet. Therefore,

$$F_n = F(a_0, \cdots, a_m | \Phi) = \{y \in G_n; \forall a \in \Phi \setminus \{a_0, \cdots, a_m\}, T(y, a_0) \leq T(y, a)\}.$$

So $F_n = G_n$ if $\Phi = \{a_0, \cdots, a_m\}$, yet they will not be equal in general, since one set does not take into account the whole configuration, while the second one does. The fourth condition is equivalent to assuming that $G(a_0, \cdots, a_m) = \emptyset$ whenever $a_0, \cdots, a_m$ are distinct nuclei with $m > d + 1$. It follows that F_n itself is either an empty set or with dimension n. Let us go further in the Poisson model. The key result is due to Slivnyak [12].

Proposition 1 (Slivnyak formula). *For any non-negative measurable function f and all $m = 0, 1, \cdots,$*

$$\mathbb{E}\left[\sum_{a_0, \cdots, a_m \in \Phi} {}^{\neq} f(a_0, \cdots, a_m, \Phi \setminus \{a_0, \cdots, a_m\}) \right]$$

$$= \int \cdots \int \mathbb{E}[f((x_0, t_0), \cdots, (x_m, t_m), \Phi)] dx_0 \cdots dx_m \Lambda(dt_0) \cdots \Lambda(dt_m).$$

Here $\sum^{\neq}$ denotes the summation over tuples of distinct arrivals.

We write here the proof given by Møller [10]. Another proof can be found in the book of Stoyan et al. [11] Both are given in the homogeneous case. The non-homogeneous extension is not difficult to derive. We start with the definition of the Palm distribution and the Campbell measure.

Let $(N, \mathcal{N})$ be a measurable space where N is the family of all subsets ϕ in $\mathbb{R}^d$ that are locally finite and simple (they do not contain multiple points). In other words, ϕ is any configuration of Φ. To understand this notation, let us define the expectation of $\Phi(B)$ for any Borel subset B. One has $\mathbb{E}[\Phi(B)] = \int \phi(B) \mathbb{P}(d\phi) = \mathbb{E} \sum_{x \in B} \mathbb{1}_B(x) = \int \sum_{x \in \phi} \mathbb{1}_B(x) \mathbb{P}(d\phi) = \int \int \mathbb{1}_B(x) \phi(dx) \mathbb{P}(d\phi)$.

The Campbell measure $\mathcal{C}$ is a measure defined on $\mathbb{R}^d \times N$, by

$$\int \sum_{x \in \phi} f(x, \phi) \mathbb{P}(d\phi) = \int f(x, \phi) \mathcal{C}(d(x, \phi))$$

where f is any non-negative measurable function on $\mathbb{R}^d \times N$. It is easy to see that $\mathcal{C}(B \times Y) = \int \phi(B) \mathbb{1}_Y(\phi) \mathbb{P}(d\phi)$, for B Borel set and $Y \in \mathcal{N}$. Therefore $\mathcal{C}(B \times Y) = \mathbb{E}[\Phi(B); \Phi \in Y]$. The reduced Campbell measure $\mathcal{C}^!$ is defined when we deal with a subset of Φ, by

$$\int \sum_{x \in \phi} f(x, \phi \setminus \{x\}) \mathbb{P}(d\phi) = \int \sum_{x \in \Phi} f(x, \phi - \delta_x) \mathbb{P}(d\phi) = \int f(x, \phi) \mathcal{C}^!(d(x, \phi)).$$

$\phi \setminus \{x\}$ and $\phi - \delta_x$ refer to ϕ with the point $x \in \phi$ deleted. We suppose now that Λ is σ-finite. The measure $B \mapsto \mathcal{C}(B \times Y)$ is absolutely continuous with respect to Λ. Therefore we can write $\mathcal{C}(B \times Y) = \int_B P_x(Y)\Lambda(dx)$, where P_x is the Radon-Nikodym derivative of $\mathcal{C}$ with respect to Λ. For each given x, $P_x(\cdot)$ is a distribution on $(N, \mathcal{N})$, called the *Palm distribution*. What is the meaning of this distribution? We follow [11, page 110]. Suppose for example, we want to compute the probability $\mathbb{P}(\Phi(b(x,r)) = 1|x)$ which is the probability conditioned on $\{x \in \Phi\}$ that Φ does not have any other point within the sphere of radius r centered at x. Since we condition on an event of zero probability, this conditional probability has to be explained. First, suppose the process to be spatially homogeneous. Then $\mathbb{P}(\Phi \in Y|x) = \mathbb{P}(\Phi \in Y_{-x}|0)$ where $Y_x = \{\phi_x, \phi \in Y\}$ with $\phi_x = \{x_n + x\}$ whenever $\phi = \{x_n\}$. Now, we have seen that $\mathbb{E}\left[\sum_{x \in \Phi} h(x, \Phi)\right] = \int \sum_{x \in \phi} h(x, \phi)\mathbb{P}(d\phi)$. Therefore, if we partition $\mathbb{R}^d$ into the domains $D_1, D_2, \cdots$, we get $\mathbb{E}\left[\sum_{x \in \Phi} h(x, \Phi)\right] = \sum_k \mathbb{E}\left[\sum_{x \in \Phi \cap D_k} h(x, \Phi)|\Phi(D_k) > 0\right]\mathbb{P}(\Phi(D_k) > 0)$. Suppose that each D_k tends to an infinitesimal volume element dx. Then $\mathbb{P}(\Phi(D_k) > 0)$ should converge to $\Lambda(dx)$ while the conditional mean would converge to the mean of $h(x, \phi)$ with respect to $\mathbb{P}(\cdot|x)$. So $\mathbb{E}[\sum_{x \in \Phi} h(x, \Phi)] = \int \mathbb{E}[h(x, \Phi)|x]\Lambda(dx)$. Actually, if the process is stationary, then the relation becomes $\mathbb{E}[\sum_{x \in \Phi} h(x, \Phi)] = \lambda \int \mathbb{E}[h(x, \Phi_x)|0]dx$, since $\Lambda = \lambda\nu_d$.

Set $P_0(Y) = \mathbb{P}(\Phi \in Y|0)$ so $\int \sum_{x \in \phi} h(x, \phi)\mathbb{P}(d\phi) = \lambda \int \int h(x, \phi_x)P_0(d\phi)dx$. Taking $h(x, \phi) = \mathbb{1}_B(x)\mathbb{1}_Y(\phi - x)$, we get the definition of P_0 namely,

$$P_0(Y) = \int \sum_{x \in \phi \cap B} \mathbb{1}_Y(\phi - x)\mathbb{P}(d\phi)/\lambda\nu_d(B) \text{ for } Y \in \mathcal{N}.$$

In the stationary case, it can be shown that $P_0(Y) = P_x(Y_x)$. In fact, $\lambda \int_B P_z(Y)dz = \mathcal{C}(B \times Y) = \mathcal{C}(B_x \times Y_x) = \lambda \int_{B_x} P_y(Y_x)dy = \lambda \int_B P_{x+z}(Y_x)dz$, for all B, x and Y. It follows that the Campbell Theorem is a consequence of the Palm measure since $\mathbb{E}[\sum_{x \in \Phi} h(x, \Phi)] = \int h(x, \phi)\mathcal{C}(d(x, \phi)) = \lambda \int \int h(x, \phi)P_x(d\phi)dx = \lambda \int \int h(x, \phi_x)P_0(d\phi)dx$.

Actually, there is also a connection between the reduced Campbell measure and the reduced Palm distribution defined as follows $P_0^!(Y) = \mathbb{P}(\Phi \setminus \{0\} \in Y)|0)$ for $Y \in \mathcal{N}$. Following the same computation as before, we get that $\int \sum_{x \in \phi} f(x, \phi \setminus \{x\})\mathbb{P}(d\phi) = \int f(x, \phi)\mathcal{C}^!(d(x, \phi)) = \lambda \int \int f(x, \phi)P_x^!(d\phi)dx = \lambda \int \int f(x, \phi_x)P_0^!(d\phi)dx$. If we manage to replace the reduced Palm measure in the equation by the probability measure $\mathbb{P}$ then we get exactly the Slivnyak equation. This is the background of the following proof.

Proof. (of Slivnyak formula), [10]. When Φ is a Poisson process, then $P_x = \mathbb{P} * \delta_{\delta_x}$. Here δ_{δ_x} denotes the distribution of the point process that consists solely of the point $\{x\}$. This convolution of distributions corresponds to the superposition of the two processes $\Phi \setminus \{x\}$ and $\{x\}$. The previous equation can be written as $P_x(Y) = \mathbb{P}(\Phi \in Y|x) = \mathbb{P}(\Phi \cup \{x\} \in Y)$ that is $\int f(\phi)P_x(d\phi) = \int f(\phi \cup \{x\})\mathbb{P}(d\phi)$ for all measurable non-negative function f. Therefore, this equality boils down to $P_x^! = \mathbb{P}$, which is exactly the identity we need to state.

The equality of $\mathbb{P} * \delta_{\delta_x}$ and P_x is established if $\mathbb{P} * \delta_{\delta_x}(V_K) = P_x(V_K)$, for all compact K in $\mathbb{R}^d$ and $V_K = \{\phi \in N; \phi(K) = 0\}$. Suppose A is a bounded Borel set. Then $\int_A \mathbb{P} * \delta_{\delta_x}(V_K)\Lambda(dx) = \int_{A \setminus K} \mathbb{P}(V_K)\Lambda(dx) = \mathbb{P}(V_K)\Lambda(A \setminus K) = \mathbb{E}[\Phi(A \setminus K); \Phi(K) = 0]$ since the Poisson process is with independent increments. This is equal to $\mathcal{C}((A \setminus K) \times V_K)$. Obviously, $\mathcal{C}((A \cap K) \times V_K) = \mathbb{E}[\Phi(A \cap K); \Phi(K) = 0] = 0$ and therefore, $\int_A \mathbb{P} * \delta_{\delta_x}(V_K)\Lambda(dx) = \mathcal{C}(A \times V_K)$ $= \int_A P_x(V_K)\Lambda(dx)$. $\square$

We go back now to the paper of Møller. Recall that the intensity of the Poisson birth process is given by $dx\Lambda(dt)$, where Λ represents the mean number of new nucleations per unit volume that occur during the time interval $[t, t + dt)$. Suppose that $\Lambda([0, \infty)) > 0$ and set $\lambda = \int S(t)\Lambda(dt) < \infty$, where $S(t) = \exp\{-v^d\omega_d \int_0^t (t - s)^d\Lambda(ds)\}$ is the probability that an arbitrary point in $\mathbb{R}^d$ is not reached by any growing nuclei at time t, and $\omega_d = \pi^{d/2}/\Gamma(\frac{d}{2} + 1)$ is the volume of the unit ball in $\mathbb{R}^d$. The quantity inside the exponential function represents the volume of the causal cone of any point and is accordingly space homogeneous. From the Slivnyak formula applied to $\int \int \mathbb{E}[\mathbb{1}_{A(x,t)=\emptyset}\mathbb{1}_{x \in B}]\Lambda(dt)dx$ we obtain that

$$\lambda = \mathbb{E}[\#\{i|C_i \neq \emptyset, x_i \in B\}]/|B|.$$

According to this latter definition, one can refer to λ as the intensity of crystals, that is the mean number of crystals per unit of volume. This quantity is independent of the choice of B because the process is assumed to be space homogeneous.

Remark 2 (see [2]). The definition of λ leads to $\lambda|B| = \int_0^\infty \int_B S(t)\Lambda(dt)dx$. Now if we combine the two points of view, then $S(t) = \mathbb{P}(x \notin \Theta^t)$ no matter where point x is in the plane. Therefore, if we set $\xi(t) = \mathbb{P}(x \in \Theta^t)$ in the stationary case, we get that $\lambda|B| = \int_0^\infty \int_B (1 - \xi(t))\Lambda(dt)dx$, which is equal to $\mathbb{E} \int_0^\infty \int_B \mathbb{1}_{(\Theta^t)^c}(x)\Lambda(dt)dx = \mathbb{E}[\sum_x \mathbb{1}_B(x)\mathbb{1}_{(\Theta^t)^c}(x)]$. This leads to a dynamic definition of λ, and $\lambda(t)$ refers to the mean number of crystals per volume up to time t, that is

$$\lambda(t) = \int\int \mathbb{1}_B \mathbb{E}[\mathbb{1}_{A(x,s)=\emptyset}; \mathbb{1}_{[0,t]}(s)]\Lambda(dt)dx = \sum_{(x_i,t_i) \in \Phi} \mathbb{E}[\mathbb{1}_{A_{a_i}=\emptyset}; t_i \leq t; x_i \in B].$$

If C is a typical crystal, its Palm distribution is defined by $\mathbb{E}[h(C)] = \mathbb{E} \sum_{i;x_i \in B, C_i \neq \emptyset} h(C_i - x_i)/\lambda|B|$, for any non-negative measurable functions h. In particular when $h = \mathbb{1}_Y$ we obtain the definition given above. Using the formula of Slinvyak, we get that

$$\mathbb{E}[h(C)] = \int \mathbb{E}\left[h\Big(C((0,t)|\Phi_t \cup \{(0,t)\})\Big)\right]\frac{p(t)}{\lambda}\Lambda(dt),$$

where $\Phi_t = \{a \in \Phi; T(0, a) > t\}$, the collection of points that have not yet been captured 0 by time t. According to this equation, $\frac{S(t)}{\lambda}\Lambda(dt)$ is interpreted as the density of the birth time τ of C.

In order to estimate the way the crystals are making a tessellation, it is useful to compute several characteristics. Towards this end, we denote by L_k the k-dimensional affine subspace of $\mathbb{R}^d$, with $0 < k \leq d$.

Definition 3. *The* mean $(k - m)$-content *of* n-interfaces intersected with a Borel set $B \subseteq L_k$ is defined by

$$\mu_{k,k-m}(B) = \frac{1}{(m+1)!}\mathbb{E}\Big[\sum_{a_0,\cdots,a_m \in \Phi} {}^{\neq}\lambda_{k-m}(B \cap F(a_0,\cdots,a_m|\Phi))\Big],$$

for $m = 0,\cdots k$. λ_{k-m} *denotes the* $(k - m)$*-dimensional Hausdorff measure.*

Recall that if d is the dimension of the space then $n = d - m$ is the dimension of the interface of $m + 1$ intersecting crystals. Consider a subspace of dimension k, then $B \cap F(a_0, \cdots, a_m | \Phi)$ corresponds to the portion of B that is occupied by this interface. This object is of Hausdorff dimension $k - m$. Indeed Møller proved that the $(k - m)$-facet $F_n \cap L_k$ is of Hausdorff dimension $k - m$. (In the case of the Voronoi tessellation, it is easy to show that $G(x_0, \cdots, x_m) = z_{0\cdots m} + L_{d-m}$ where if L_m is the m-dimensional linear subspace generated by $(x_1 - x_0, \cdots, x_m - x_0)$ then $L_{d-m} = L_m^\perp$ and $z_{0\cdots m}$ is the center of the sphere in $x_0 + L_m$, which contains $x_0, \cdots, x_m$. Therefore, the dimension of G_m is $d - m$. Now, if we deal with $G(x_0, \cdots, x_m) \cap L_k$, then we define $\mathcal{L}_m$ the linear subspace generated by $(x_1 - x_0, \cdots, x_m - x_0)$ and we denote by $\mathcal{L}_{k-m}^\perp$ its orthogonal in L_k. It follows that $G(x_0, \cdots, x_m) \cap L_k = z_{0\cdots m} + \mathcal{L}_{k-m}^\perp$ which implies that this set is of dimension $k - m$). Actually, because the Poisson process is stationary in space, the measure μ is translation-invariant and does not depend on the choice of B. Therefore, $\mu_{k,k-m}(B) = \mu_{k,k-m}\lambda_k(B)$, where $\mu_{k,k-m}$ is a non-negative constant that corresponds to the mean $(k - m)$-content of $(k - m)$-interfaces per unit volume in L_k. $\mu_{k,k-m}$ is called the density of $(k - m)$-interfaces in L_k.

Theorem 1 (Møller). *For each of the cases*

1. $0 < k = m \leq d$, that concerns the vertices in L_k
2. $1 \leq k = m + 1 \leq d$ that concerns the edges in L_k
3. $k = d$ and $m = 1$ that concerns the faces in $\mathbb{R}^d$
4. $1 \leq k \leq d$ and $m = 0$ that concerns the k-interfaces in L_k

it holds that

$$\mu_{k,k-m} = v^{md+n}c_{kn}\int_0^\infty \Big\{\int_0^t (t - s)^{d-1}\Lambda(ds)\Big\}^{m+1}S(t)dt$$

where

$$c_{kn} = \frac{2^{m+1}\pi^{(m+1)d/2}\Gamma(\frac{dm+n+1}{2})\Gamma(\frac{k+1}{2})}{(m+1)!\Gamma(\frac{dm+n}{2})\Gamma(\frac{d+1}{2})^{m+1}\Gamma(\frac{k-m+1}{2})}.$$

An interesting point is the connection between this function and the hazard function, since $\mu_{k,k-m} = \text{constant} \int_0^\infty h(t)^{m+1} S(t) dt$, where $h(t)$ is the hazard function in the homogeneous case.

In particular $\mu_{d,d}$ is the mean local volume density, and $\mu_{d,d-1}$ is the mean local surface density of the crystallized region. This formula is extended by Capasso et al. to the dynamic case. Define $C(a_i, t|\Phi)$ to be the crystal generated by the nucleus a_i, viewed when it is $t - t_i$ units of times old. Also, define the amorphous region at time t, $C_e(t|\Phi) = \{y; T(y, a_i) > t, \forall i \in \mathbb{N}\}$. Denote by $F(t, a_0, \cdots, a_m|\Phi)$ the dynamic n-interface at time t. $F(t, a_0, \cdots, a_m|\Phi) = \cap_{i=0}^m C(a_i, t|\Phi)$. In fact one of the a_i's can be equal to e.

The mean $(k - m)$-content of n-interfaces intersected with a Borel set $B \subseteq L_k$ at time t is defined by

$$\mu_{k,k-m}(t, B) = \frac{1}{(m+1)!} \mathbb{E}\left[\sum_{a_0, \cdots, a_m \in \Phi} {}^{\neq} \lambda_{k-m}(B \cap F(t, a_0, \cdots, a_m|\Phi)) \right],$$

for $m = 0, \cdots k$. Again, following the space stationarity argument, we obtain that $\mu_{k,k-m}(t, B) = \mu_{k,k-m}(t) \lambda_k(B)$, where if the rate of growth is constant

$$\mu_{k,k-m}(t) = c_{d,n} \int_0^t \left(\int_0^\tau (\tau - s)^{d-1} \Lambda(ds) \right)^{m+1} S(\tau) d\tau.$$

5 Estimators

As a crystallization process is characterized at any time t by the already covered space and by the geometrical characteristics of this covered space, a better understanding of the model may be obtained if we estimate the corresponding parameters. We follow here Aletti and Saada [2]. Let $(\Omega, \mathcal{F}, \{\mathcal{F}_t\}_{t \in \mathbb{R}_+}, \mathbb{P})$ be a filtered probability space (the filtration $\{\mathcal{F}_t\}_{t \in \mathbb{R}_+}$ is assumed to have the usual properties) and let $(E, \mathcal{E}, |\cdot|)$ be a nonnegative measure space.

Definition 4. *A $\mathbb{R}_+ \times E$-indexed stochastic process $N : \Omega \to \{0, 1\}$ is a crystallization on E if*

- *$\{(t, x, \omega) \in \mathbb{R}_+ \times E \times \Omega : N_{t,x}(\omega) = 1\} \in \mathcal{B}_{\mathbb{R}_+} \otimes \mathcal{E} \otimes \mathcal{F}$, where $\mathcal{B}_{\mathbb{R}_+}$ is the Borel σ-algebra on $\mathbb{R}_+$ (i.e. the process is measurable),*
- *For any $t \in \mathbb{R}_+$, $\{(x, \omega) \in E \times \Omega : N_{t,x}(\omega) = 1\} \in \mathcal{E} \otimes \mathcal{F}_t$ (which implies that the process is $(\mathcal{F}_t)$-adapted),*
- *$\mathbb{P}(\{N_{0,x} = 0, \forall x \in E\}) = 1$,*
- *$\mathbb{P}(\{N_{s,x} \leq N_{t,x}, \forall x \in E, \forall s \leq t\}) = 1$.*

Given a crystallization N, the *crystalline phase* Θ_t at time t is the $\mathcal{E}$-valued stochastic process defined as $\Theta_t^{(N)}(\omega) := \{x \in E : N_{t,x}(\omega) = 1\}$. Denote by $A_x(t) = \int_0^t h(x, s) ds$ the cumulative hazard function at point x and time t. We provide here three alternative estimators for the survival function in the spirit of the Kaplan-Meier estimator, adapted to this context. The use of each of them depends on the kind of data available. These estimators are obviously used to estimate the degree of crystallinity since $\xi(x,t) = 1 - S(x,t)$. We first introduce some notation and then define the estimators.

- $(N_{t,x}^{(i)})_{i=1,\dots,n}$ are n i.i.d. *crystallization processes* on E;
- the censoring times $(U_i)_{i=1,\dots,n}$ are assumed to be n stopping times;
- $\mathfrak{N}_x(t) := \sum_1^n \widetilde{N}_{t,x}^{(i)}$, where $\widetilde{N}_{t,x}^{(i)} := N_{t \wedge U_i, x}^{(i)} = \mathbb{1}_{U_i \geq t} N_{t,x}^{(i)} + \mathbb{1}_{U_i < t} N_{U_i,x}^{(i)} = \int_0^{U_i} N_{dt,x}^{(i)}$ is the underlying *censored sample*;
- the common observation window $B \in \mathcal{E}$ is assumed without edge effects and with $|B| < \infty$;
- the *uncensored covered fraction* $(P^{(i)}(t))_{i=1,\dots,n}$ of the sample in the window B is defined by $P^{(i)}(t) := P^{(i),B}(t) = \frac{1}{|B|} \int_B N_{t,x}^{(i)} \, dx$;
- $\mathfrak{P}(t) := \sum_1^n \widetilde{P}^{(i)}(t)$, where $\widetilde{P}^{(i)}(t) := P^{(i)}(t \wedge U_i) = \int_0^t \mathbb{1}_{U_i \geq s} \, dP^{(i)}(s)$ is the *censored covered fraction* of the sample in B;
- $Y(t,x) := \sum_1^n Y^{(i)}(t,x)$ where $Y^{(i)}(t,x) = \mathbb{1}_{U_i \geq t}(1 - N_{t,x}^{(i)}) = \mathbb{1}_{U_i \geq t}(1 - \widetilde{N}_{t,x}^{(i)})$ is the *censored uncovered sample*;
- $Y(t) := \sum_1^n \mathfrak{Y}^{(i)}(t)$ where $\mathfrak{Y}^{(i)}(t) = \mathbb{1}_{U_i \geq t}(1 - P^{(i)}(t)) = \mathbb{1}_{U_i \geq t}(1 - \widetilde{P}^{(i)}(t))$ is the *censored uncovered fraction*;

The first estimator for the survival function has to be used when the available data are the $(\widetilde{N}_{t,x}^{(i)})_{i=1,\dots,n}$.

Theorem 2. *By using the previous notations and by defining* $J(t,x) := \mathbb{1}_{Y(t,x)>0}$, *the Nelson–Aalen estimator for the cumulative hazard function* $A_x(t)$ *is*

$$\hat{A}_x(t) := \int_0^t \frac{J(s,x)}{Y(s,x)} \, d\mathfrak{N}_x(s) \, .$$

If the processes $(N_{t,x}^{(i)})_{i=1,\dots,n}$ *are homogeneous* $(h(t,x) = h(t))$, *then the N–A estimator is defined by* $\hat{A}(t) := \frac{|\hat{A}_x(t)|}{|B|}$.

Recall that $S(t) = \boldsymbol{\pi}_{s<t}(1 - dA(s))$ and $A(t) = \int_0^t dS(s)/S(s)$ are the links between the cumulative hazard function A and the survival one S, see [1] or [7]. Here $\boldsymbol{\pi}$ stands for the product-integral.

Corollary 1. *The Kaplan-Meier estimator for the survival function is* $\hat{S}_x(t) = \boldsymbol{\pi}_{s<t}(1 - d\hat{A}_x(s))$. *In the homogeneous case it is equal to* $\hat{S}(t) = \boldsymbol{\pi}_{s<t}(1 - d\hat{A}(s))$.

The second estimator is used when the available data are the $(\widetilde{P}_{t,x}^{(i)})_{i=1,\dots,n}$.

Theorem 3. *Under the previous notation, and with* $J^{(\varepsilon)}(t) := \mathbb{1}_{Y(t)>\varepsilon}$, *the Nelson–Aalen estimator for the ε-cumulative hazard function* $A^{(\varepsilon)}(t) = \int_0^t h(s) J^{(\varepsilon)}(s) ds$ *is defined as* $\breve{A}^{(\varepsilon)}(t) := \int_0^t \frac{J^{(\varepsilon)}(s)}{Y(s)} \, d\mathfrak{P}(s) \, .$

Corollary 2. *The Kaplan-Meier estimator for the survival function is defined in this case by* $\check{S}^{(0)}(t) = \boldsymbol{\pi}_{s<t}(1 - \check{A}^{(0)}(s))$.

The third one is used in case of a lack of data. It is defined by means of a randomization method and leads to $\check{S}(t) := \int_0^1 \bar{S}_r(t)\,dr$, where $\bar{S}_r(t)$ is the usual Kaplan-Meier estimator for the survival function $S_r(t)$ associated with the time $T(r) = \inf\{t\colon P(t) \geq r\}$.

As seen before, the geometrical aspect of the phenomenon is also of main interest. It is described in particular by the mean $(k-m)$-content of $(k-m)$-interfaces per unit volume in L_k, $\mu_{k,k-m}$. A "natural" unbiased estimator for the density of $(k-m)$-interfaces in L_k based on the observations on a region $B \subseteq L_k$, is

$$\widehat{\mu}_{k,k-m} = \frac{\sum_{a_0,\cdots,a_m \in \Phi}^{\neq} \lambda_{k-m}(B \cap F(a_0,\cdots,a_m|\Phi))}{(m+1)!\lambda_k(B)},$$

provided that $0 < \lambda_k(B) < +\infty$, as a consequence of the Slivnyak formula. Note that each $\widehat{\mu}_{k,k-m}$ (and hence $\widehat{\widehat{\mu}}_{k,k-m}$) is consistent when $\lambda_k(B) \to \infty$. As a consequence,

$$\widehat{\mu}_{k,k-m} \xrightarrow[\lambda_k(B)\to\infty]{L^1,L^2,\text{a.s.}} \mu_{k,k-m}.$$

6 Simulations and New Results

In nucleation-*exclusion* models (i.e., when the starting radius of a germ is $\delta > 0$, see [9]), a new germ cannot be born at x if the entire ball of center x and radius δ is not completely "free". We present here a simple proof of an asymptotic confidence interval for the degree of crystallinity (namely, $\mu_{d,d}$), when $\delta = 0$ (classical J-M incomplete tessellation). Extensions are left to subsequent papers.

Given $T > 0$, $\sigma(N(T,x), x \in B_1)$ is independent of $\sigma(N(T,x), x \in B_2)$ if the "distance" between B_1 and B_2 is sufficiently large. In Møller's models, since $v = 1$, it is sufficient to take this distance greater than $vT + 2\delta$. Now, divide the entire space $\mathbb{R}^d$ into disjoint cubes whose edge length is $l \geq vT + 2\delta$, mark each of them with a reference point $z \in \mathbb{Z}^d$, and consider the $\mathbb{Z}^d$-indexed process $X_z := (\int_{lz}^{l(z+1)} N(T,x)\,dx)/l^d = \widehat{\mu}_{d,d}(B_z)$, where $B_{(z_1,\ldots,z_d)} = \{(x_1,\ldots,x_d) \in \mathbb{R}^d\colon z_i \leq x_i \leq z_i + 1, \forall i\}$. Following the notations in [3, 8], the process $\{X_z, z \in \mathbb{Z}^d\}$ is 1-dependent. Now, take an increasing sequence A_n of subset of $\mathbb{Z}^d$. Denote by $|A_n| := \#\{A_n\}$ the cardinality of A_n. Assume $\lim_n |A_n| = \infty$ and $\lim_n |A_n \setminus A_{n-1}|/|A_{n-1}| = 0$. As a consequence, since $0 \leq X_z \leq 1$, we have the following results.

Theorem 4 (cfr. [8]). *Assume* $\liminf_n Var(S_n)/|A_n| = \alpha > 0$, *where* $S_n = \sum_{z \in A_n}(X_z - \mathbb{E}[X_z])$. *Then*

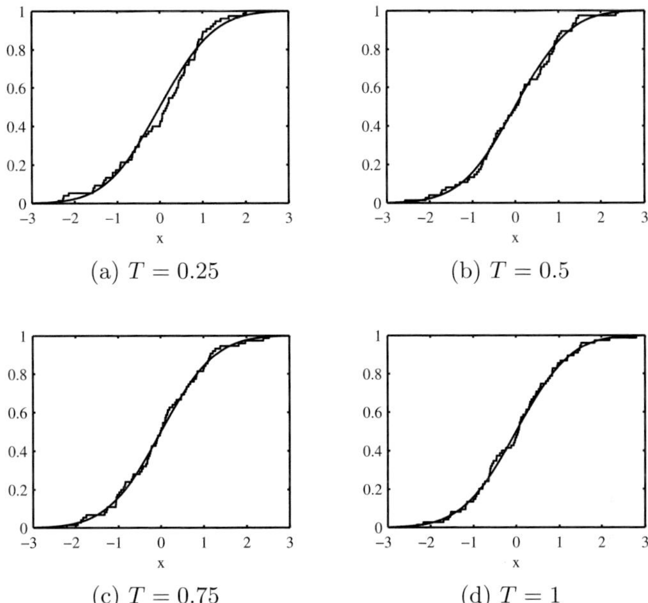

(a) $T = 0.25$

(b) $T = 0.5$

(c) $T = 0.75$

(d) $T = 1$

Fig. 2: Comparison between cumulative function of standardized data and $\Phi(x)$ (sample size $N = 50$, $\Delta x = 10$).

$$Y_n := \frac{S_n}{\sqrt{Var(S_n)}} \xrightarrow[n \to \infty]{Law} N(0,1), \quad \sup_{x \in \mathbb{R}} |F_{Y_n}(x) - \Phi(x)| = O(\sigma_n^{-1}(\log(\sigma_n))^{(d-1)/2}$$

where $\sigma_n := \sqrt{Var(S_n)}$ and $F_{Y_n}(x)$, $\Phi(x)$ denote the cumulative distribution functions of Y_n and of a standard gaussian variable, respectively.

Another version of this theorem is given by [3] in the case of a stationary process. Unfortunately, this theorem can be applied to build a confidence interval only when $\sigma^2 > 0$.

We propose here a simple and new proof when the process has a positive correlation.

Lemma 1. *The previous theorems hold when*

1. $cov(X_{z_1}, X_{z_2}) \geq 0$;
2. $\inf_z Var(X_z) = a > 0$.

Remark 3. Assumption 2 is always satisfied when the process is stationary (see [3]), and it is a reasonable assumption in general situations for CLT.

Proof (of Lemma 1). We assume here, without loss of generality, that $\mathbb{E}[X_z] = 0$ and $|X_z| \leq 1$. We write $z \sim z'$ if $\sup_i |z_i - z_i'| \leq 1$ (i.e. X_z and $X_{z'}$ are not independent). Now, $\#\{z' : z' \sim z\} = 3^d$, and hence $Var(S_n)/|A_n| \leq 3^d$. We have

$$Var(S_n) = \underbrace{\sum_{z \in \partial A_n} \mathbb{E}[X_z \sum_{z' \sim z, z' \in A_n} X_{z'}]}_{V_1} + \underbrace{\sum_{z \in A_n \setminus \partial A_n} \mathbb{E}[X_z \sum_{z' \sim z} X_{z'}]}_{V_2}.$$

Again, since $\#\{z' : z' \sim z\} = 3^d$, it follows that

$$\left| \frac{V_1}{|A_n|} \right| \leq \frac{|\partial A_n| 3^d}{|A_n|} \left(\xrightarrow[n \to \infty]{} 0 \right).$$

For V_2, we have

$$\frac{V_2}{|A_n|} = \frac{\sum_{z \in A_n \setminus \partial A_n} E(X_z \sum_{z' \sim z} X_{z'})}{|A_n|} \geq$$

$$\frac{\sum_{z \in A_n \setminus \partial A_n} E(X_z^2)}{|A_n|} \geq a \frac{|A_n| - |\partial A_n|}{|A_n|} \left(\xrightarrow[n \to \infty]{} a > 0 \right).$$

$\square$

Lemma 1 and Theorem 4 imply the CLT for $\widehat{\mu}_{d,d}$.

Proposition 2. *The process* $X_z := \widehat{\mu}_{d,d}(B_z)$ *satisfies* $cov(X_{z_1}, X_{z_2}) \geq 0$ *under* $\delta = 0$.

Proof. For any $x_1, x_2 \in \mathbb{R}^d$, we have that

$$\mathbb{P}(N(T, x_1) = 0, N(T, x_2) = 0) = \exp(-\nu_0[A(x_1, T) \cup A(x_2, T)])$$
$$\geq \exp(-\nu_0[A(x_1, T)]) \exp(-\nu_0[A(x_2, T)])$$
$$= \mathbb{P}(N(T, x_1) = 0)\mathbb{P}(N(T, x_2) = 0)$$

which implies $cov(N(T, x_1), N(T, x_2)) \geq 0$, i.e. $\mathbb{P}(N(T, x_1) = 1, N(T, x_2) = 1) \geq \mathbb{P}(N(T, x_1) = 1)\mathbb{P}(N(T, x_2) = 1)$. Now,

$$\mathbb{E}[X_{z_1} X_{z_2}] = \mathbb{E}\left[\frac{\int_{lz_1}^{l(z_1+1)} N(T, x_1)\, dx_1 \int_{lz_2}^{l(z_2+1)} N(T, x_2)\, dx_2}{l^{2d}} \right]$$

$$= \frac{\int_{lz_2}^{l(z_2+1)} \int_{lz_1}^{l(z_1+1)} \mathbb{E}[N(T, x_1)N(T, x_2)]\, dx_1 dx_2}{l^{2d}}$$

$$\geq \frac{\int_{lz_2}^{l(z_2+1)} \int_{lz_1}^{l(z_1+1)} \mathbb{E}[N(T, x_1)]\mathbb{E}[N(T, x_2)]\, dx_1 dx_2}{l^{2d}}$$

$$= \mathbb{E}[X_{z_1}]\mathbb{E}[X_{z_2}].$$

$\square$

Remark 4. We leave to subsequent papers the investigation of the possibility of proving the same kind of results for the asymptotic law of the joint distribution of $\widehat{\mu}_{k,n-k}, k = 0, \ldots, n$ stating more general assumptions, since these estimators need not have a positive correlation

Table 1: Confidence intervals for $\mu_{d,d}$ for different simulations. T is the time of simulations, N the sample size, Δx the edge of the window, $\mu_{d,d}$ the theoretical value, $\widehat{\mu}_{d,d}$ the point estimator ($\alpha = 2.5$, $\beta = 1.5$, $\delta = 0$, $d = 2$).

T	N	Δx	$\mu_{d,d}$	$\widehat{\mu}_{d,d}$	CI (99%) for $\mu_{d,d}$
0.25	250	10	0.0093	0.0093	0.0088 − 0.0099
0.50	250	10	0.1004	0.0998	0.0966 − 0.1029
0.75	250	10	0.3542	0.3530	0.3457 − 0.3602
1.00	250	10	0.6978	0.6969	0.6888 − 0.7050
0.25	75	30	0.0093	0.0093	0.0090 − 0.0096
0.50	75	30	0.1004	0.1008	0.0990 − 0.1025
0.75	75	30	0.3542	0.3552	0.3513 − 0.3590
1.00	75	30	0.6978	0.6989	0.6945 − 0.7032

6.1 Simulations

We have performed computer simulations of Johnson–Mehl crystallization processes for the following values of the parameters: $d = 2$ (dimension), $\alpha = 0.25$ and $\beta = 1.5$ (parameters of the free-rate nucleation $\Lambda(t) = \alpha t^{\beta-1}$) and $\delta = 0$ (radius of nucleation), $v = 1$ (speed of growth) at different values of $T = \{0.25, 0.5, 0.75, 1\}$ in different windows $A = [0, \Delta x]^2$. Figure 1 shows a typical simulation for different times. Edge effects were controlled by simulating the process on the larger window ($[0 - Tv - 2\delta, \Delta x + Tv + 2\delta]^2$). The window is divided into Δx^2 unit squares and the process $\{X_z, z \in [1, \Delta x]^2 \cap \mathbb{Z}^2\}$ is sampled. SAS© 9.0 was used to perform the goodness of fit with the gaussian distribution with different test of normality (Shapiro–Wilk, Kolmogorov–Smirnov, Cramer–von Mises, Anderson–Darling). No test has shown significant differences between gaussian distributions and our samples. Figure 2 compares the cumulative distribution function of the standardized data with the cumulative distribution function $\Phi(x)$ of a standard gaussian variable. Point estimators and confidence intervals for $\mu_{d,d}$ are shown in Table 1.

Acknowledgments

The research of Diane Saada is supported in part by the Israel Science Foundation (grant no. 032-1585).

References

1. Andersen, P.K. Borgan, Ø., Gill, R.D., Keiding, N.: Statistical models based on counting processes. Springer Series in Statistics. Springer-Verlag, New York, 1993.

2. Aletti, G., Saada, D.: Survival analysis in Johnson-Mehl tessellation. To appear on Stat. Inference Stoch. Process, 2006.
3. Bolthausen, E.: On the central limit theorem for stationary mixing random fields. Ann. Probab., 10(4):1047–1050, 1982.
4. Capasso, V., Burger, M., Micheletti, A.: An extension of the Kolmogorov-Avrami formula to inhomogeneous birth-and-growth processes. This volume.
5. Capasso, V., Burger, M., Micheletti, A., Salani, C.: Mathematical models for polymer crystallization processes. In Mathematical modelling for polymer processing, volume 2 of Math. Ind., pages 167–242, 313–315. Springer, Berlin, 2003.
6. Capasso, V., Micheletti, A.: On the hazard function for inhomogeneous birth-and-growth processes. This volume.
7. Gill, R.D.: Lectures on survival analysis. In Lectures on probability theory (Saint-Flour, 1992), volume 1581 of Lecture Notes in Math., pages 115–241. Springer, Berlin, 1994.
8. Guyon, X., Richardson, S.: Vitesse de convergence du théorème de la limite centrale pour des champs faiblement dépendants. Z. Wahrsch. Verw. Gebiete, 66(2):297–314, 1984.
9. Møller, J.: Random Johnson-Mehl tessellations. Adv. in Appl. Probab., 24(4):814–844, 1992.
10. Møller, J.: Topics in Voronoi and Johnson-Mehl tessellations. In Stochastic geometry (Toulouse, 1996), volume 80 of Monogr. Statist. Appl. Probab., pages 173–198. Chapman & Hall/CRC, Boca Raton, FL, 1999.
11. Stoyan, D., Kendall, W.S., Mecke, J.: Stochastic geometry and its applications. John Wiley & Sons Ltd., Chichester, 1987. With a foreword by D.G. Kendall.
12. Slivnjak, I.M.: Some properties of stationary streams of homogeneous random events. Teor. Verojatnost. i Primenen., 7:347–352, 1962.

Optimal Marketing Decision in a Duopoly: A Stochastic Approach

Luigi De Cesare and Andrea Di Liddo

Dipartimento di Scienze Economiche, Matematiche e Statistiche,Università di Foggia, Via IV Novembre 1, 71100 Foggia , Italy
{l.decesare,a.diliddo}@unifg.it

Summary. Let us consider two new perfect substitute durable products which are produced and sold in a market by two competing firms.

Looking at a potential buyer, we build a stochastic rule by which she purchases the good from one of the two firms (so that she becomes an *adopter*). The model is considered discrete in time and space. The probability of transition from the non adopter state to the adopter one depends on an imitation mechanism (*word-of-mouth*) as well as on the pricing and advertising policies of the producers/sellers. It is assumed that only actual information about the market determine the evolution in the subsequent time step so that a Markov process arises. Both firms maximize their expected discounted profits by choosing optimal marketing strategies. Suitable equilibria are characterized and, because of the lack of convexity in the model, the simulated annealing algorithm is proposed to compute them.

1 Introduction

The diffusion of a new product (innovation) in a market has been modelled firstly in the seminal paper by [1].

The population of potential consumers is divided into two classes: the class of the adopters - i.e. individuals which have already bought the new product and which spread information about it; the non-adopters or uninformed - i.e. individuals which are not yet informed about the innovation. The Bass equation gives the dynamic of cumulative adopters as a function of advertising and interpersonal communication. The Bass model and its early generalizations have been used, since the 1980, to address and solve optimal-control problems governed by differential equations. For a review of the decision problems related to the diffusion of new products in a market see [2] and [4].

In this paper we firstly discuss a duopoly model of innovation diffusion. There are two competing firms which produce and sell two versions of the new product which are perfect substitutes and differ only for the brand of the producer. Advertising and interpersonal contacts also contribute to the diffusion of the new product. Moreover consumer's decisions depend on the price of the product and, since the two products are substitutes, consumers react also to the difference between the prices. The model in this paper is presented in Section 2 as a stochastic rule by which a potential buyer can become an adopter of one of the two products. The model is considered discrete in time and space. The probability of transition from the state of non-adopter to the state of adopter of one kind of products depends on an imitation mechanism (*word-of-mouth*) as well as on the pricing and advertising policies of the producer/seller. Since it is assumed that only actual information about the market determines the evolution in the next time step, then the process is a Markov one. After a brief discussion about the features of innovation diffusion dynamics, a noncooperative game between the two firms is treated.

2 The Model

We consider a population of M (potential) consumers each of which can buy at most one copy of a new durable product (innovation) choosing between two perfect substitutes P_1 and P_2. The innovation is produced and sold by two firms which can practise discrimination in prices since the two brands are differently perceived by the consumers. Let us denote by $A_{n,i}$ the number, at time n, of the individuals who have already bought the product P_i manufactured by the firm F_i, $i = 1, 2$. It is $A_{0,i} = 0$.

We assume that potential consumers are convinced to buy the new product through the advertising given by the two firms. The advertising performed by the firm F_i has a (nonnegative) influence on both the sales of the firm F_i and F_j and viceversa.

Let us denote by $\gamma_{i,n}$, $i = 1, 2$ the quantities (normalized to one) of the advertising produced by the firm F_i at time n. The effectiveness of the advertising is measured through the functions g_i and h_i. Precisely $g_i(\gamma_{i,n})$ represents the effect on the sales of the firm F_i of the advertising made by the firm F_i; whereas $h_i(\gamma_{j,n})$ measures the influence on the sales of the firm F_i given by the advertising made by the firm F_j, $i \neq j$.

Furthermore people are convinced to buy the new product through interpersonal contacts with previous adopters. This effect is modelled by parameter $k_{i,j}$ which represents the effect of word-of-mouth of P_i adopter's to convince a non adopter to buy the product P_j.

Obviously, price also influences the decision of a potential customer. Higher it is the price, lower the probability that the product is purchased. A measure of this effect is given by a so-called *price-response function* $q_i(p_{1,n}, p_{2,n})$ where $p_{i,n}$ is the price of the product P_i at time n.

The following properties are assumed to hold about the functions g_i, h_i:

1. $g_i(0) = 0;$ $i = 1, 2;$

2. $h_i(0) = 0;$ $i = 1, 2;$

3. $0 \leq g_i(\gamma_{i,n}) + h_i(\gamma_{j,n}) \leq 1$ $i, j = 1, 2$

Moreover the functions g_i and h_i are assumed to be increasing and concave in their arguments to incorporate decreasing advertising returns.

We assume that the *price-response function* $q_1(p_1, p_2)$ is increasing with respect to p_2 and that it is decreasing with respect to p_1. Furthermore $0 \leq q_1(p_1, p_2) \leq 1$. The analogous properties hold for q_2. In the rest of the paper we choose price-response function as follows

$$\begin{cases} q_1(p_1, p_2) = \exp(-\alpha_1 p_1)\varphi_1(p_2 - p_1) \\ q_2(p_1, p_2) = \exp(-\alpha_2 p_2)\varphi_2(p_1 - p_2) \end{cases}$$

where α_i are positive constants and φ_i are increasing functions. So, potential consumers react to the price of the product they are going to buy but they also react to the difference between the prices of the two products.

We provide a stochastic rule for a potential buyer to become an adopter of one of the two products P_1, P_2. The process is considered discrete in time and we assume that decisions are taken at time $n \in \{0, 1, ..., T - 1\}$, where $T \in \mathbb{N}$.

Let us define, for $j = 1, \ldots, M$ and $n = 0, \ldots, T$, $i = 1, 2$, the random variables $X_{n,i}^j$ as follows:

$$X_{n,i}^j = \begin{cases} 1 & \text{if the } j\text{-th individual is an adopter} \\ & \text{of product } P_i \text{ at time } n \\ \\ 0 & \text{if the } j\text{-th individual is not yet an adopter} \\ & \text{of product } P_i \text{ at the time } n. \end{cases}$$

Let

$$X_n^j = (X_{n,1}^j, X_{n,2}^j).$$

Thus the number of adopters at time n is given by

$$A_n = \sum_{j=1}^{M} X_n^j.$$

where

$$A_n = (A_{n,1}, A_{n,2}).$$

If the j-th individual is not yet an adopter at time n, then she becomes an adopter at time $n + 1$ with probabilities

$$r_{n,A_n,1} := P\left(X_{n+1}^j = (1,0) | X_n^j = (0,0), X_n^1, \ldots, X_n^M\right) =$$

$$q_1(p_{1,n}, p_{2,n}) \left(1 - (1 - g_1(\gamma_{1,n}) - h_1(\gamma_{2,n})) \left(1 - \frac{k_{1,1}}{M} \right)^{A_{n,1}} \left(1 - \frac{k_{1,2}}{M} \right)^{A_{n,2}} \right)$$

$$r_{n,A_n,2} := P\left(X_{n+1}^j = (0,1) | X_n^j = (0,0), X_n^1, \ldots, X_n^M \right) =$$

$$q_2(p_{1,n}, p_{2,n}) \left(1 - (1 - g_2(\gamma_{2,n}) - h_2(\gamma_{1,n})) \left(1 - \frac{k_{2,1}}{M} \right)^{A_{n,1}} \left(1 - \frac{k_{2,2}}{M} \right)^{A_{n,2}} \right)$$

Moreover we have

$$\begin{cases} P\left(X_{n+1}^j = (0,0) | X_n^j = (0,0), X_n^1, \ldots, X_n^M \right) = 1 - r_{n,A_n,1} - r_{n,A_n,2} \\ P\left(X_{n+1}^j = (0,0) | X_n^j = (1,0), X_n^1, \ldots, X_n^M \right) = 0 \\ P\left(X_{n+1}^j = (0,1) | X_n^j = (1,0), X_n^1, \ldots, X_n^M \right) = 0 \\ P\left(X_{n+1}^j = (0,0) | X_n^j = (0,1), X_n^1, \ldots, X_n^M \right) = 0 \\ P\left(X_{n+1}^j = (1,0) | X_n^j = (0,1), X_n^1, \ldots, X_n^M \right) = 0 \\ P\left(X_{n+1}^j = (1,0) | X_n^j = (1,0), X_n^1, \ldots, X_n^M \right) = 1 \\ P\left(X_{n+1}^j = (0,1) | X_n^j = (0,1), X_n^1, \ldots, X_n^M \right) = 1 \end{cases}$$

The first equality means that the probability to remain non adopter for an individual who has not already adopted the innovation is $1 - r_{n,A_n,1} - r_{n,A_n,2}$. The last two equalities mean that if the j-th individual is an adopter at time n, then she remains an adopter for all the future time. The meaning of the other equalities is obvious.

The stochastic process $A = (A_n)_{n=0,\ldots,T}$ is a Markov chain. The state space is given by the set

$$S_M := \{ (l,j) \in \mathbb{N}^2 | l + j \leq M \}.$$

S_M has $\sigma_M \equiv \frac{(M+1)(M+2)}{2}$ elements.

Note that the Markov chain is nonhomogeneous: that is the transition probabilities are non-stationary because at any time n they depend on the advertising rates $\gamma_{i,n}$ and on the selling prices $p_{i,n}$, $i = 1, 2$.

Since there are no adopters at time $n = 0$, we have that the distribution of the initial state is the vector $\pi \in \mathbb{R}^{\sigma_M}$, defined by

$$\pi_{s_l} = P(A_0 = s_l) = \begin{cases} 1 & \text{if } s_l = (0,0) \\ 0 & \text{if } s_l \neq (0,0). \end{cases}$$

Setting $\mathbf{i} = (i_1, i_2) \in S_M$ and $\mathbf{j} = (j_1, j_2) \in S_M$, the transition probabilities are

$$P(A_{n+1} = \mathbf{j} | A_n = \mathbf{i}) = \begin{cases} \pi_{i,j}^n & \text{if } i_1 \leq j_1 \text{ and } i_2 \leq j_2 \\ 0 & \text{otherwise} \end{cases}$$

where $\pi_{i,j}^n$ are given by

$$\frac{(M - i_1 - i_2)!}{(j_1 - i_1)!(j_2 - i_2)!(M - j_1 - j_2)!} \; r_{n,i,1}^{j_1 - i_1} \; r_{n,i,2}^{j_2 - i_2} \left(1 - r_{n,i,1} - r_{n,i,2}\right)^{M - j_1 - j_2}$$

If the advertising levels and the selling prices are constant in time, then the Markov chain is homogeneous. In this case let $\gamma_{i,n} \equiv \gamma_i$. If $\gamma_1 + \gamma_2 > 0$, then, by standard Markov chain asymptotic properties, it follows that

$$\lim_{n \to +\infty} P(A_{n,1} + A_{n,2} = M) = 1.$$

This means that, as the time horizon tends to infinity, the whole population adopts one of the two new products with probability one. If $\gamma_1 + \gamma_2 = 0$, then nobody becomes an adopter.

3 The Dynamic Game

Let $c_{p,i}$ be the per unit cost of the product P_i. Moreover let us indicate by $c_{\gamma,i}$ the unitary costs, paid by the firm F_i for the advertising made during the period $[0, T]$. Here $c_{p,i}$ and $c_{\gamma,i}$ are given positive constants. Let $\delta_i > 0$ be the (constant in time) one period instantaneous discount rate. The stochastic discounted returns to the firm F_i in the planning period, given a price-advertising policy, are then

$$\sum_{k=0}^{T-1} e^{-\delta_i k} (p_{i,k} - c_{p,i})(A_{k+1,i} - A_{k,i}) - c_{\gamma,i}\gamma_{i,k}.$$

The firms perform control of a common stochastic discrete time dynamic system which is a non-homogeneous Markov chain with one-step transition matrix depending on control parameters. At every time step, each player makes decision in order to maximize her total discounted payoff for the planning period assuming that the other player does the same. We suppose that each player knows the current state of the system (symmetric complete information). We describe the game by the dynamic Nash equilibrium.

The random transition from the current state A_n to the next one A_{n+1} depends only on the actions of players:

$$\Phi_{i,n} := (\gamma_{i,n}(A_n), p_{i,n}(A_n))$$

and the current state A_n. We denote by

$$u_{i,n}(A_{n+1} - A_n, \Phi_{1,n}, \Phi_{2,n}) := (p_{i,n} - c_{p,i})(A_{n+1,i} - A_{n,i}) - c_{\gamma,i}\gamma_{i,n} \qquad (1)$$

the firm current payoff. We observe that the strategies of the firms at every time step depend only on the current state of the system.

At time step $n = 0, 1, \ldots, T-1$, each firm chooses an optimal strategy:

$$\Psi_{i,n}(s) = (\Phi_{i,n}(s), \Phi_{i,n+1}(s), \ldots, \Phi_{i,T-1}(s)) \quad \forall s \in S_M$$

where

$$\Phi_{i,n}(s) = (\gamma_{i,n}(s), p_{i,n}(s)), \quad \forall s \in S_M,$$

maximizing the expected discounted sum of future one-period payoffs (1), given the policy of the other firm:

$$U_{i,n}(s, \Psi_{1,n}, \Psi_{2,n}) = E_{n,s} \sum_{k=n}^{T-1} e^{-\delta_i(k-n)} u_{i,k}(A_{k+1} - A_k, \Phi_{1,k}, \Phi_{2,k}). \quad (2)$$

Here $E_{n,s}$ is the expected value conditioned on $[A_n = s]$, that is the firms make decisions observing the state of the system at time n.

The game solution consists in a dynamic Nash equilibrium. At time n, a pair $(\hat{\Psi}_{1,n}, \hat{\Psi}_{2,n})$ is a Nash equilibrium if, for all $s \in S_M$,

$$\begin{cases} U_{1,n}(s, \hat{\Psi}_{1,n}, \hat{\Psi}_{2,n}) = \max_{\Psi_{1,n}} U_{1,n}(s, \Psi_{1,n}, \hat{\Psi}_{2,n}) \\ U_{2,n}(s, \hat{\Psi}_{1,n}, \hat{\Psi}_{2,n}) = \max_{\Psi_{2,n}} U_{2,n}(s, \hat{\Psi}_{1,n}, \Psi_{2,n}) \end{cases} \quad (3)$$

From the elementary properties of Markov chains, we have

$$E_{n,s} f(s, A_{n+1}, \ldots, A_T) =$$

$$\sum_{i_{n+1}, \ldots, i_T} f(s, A_{n+1}, \ldots, A_T) \pi^n_{s,i_{n+1}} \pi^{n+1}_{i_{n+1}, i_{n+2}} \cdots \pi^{T-1}_{i_{T-1}, i_T} =$$

$$\sum_{i_{n+1}} \pi^n_{s,i_{n+1}} \sum_{i_{n+2}} \pi^{n+1}_{i_{n+1}, i_{n+2}} \cdots \sum_{i_T} \pi^{T-1}_{i_{T-1}, i_T} f(s, A_{n+1}, \ldots, A_T)$$

where $\pi^n_{i,j} = P(A_{n+1} = \mathbf{j} | A_n = \mathbf{i})$. Let's

$$g_{T-n-1}(s, \mathbf{i_n}, \ldots, \mathbf{i_{T-1}}) := E_{T-1, i_{T-1}} f(s, \mathbf{i_n}, \ldots, \mathbf{i_{T-1}}, A_T)$$

$$g_{T-n-2}(s, \mathbf{i_n}, \ldots, \mathbf{i_{T-2}}) := E_{T-2, i_{T-2}} g_{T-n-1}(s, \mathbf{i_n}, \ldots, \mathbf{i_{T-2}}, A_{T-1})$$

$$\vdots$$

$$g_1(s, \mathbf{i_{n+1}}) := E_{n+1, i_{n+1}} g_2(s, \mathbf{i_{n+1}}, A_{n+2}).$$

Then we have

$$E_{n,s} f(s, A_{n+1}, \ldots, A_T) = E_{n,s} g_1(s, \mathbf{i_{n+1}})$$

and hence

$$E_{n,s} f(s, A_{n+1}, \ldots, A_T) = E_{n,s} E_{n+1, A_{n+1}} \cdots E_{T-1, A_{T-1}} f(s, A_{n+1}, \ldots, A_T).$$

From (2) we have (we omit some functional dependencies)

$$U_{i,n}(s) = E_{n,s}\left(u_{i,n}(A_{n+1} - s) + e^{-\delta_i}\sum_{k=n+1}^{T-1} e^{-\delta_i(k-(n+1))}u_{i,k}\right) =$$

$$E_{n,s}\, u_{i,n}(A_{n+1} - s) +$$

$$e^{-\delta_i}E_{n,s}\left(E_{n+1,A_{n+1}}\cdots E_{T-1,A_{T-1}}\sum_{k=n+1}^{T-1} e^{-\delta_i(k-(n+1))}u_{i,k}\right) =$$

$$E_{n,s}\, u_{i,n}(A_{n+1} - s) + e^{-\delta_i}E_{n,s}\, U_{i,n+1}(A_{n+1})$$

where $n = 0, 1, \ldots, T - 1$, $s \in S_M$ and $U_{i,T} \equiv 0$.

Hence we can try to solve the problem by a dynamic programming algorithm. Let's

$$\hat{U}_{i,n}(A_n, \Phi_{1,n}, \Phi_{2,n}) := U_{i,n}(A_n, (\Phi_{1,n}, \hat{\Psi}_{1,n+1}), (\Phi_{2,n}, \hat{\Psi}_{2,n+1}))$$

the payoff of a firm corresponding to a given policy at time t and optimal strategies for time $t + 1, \ldots, T - 1$.

If $(\hat{\Psi}_{1,n+1}, \hat{\Psi}_{2,n+1})$ is a Nash equilibrium for (3) at time $n + 1$ and $(\hat{\Phi}_{1,n}, \hat{\Phi}_{2,n})$ is a (unique) Nash equilibrium, for all $s \in S_M$, of the following problem:

$$\begin{cases}
\hat{U}_{1,n}(s, \hat{\Phi}_{1,n}, \hat{\Phi}_{2,n}) = \max_{\Phi_{1,n}} E_{n,s}\, u_{1,n}(A_{n+1} - s, \Phi_{1,n}, \hat{\Phi}_{2,n}) + \\
\qquad\qquad\qquad e^{-\delta_1}E_{n,s}\hat{U}_{1,n+1}(A_{n+1}, \hat{\Phi}_{1,n+1}, \hat{\Phi}_{2,n+1}) \\[2mm]
\hat{U}_{2,n}(s, \hat{\Phi}_{1,n}, \hat{\Phi}_{2,n}) = \max_{\Phi_{2,n}} E_{n,s}u_{2,n}(A_{n+1} - s, \hat{\Phi}_{1,n}, \Phi_{2,n}) + \\
\qquad\qquad\qquad e^{-\delta_2}E_{n,s}\hat{U}_{2,n+1}(A_{n+1}, \hat{\Phi}_{1,n+1}, \hat{\Phi}_{2,n+1})
\end{cases} \qquad (4)$$

then $(\hat{\Psi}_{1,n}, \hat{\Psi}_{2,n}) = ((\hat{\Phi}_{1,n}, \hat{\Psi}_{1,n+1}), (\hat{\Phi}_{2,n}\hat{\Psi}_{2,n+1}))$ is a Nash equilibrium for (3) at time n.

The previous expected values can be rewritten (again we omit some functional dependencies) as:

$$\eta_{i,n}(\Phi_{1,n}, \Phi_{2,n}) := E_{n,s}\left(u_{i,n}(A_{n+1} - s) + e^{-\delta_i}\hat{U}_{i,n+1}(A_{n+1})\right) =$$

$$\sum_{h_1=0}^{M_s}\sum_{h_2=0}^{M_s-h_1}\left(u_{i,n}((h_1, h_2)) + e^{-\delta_i}\hat{U}_{i,n+1}(s + (h_1, h_2))\right)\pi^n_{s,s+h}$$

where

$$s = (s_1, s_2,), \quad h = (h_1, h_2), \quad M_s = M - (s_1 + s_2)$$

$$\pi^n_{s,s+h} = P(A_{n+1} = s + (h_1, h_2)|A_n = s) =$$

$$\frac{M_s!}{h_1!h_2!(M_s - h_1 - h_2)!} \, r^{h_1}_{n,s,1} r^{h_2}_{n,s,2} (1 - r_{n,s,1} - r_{n,s,2})^{M_s - h_1 - h_2}$$

Using the dynamic programming techniques, we solve the problem (3) by backward recursion starting from the last stage. At each stage n we solve the problem (4), given that the stage $n + 1$ has already been solved. In other words at stage n, the values $\hat{U}_{i,n+1}(s)$ are known for all $s \in S_M$ and for the last stage we have $\hat{U}_{i,T} \equiv 0$.

In order to obtain a numerical solution of the problem (4), we use the following iterative algorithm (see [3]). We choose an initial policy $\Phi^{2k}_{1,n}$ (where $k = 0$) for the firm F_1 and we determine the optimal response of the firm F_2 finding

$$\Phi^{2k+1}_{2,n} := \arg \max_{\Phi_{2,n}} \eta_{2,n}(\Phi^{2k}_{1,n}, \Phi_{2,n})$$

Furthermore we compute the optimal response of the firm F_1 for this policy:

$$\Phi^{2(k+1)}_{1,n} := \arg \max_{\Phi_{1,n}} \eta_{1,n}(\Phi_{1,n}, \Phi^{2k+1}_{2,n})$$

Under suitable conditions the sequence $(\Phi^{2k}_{1,n}, \Phi^{2k+1}_{2,n})$, obtained iterating the previous steps, converges to the solution of the problem (4). Because of the complexity of the functions η_i it is hard to obtain analytical information i.e. monotonicity, convexity etc. Also the existence and uniqueness of the optimal response remains an open problem. We solve numerically the previous global maximum problems using at each step k the Simulated Annealing algorithm. We iterate on k until the differences $||\Phi^{2(k-1)}_{1,n} - \Phi^{2k}_{1,n}||$ and $||\Phi^{2(k-1)+1}_{2,n} - \Phi^{2k+1}_{2,n}||$ are small according to a given precision.

In our simulation we consider the following functions for the advertising effects:

$$g_i(\gamma_i) := \rho_i \log(1 + \gamma_i)/\log(2) \qquad h_i(\gamma_j) := \xi_i \log(1 + \gamma_j)/\log(2)$$

where $\rho_i \geq 0$, $\xi_i \geq 0$ and $\phi_i := \rho_i + \xi_i < 1$. We choose $\delta_i = 0$, $M = 20$ and $T = 10$. The other parameters are listed in table (1).

Table 1: Simulation parameters.

Figure	$c_{p,1}$	$c_{p,2}$	$c_{\gamma,1}$	$c_{\gamma,2}$	ρ_1	ρ_2	ξ_1	ξ_2	α_1	α_2
1	0.40	0.50	1.20	0.80	0.40	0.25	0.02	0.03	0.45	0.50
2	0.40	0.50	1.50	0.80	0.40	0.25	0.02	0.03	0.45	0.50
3	0.40	0.40	1.00	0.80	0.30	0.25	0.02	0.03	0.50	0.50
4	0.40	0.40	1.20	0.80	0.40	0.25	0.02	0.03	0.50	0.50

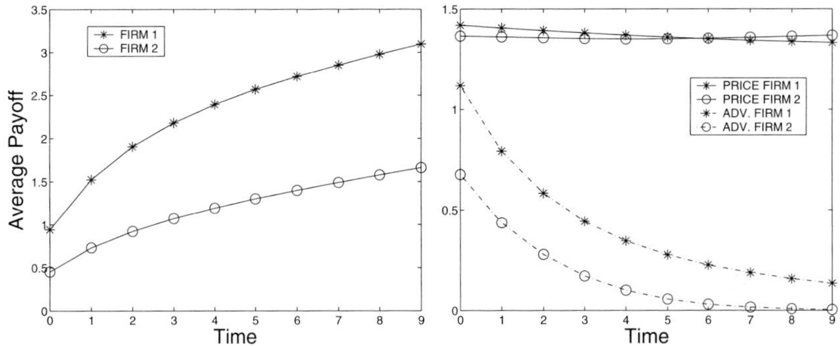

Fig. 1: Average payoffs and average price/advertising strategies.

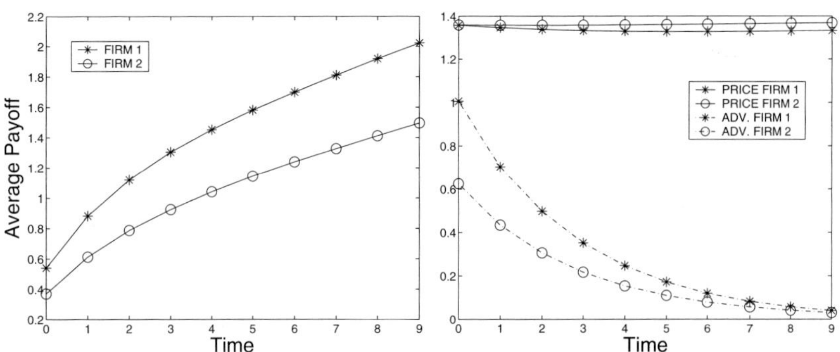

Fig. 2: Average payoffs and average price/advertising strategies.

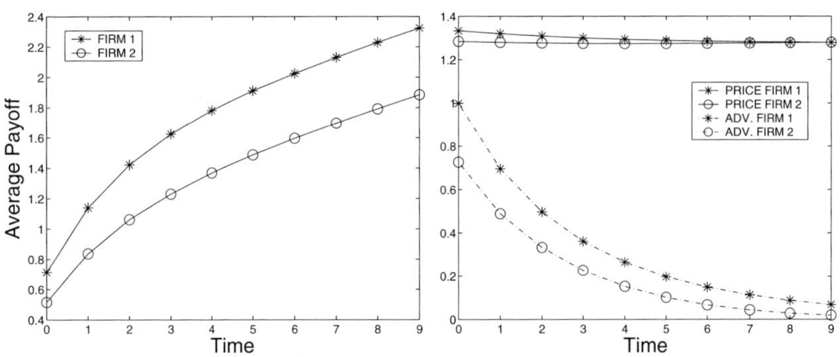

Fig. 3: Average payoffs and average price/advertising strategies.

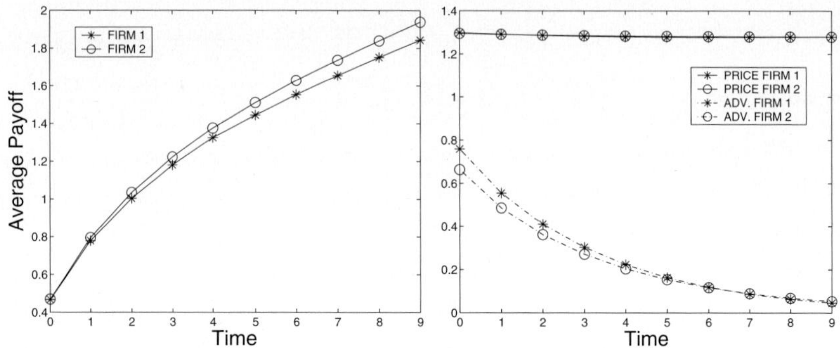

Fig. 4: Average payoffs and average price/advertising strategies.

In the following pictures the expected returns of the firms, given the information at the initial time and when optimal price/advertising strategies are performed, are plotted against the time. Precisely we can see the returns on the left figure and the price/advertising profiles on the right figure. The expected values

$$G_i(n) := E_0 \left(\sum_{k=0}^{n} e^{-\delta_i k} (\hat{p}_{i,k} - c_{p,i})(A_{k+1,i} - A_{k,i}) - c_{\gamma,i}\hat{\gamma}_{i,k} \right)$$

are computed by a Monte Carlo simulation generating a sample path of the Markov chain $(A_n)_{n=0,\ldots,T}$. Note that, according to the standard literature, the advertising profiles are decreasing in time while the price profiles are decreasing at the beginning and then are definitively increasing.

References

1. Bass, F.M. : A new product growth model for consumer durables. Management Science, **15**, 215–227 (1969)
2. Dockner, E., Jørgensen, S., van Long, N., Sorger, G.: Differential Games in Economics and in Management Science. Cambridge University Press, Cambridge (2000)
3. Golubtsov, P.V., Lyubetsky, V.A.: Stochastic Dynamic Game with Various Types of Information. Problems of Information Transmission, **39**, 266–293 (2003)
4. Jørgensen, S., Zaccour, G.: Differential Games in Marketing. Kluwer Academic Publisher, Boston (2004)

Appendix

Color Plates

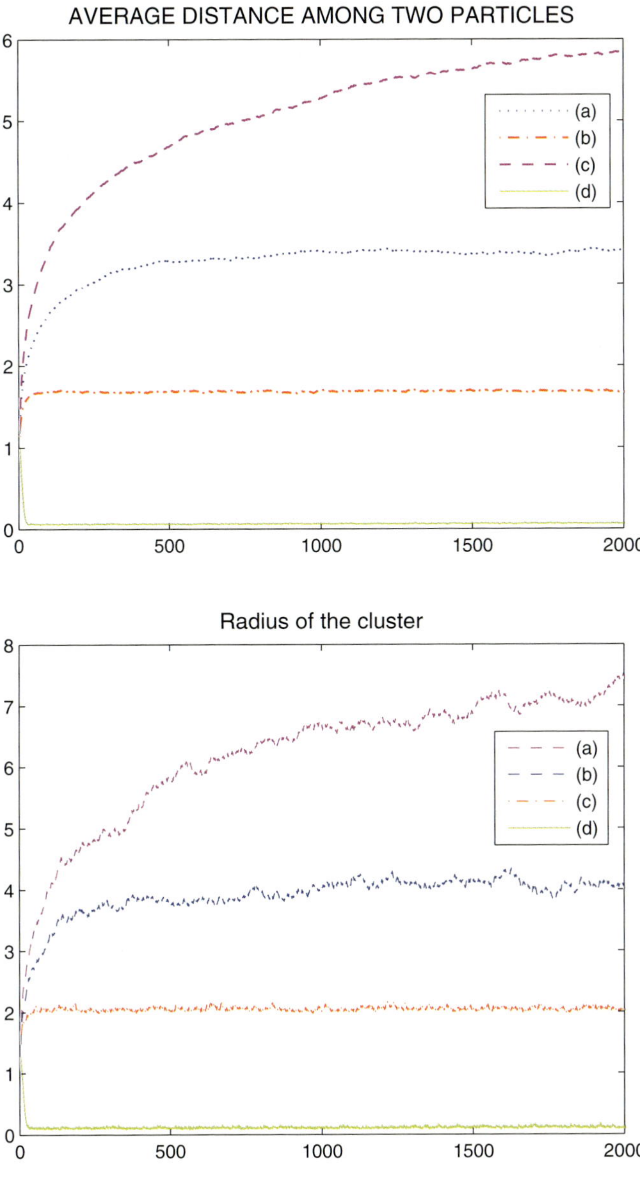

Plate 1: Comparison among the evolution of the radius of the cluster and the average distance among particles for different values of parameters: (a) $\alpha_1 = \alpha_2 = 1$; (b) $\alpha_1 = 1; \alpha_2 = 2$; (c) $\alpha_1 = 1; \alpha_2 = 0$; (d) $\alpha_1 = 0; \alpha_2 = 1$ (*V.Capasso et al., Figure 2 page 30*)

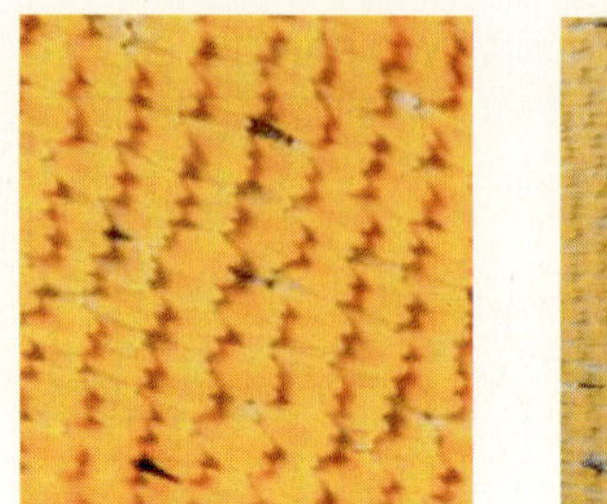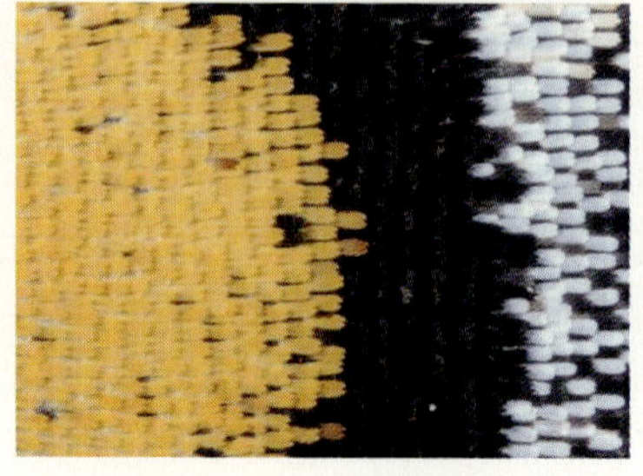

Plate 2: Parallel rows of scale cells (left) and color pattern (right)in a butterfly wing. The color pattern is a finely-tiled mosaic pattern produced by regularly arranged monochromatic scale cells (*T.Sekimura, Figure 1 page 208*)

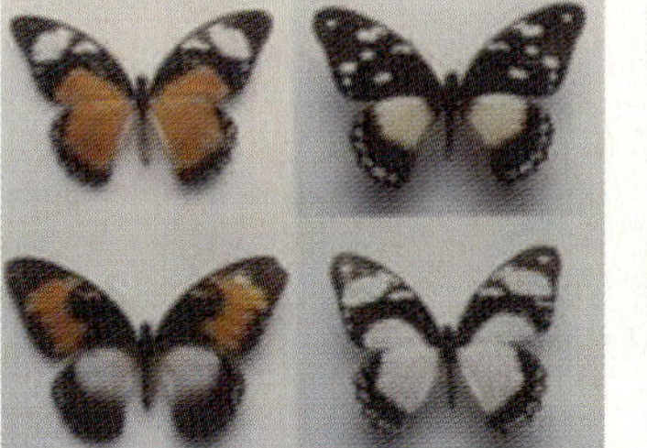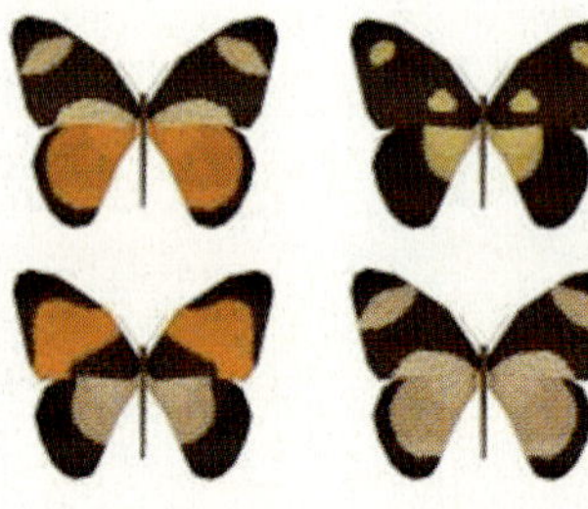

Plate 3: (a)(left) Polymorphism in mimetic females of *Papilio dardanus*. *trophonius*(top left), *cenea*(top right),*planemoides*(bottom left),*hippocoon*(bottom right). (b)(right) Numerical simulation results by the model illustrating global color patterns for *trophonius*(top left), *cenea*(top right),*planemoides*(bottom left),*hippocoon*(bottom right) (*T.Sekimura, Figure 4 page 214*)

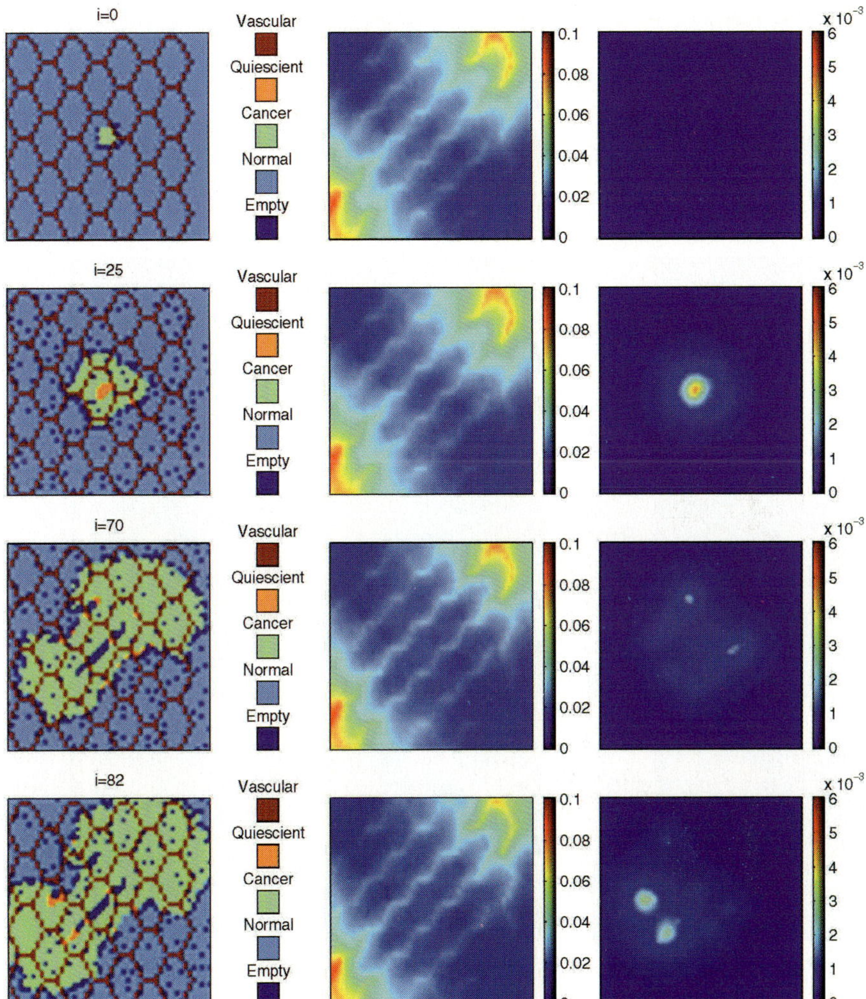

Plate 4: Four snapshots showing simulations with no VEGF coupling and no conducted stimuli. Time increases from top to bottom. The left column corresponds to the evolution of the colonies of normal and cancerous cells, the central column to the distribution of oxygen and the right column to VEGF distribution (*P.K. Maini et al., Figure 3 page 171*)

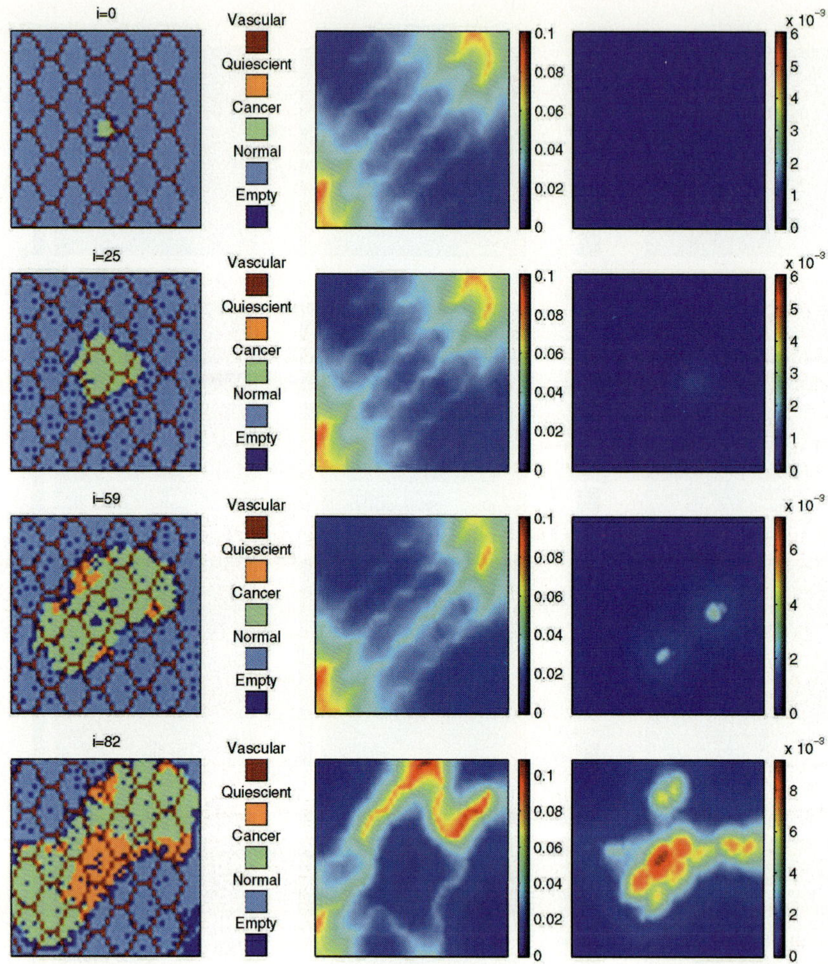

Plate 5: Four snapshots showing simulations with vascular adaptation coupled to VEGF released by hypoxic cells. Time increases from top to bottom. The left column corresponds to the evolution of the colonies of normal and cancerous cells, the central column to the distribution of oxygen and the right column to VEGF distribution (*P.K. Maini et al., Figure 4 page 172*)

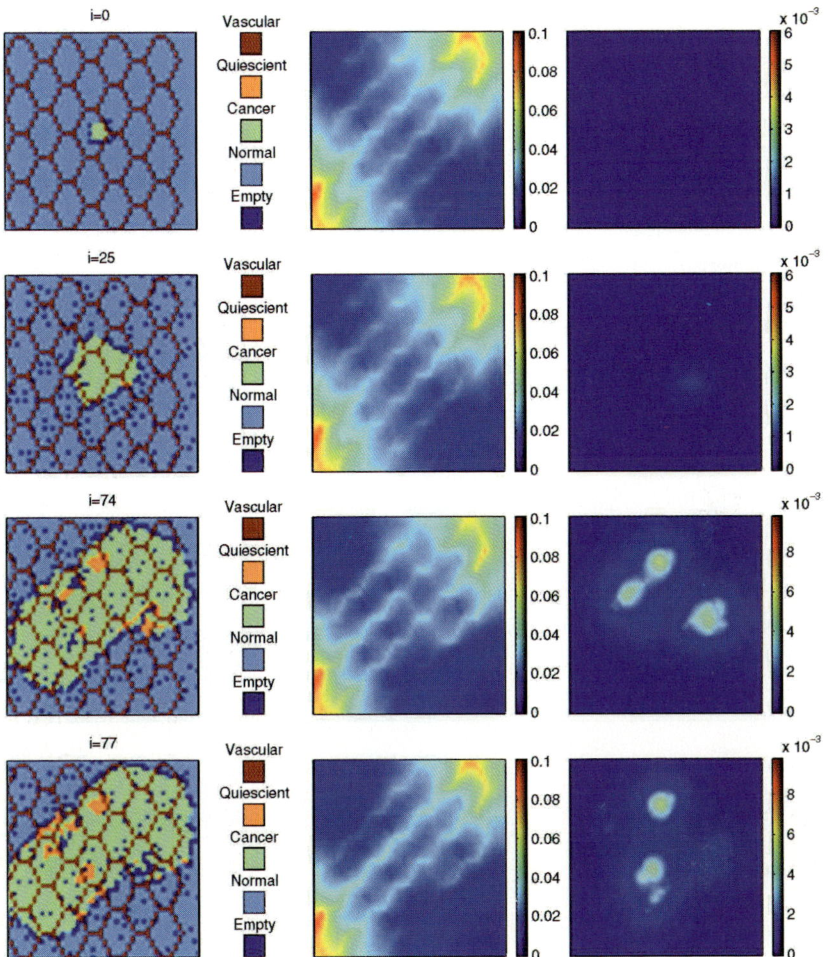

Plate 6: Four snapshots showing simulations with a structural adaptation mechanism coupled to VEGF released by hypoxic cells plus "nearest-neighbour" downstream stimulus. The left column corresponds to the evolution of the colonies of normal and cancerous cells, the central column to the distribution of oxygen and the right column to VEGF distribution (*P.K. Maini et al., Figure 5 page 174*)

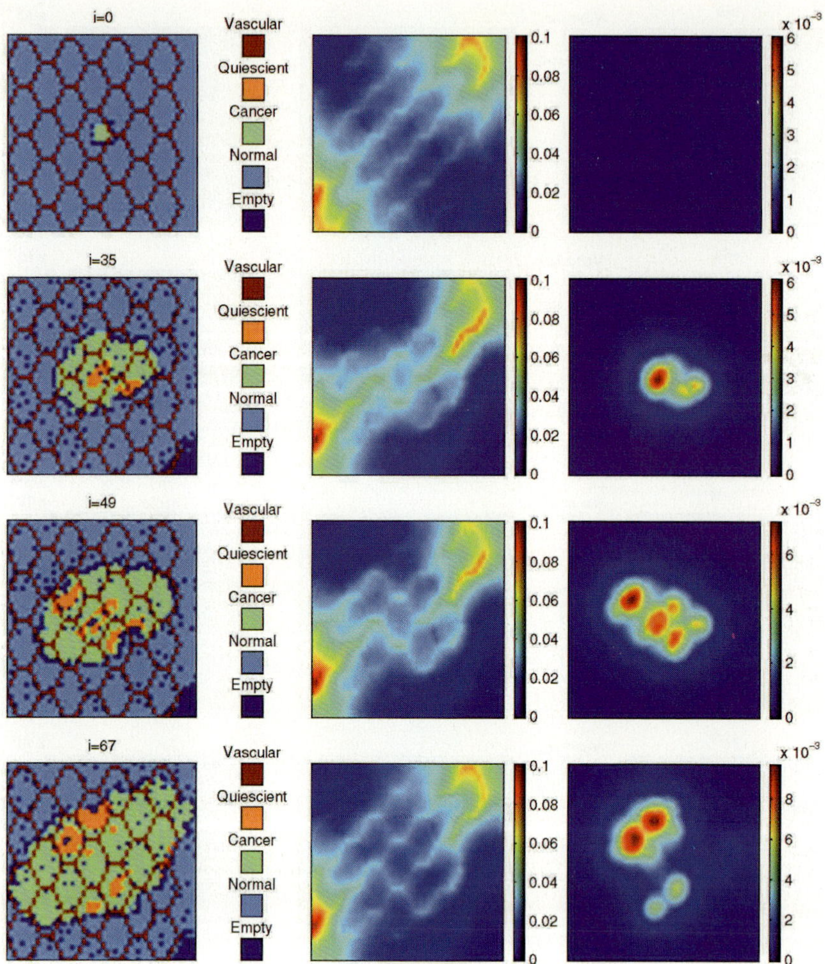

Plate 7: Four snapshots showing simulations with a structural adaptation mechanism coupled to VEGF released by hypoxic cells plus "nearest-neighbour" upstream stimulus. The left column corresponds to the evolution of the colonies of normal and cancerous cells, the central column to the distribution of oxygen and the right column to VEGF distribution (*P.K. Maini et al., Figure 6 on page 176*)

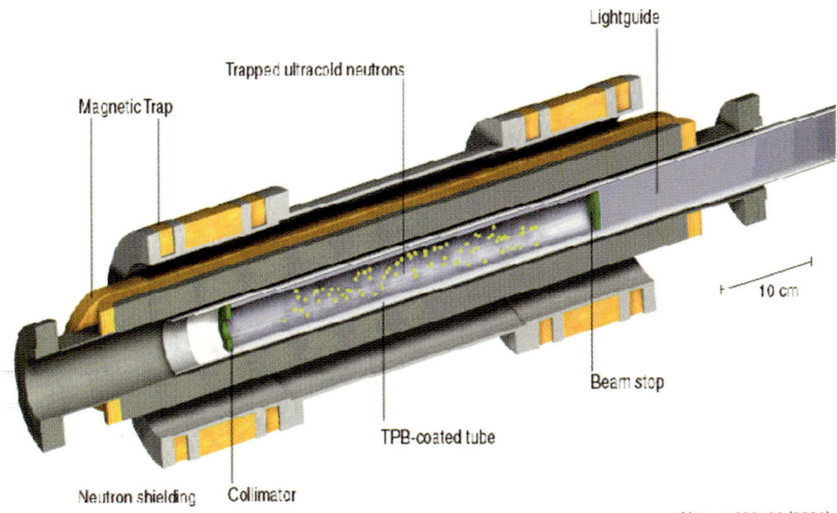

Plate 8: At the NIST Center for Neutron Research, cold neutrons from a reactor are guided into a magnetic trap and can inelastically scatter in superfluid ^{4}He to produce ultracold neutrons. Above, we show a cross sectional perspective of the magnetic trap that confines these ultracold neutrons (*G.L. Yang et al., Figure 1 page 143*)